Their Greatest Victory

# Their Greatest Victory

## 24 Athletes Who Overcame Disease, Disability and Injury

### DAVID L. PORTER

McFarland & Company, Inc., Publishers

*Jefferson, North Carolina, and London*

ISBN 978-0-7864-7305-2

softcover : acid free paper ∞

LIBRARY OF CONGRESS CATALOGUING DATA ARE AVAILABLE

BRITISH LIBRARY CATALOGUING DATA ARE AVAILABLE

On the cover: *clockwise from top center* Alice Marble, 1940 (International
Tennis Hall of Fame & Museum); Babe Didrikson Zaharias (Babe Didrikson
Zaharias Foundation); Dummy Hoy c. 1888 (National Baseball
Hall of Fame Library); Alonzo Mourning c. 1990 (Georgetown University
Sports Information); Harry Greb (collection of Bill Paxton, www.harrygreb.com);
Wilma Rudolph, May 1963 (Tennessee State University Sports Information)

Manufactured in the United States of America

*McFarland & Company, Inc., Publishers
Box 611, Jefferson, North Carolina 28640
www.mcfarlandpub.com*

I dedicate this book to the 24 athletes, who demonstrated remarkable mental toughness, unyielding passion, competitive drive, courage, a strong work ethic, self-discipline, determination, perseverance, and other admirable qualities in recording their greatest victory by overcoming seemingly insurmountable adversities to attain athletic success.

I especially dedicate this book to my late older brother, Marvin, who exhibited many of the above qualities in his 46-year battle with Type 1 diabetes and whose ideas inspired this book. Marvin died on March 8, 2007, at age 69 of complications related to diabetes.

# Acknowledgments

I thank Jim Abbott, Rocky Bleier, Glenn Cunningham, Scott Hamilton, Doris Hart, Ben Hogan, Tommy John, Bobby Jones, Alice Marble, Alonzo Mourning, Wilma Rudolph, Ron Santo, and Babe Didrikson Zaharias, whose autobiographies helped me better understand the medical adversities they faced and how they coped with them. John also kindly let me interview him at the Bob Feller Museum in Van Meter, Iowa, while Cunningham shared his remarkable experiences with me several decades ago.

This work also benefited from the perceptive insights of those who wrote biographies of the 24 athletes or helped those athletes write their autobiographies. I am indebted to Samuel Abt, Lorenz Benet, Ira Berkow, Scott Brown, Susan Cayleff, James Dodson, Mark Frost, Bill Gutman, William Oscar Johnson, O.B. Keeler, Dale Leatherman, Sidney L. Matthew, Randy Minkoff, Terry O'Neal, Bill Paxton, Harry Paxton, Martin Ralbovsky, Grantland Rice, Curt Sampson, George X. Sand, Maureen M. Smith, Cindy Thomson, Don Van Natta Jr., Dan Wetzel, Nancy P. Williamson, and Richard Worth.

I also thank the many sportswriters, especially those whose articles appeared in *Sports Illustrated* and *Sport*, and recounted the struggles the various athletes faced and their remarkable comebacks.

Pete Cava, sportswriter and former press information director of USA Track and Field, Indianapolis, Indiana, gave me many valuable suggestions for sources to contact in regard to photographs.

Many people helped with photographs for the book. They include Paige Adair of Kenan Research Center, Atlanta History Center, Atlanta, Georgia; Kelly Barnes of the World Golf Hall of Fame and Museum, St. Augustine, Florida; Bill Bennett of UCLA Athletics, Los Angeles, California; James Calsyn of Icon Sports Media; Max Carey of Georgetown University Sports Information, Washington, D.C.; Carol Copley and John Heisler of the University of Notre Dame Athletics, South Bend, Indiana; Candace Dunback and Abbi Huderle of the Booth Family Hall of Athletics, University of Kansas, Lawrence, Kansas; John Horne of the National Baseball Hall of Fame Library, Cooperstown, New York; Russell Luna of Tennessee State University Sports Information, Nashville, Tennessee; Meredith Miller of the International Tennis Hall of Fame, Newport, Rhode Island; W.L. Pate Jr. of the Babe Didrikson Zaharias Museum, Beaumont, Texas; Bill Paxton, operator of the Harry Greb web site and author of

*The Fearless Harry Greb*; Dr. Ivonne Schmid of the International Swimming Hall of Fame, Fort Lauderdale, Florida; the Shutterstock Team, www.shutterstock.com; Shannon Smith, National Wrestling Hall of Fame and Museum, Stillwater, Oklahoma; and Linda Sprouse of University of Colorado Sports Information, Boulder, Colorado. Don Cuoco, the director of the International Boxing Research Organization, facilitated the securing of the Harry Greb photographs.

Scott Harvick of the Bob Feller Museum helped make possible my interview with Tommy John. Chris Louderback of the William Penn University Library secured several interlibrary loan books for me. David Wright of William Penn University, who had heard Rocky Bleier give a motivational speech, suggested that I include him in the book. Dr. Fred Allen, Dr. Noel Stahle, and Dr. Michael Collins of William Penn University gave their encouragement at various stages. Bob Barnes at William Penn University helped in the selection of a few photographs.

I am indebted to my son, Kevin, who helped to secure and edit photographs for the book, proofread two chapters for grammatical errors, and provided information on documenting Internet sources.

I wish to thank my wife, Marilyn, who helped me with the book title and read through portions of the manuscript for grammatical errors.

# Table of Contents

# *Preface*

In 1961 my older brother, Marvin, suddenly collapsed while walking in Philadelphia, Pennsylvania. He had graduated a year earlier from Bucknell University with B.A. and B.S. degrees in civil engineering and had begun working as an engineer for the Philadelphia Electric Company. Marvin was rushed to the University of Pennsylvania Hospitals, where he was diagnosed with Type 1 diabetes. Although a distant relative on my father's side had Type 1 diabetes, Marvin attributed his diabetes to an infection he had contracted while our family was visiting relatives in Toccoa, Georgia, in July 1952. During the six-week trip, our family also visited other relatives in Tennessee, Kentucky, Illinois, and Wisconsin. A doctor did not check Marvin's infection until we returned home to Nashua, New Hampshire.

Marvin battled his diabetes courageously for 46 years, following a strict diet and taking daily doses of insulin. He completed a master's degree in engineering management in 1970 from Drexel University and worked more than four decades for Philadelphia Electric Company.

His health, however, declined markedly after he suffered a heart attack and fell down a flight of stairs at his Wallingford, Pennsylvania, home in December 2006. The following month, he developed a staph infection in one foot. Doctors removed part of that foot to stop the infection from spreading. Marvin's mind remained sharp, but he became quite depressed and anxious. Marvin suffered considerable pain and faced the prospect of further complications related to diabetes.

In February 2007, Marvin asked me if I would write an inspirational book about athletes who overcame major health problems. I had already authored or edited numerous sports books and was completing a biography of basketball star Michael Jordan.[1] We discussed how Hamilton Richardson, Ron Santo, Gary Hall Jr., and other diabetics had distinguished athletic careers. I promised Marvin that I would write this book after completing the Jordan biography. Marvin died a month later at age 69 from complications related to diabetes.

Since 2008 I have researched the experiences of 24 athletes who overcame seemingly insurmountable medical odds to attain athletic success. I refer collectively to their conquering or overcoming the adversity as their greatest victory. The 24 athletes represent various team and individual sports, with slightly more than half from baseball (7), track and field (4), and golf (3). The remainder are spread among swimming (2), tennis (2), basketball (1), boxing (1), cycling (1), figure skating (1), football (1), and wrestling (1). Nearly all performed primarily in the twentieth century.

The athletes battled life-threatening diseases, major childhood illnesses, challenging physical disabilities, near-fatal or life-changing accidents, or career-threatening injuries. Jeff Blatnick, Jon Lester, and Babe Didrikson Zaharias battled cancer, while Hall and Santo faced Type 1 diabetes. Gail Devers was confronted with Graves' disease, Alice Marble with tuberculosis, Alonzo Mourning with kidney disease, and Wilma Rudolph with polio. Scott Hamilton suffered from a pancreatic disorder, Bobby Jones from a digestive ailment, and Doris Hart from a serious knee infection as children. Jim Abbott was born with only one hand, while Dummy Hoy was deaf as a result of meningitis and Harry Greb suffered blindness from a boxing match. Glenn Cunningham, Three-Finger Brown, Bill Toomey, and Mike Burton were victims of childhood accidents. Ben Hogan and Greg LeMond survived horrendous accidents during the prime of their athletic careers. Lou Brissie and Rocky Bleier suffered severe military combat injuries, while Tommy John tore ligaments in his pitching elbow.

One chapter is devoted to each of the 24 athletes, describing the problem, the medical issues he or she faced, how success was achieved despite the setback, and the personal qualities that helped the athlete to prevail.

The book is divided into two parts. Part I includes 15 athletes who dealt with diseases and physical disabilities. Part II includes nine athletes who were involved in near-fatal or life-changing accidents or suffered career-threatening injuries as adults. They were hurt in vehicular mishaps, hunting accidents, explosions, combat, and even sports.

Some athletes could have been included in either the first or second part. In each instance, the athlete was placed in the category I deemed most appropriate. Hamilton suffered from both a pancreatic disorder and cancer, but the former came before his illustrious skating career. Hoy's deafness derived from meningitis, but his condition was primarily considered a physical disability. Greb's blindness came from a boxing match, but his injury was also primarily considered a physical disability. Rudolph's polio was a physical disability, but stemmed primarily from a viral disease. Abbott did not consider being born with one hand a physical handicap, but his remarkable life merits inclusion.

It is my fervent hope that the stories of these 24 courageous athletes will inspire others who are facing difficult health challenges.

# Part I. Diseases and Physical Disabilities

## *Cancer*

## JEFF BLATNICK

"If you can win in adversity, you can win anywhere" typified the saga of Jeff Blatnick, who made a remarkable comeback from a major disease to attain wrestling stardom. Blatnick was diagnosed with Hodgkin's disease, cancer of the lymph nodes. When the cancer went into remission, he made the 1984 U.S. Olympic Greco-Roman wrestling team and became only the second U.S. Greco-Roman wrestler to win an Olympic gold medal.

Blatnick grew up in a middle-class family. Jeffery Carl Blatnick, the son of Carl Blatnick, a General Electric Company draftsman, and Angela Blatnick, was born in Niskayuna, New York, on July 26, 1957, and starred in athletics at Niskayuna High School, near Schenectady, where he participated in football, basketball, cross-country, and wrestling. He began wrestling in tenth grade in 1975 because of several bomb scares. Wrestling coach Joseph Bena convinced Blatnick and his brother Dave to stop playing other sports and "to substitute mat burns for bench splinters."[1] Blatnick lacked physical strength, however, being pinned in his first two matches and losing nine of 16 matches as a sophomore.

Blatnick improved markedly the next two years and finished his scholastic career with 64 wins and 21 losses. He swept all 33 matches as a senior and captured the New York State wrestling championship in the 215-pound weight class. "Bena was a real motivator," Blatnick recalled. "He managed to get a lot of us to think for ourselves." The Niskayuna wrestlers practiced in the school cafeteria, moving all the tables aside. Only half of the wrestlers scrimmaged at one time.

After graduating from Niskayuna High School in 1975, Blatnick entered Springfield College in Massachusetts that fall on a football scholarship. He enjoyed wrestling much more than football, however, and attended the summer national wrestling camps of Dan Gable, legendary University of Iowa wrestling coach. "Gable has this ability to push you beyond what you think you can do."[2]

Springfield coach Doug Parker recruited Blatnick for wrestling. Blatnick garnered NCAA Division II All-America wrestling honors at heavyweight from 1977 to 1979, placing second in the 1977 NCAA Division II Championships and capturing the

1978 and 1979 NCAA Division II titles. He also earned NCAA Division I All-America honors twice, finishing sixth at the 1978 NCAA Division I Nationals and third at the 1979 Division I Nationals. He student taught in Boston and trained with Jim Peckham, athletic director at Emerson College and Greco-Roman coach of the 1976 Olympic team. In 1979, he graduated from Springfield College with a bachelor of science degree in physical education and coaching.

After completing his collegiate wrestling eligibility, the 6-foot 2-inch, 248-pound Blatnick switched from freestyle to Greco-Roman wrestling, a technique that prohibits the use of the legs and holds below the waist. As a free stylist, he demonstrated great potential for Greco-Roman wrestling because he chiefly relied on upper-body strength rather than leg strength. Blatnick, who explained, "I had great hand speed and great endurance,"[3] also benefited from his wide hips, extremely flexible back, and long arms.

Blatnick worked on a master's degree at North Dakota State University in Fargo

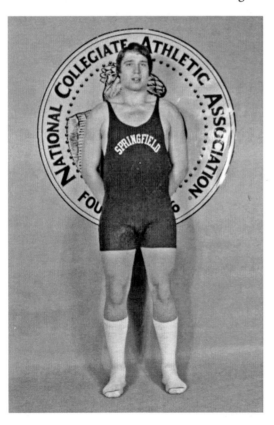

and spent the next four years as graduate assistant wrestling coach under Bucky Maughan. Blatnick trained with Brad Rheingans of the Minnesota Wrestling Club for the 1980 U.S. Olympic Greco-Roman wrestling team at North Dakota State. Rheingans had finished fourth at the 1976 Olympic Games in Montreal and won a bronze medal in the 1979 World Cup. He bested Blatnick in the 220-pound class at the 1979 Amateur Athletic Union (AAU) Greco-Roman National Championships.[4]

Rheingans asked Blatnick to try out for the 1980 American Greco-Roman world championship team. At the trials, Blatnick finished second to Bob Walker in the heavyweight division. Walker defeated Blatnick in two of three matches, recording two 30-second pins. Blatnick, however, edged Walker 8–7 in the middle match. He learned, "I could win the matches that went the distance," but needed "to avoid getting caught in an early move." The Walker match encouraged him to switch permanently to Greco-Roman wrestling.

Jeff Blatnick, pictured in front of the NCAA logo while a wrestler at Springfield College in the late 1970s, captured the 1978 and 1979 NCAA Division II heavyweight titles (courtesy National Wrestling Hall of Fame and Museum).

Rheingans and Blatnick in February 1979 joined the rest of the American wrestling squad training in Minneapolis for the 1980 Olympics. Seven Olympians trained exclusively in Greco-Roman wrestling. Blatnick believed that his wrestling skills improved. "These guys passed their knowledge on to me, and I still had the best workout partner in the country."[5]

At the Olympic Trials, Blatnick qualified for the 1980 U.S. Greco-Roman wrestling team in the super-heavyweight class, "only to have the American boycott postpone his dream four years." The United States boycotted the 1980 Summer Olympic Games at Moscow because of the invasion of Afghanistan by the then–Soviet Union. "Blatnick lost his first shot at Olympic gold without ever putting his knee on a mat." Although disappointed, he vowed to return because "I hadn't peaked yet."[6]

Blatnick fared well in Greco-Roman wrestling while competing for the Adirondack Three-Style Wrestling Association from 1980 to 1982. In 1980, he captured the AAU national championship in the heavyweight class and a silver medal in the World Cup super heavyweight class. Two years later, Blatnick won the AAU crown in the 220-pound class. He felt in top physical condition, and was getting closer to fulfilling his Olympic dream. "But 18 months shy of realizing that dream, Blatnick's goal became simply living."[7]

After returning to North Dakota in 1982, 24-year-old Blatnick discovered several bumps on his neck. "I knew something was wrong," he recalled. Doctors diagnosed him in July 1982 with Hodgkin's disease, a cancer of the lymph nodes. Blatnick explained, "It's a shock when you first hear it simply because you don't understand how you could have contracted it."[8] He did not know much about Hodgkin's disease, feared it, and did not know how to tell his parents. His parents had lost their oldest son, Dave, in a motorcycle accident in 1977 and had encouraged Blatnick to try out for the 1980 Greco-Roman Olympic team. Blatnick embarked on "a solitary journey," not disclosing his cancer to anyone for a while. "The hardest thing," he discovered, "was not knowing what would happen."[9]

Although "many in the wrestling community gave up on him," Blatnick was determined to conquer the Hodgkin's disease, but first needed to conquer his fear. He wondered, "Am I going to die? Why did this happen?" But Blatnick's fears gradually subsided, especially after doctors prescribed treatments, and he returned to focusing on his job, relationships, and wrestling. Blatnick added, "I really do enjoy life" and "am not afraid of losing." He insisted, "I could beat this thing," and he vowed "to attack everything with a lot of optimism."[10]

After surgeons removed his spleen and appendix in August 1982, Blatnick underwent "rigorous" radiation treatments from October 1982 to March 1983. He recalled, "The radiation treatments really knocked me down physically," but realized, "Radiation was the ticket home."[11] Blatnick applied a three-pronged formula for conquering cancer and achieving wrestling success, refusing "to indulge in self-pity," keeping "his problems to himself," and viewing himself as "a proud medieval knight out to slay the cancer dragon."[12]

In November 1983, doctors told Blatnick his disease was in remission. Blatnick needed to start all over again with his wrestling and learn not to fear losing. He neglected the advice of doctors and resumed training too quickly. Blatnick began riding a stationary bicycle two weeks after his initial operation and was wrestling one week later. "I hadn't been on a mat in a while and I threw myself back into it too fast," he realized. At this point, "the New York native wasn't a good bet to even become an Olympian."[13]

Nevertheless, the determined Blatnick valiantly pursued his dream of training for the Olympic team. "His first bout with cancer then delayed, but didn't deter, his courageous route to the gold." "I never lost sight of 1984,"[14] he recalled. According to Blatnick, "It was simply believing that I could do that." Blatnick found it very difficult mentally and physically to concentrate on training. The training, however, gave him "a release — a way to not think about what I was battling through." He considered the cancer "an inconvenience," and vowed, "I wasn't going to take myself out of the game. At the time, my body might not have been able to keep up, but my mind kept flying."[15]

Blatnick soon regained his form and defeated 6-foot 2-inch, 331-pound William "Pete" Lee, who had finished fifth at the 1976 Olympic Games and the 1982 World Championship, at the Olympic Trials at Grand Valley State University to qualify for the 1984 U.S. Olympic team in the super-heavyweight division. The media, however, did not know about Blatnick's Hodgkin's disease until he told a Schenectady-area reporter about it shortly before leaving for the 1984 Los Angeles Olympic Games. He deliberately kept the news from the media until after the Olympic Trials. "I wanted to stay focused on wrestling," he insisted. "I wanted to talk about wrestling, not cancer." Upon completing his training, though, he decided to tell the media about his cancer. Blatnick's compelling story made him "a media darling" at the Olympics.[16]

Before 1984, American wrestlers had never garnered an Olympic medal in Greco-Roman wrestling. No one expected Blatnick to change that because of his battle with Hodgkin's disease and the removal of his spleen. Blatnick relished being the underdog, citing, "No pressure, no fear of losing. It was just a matter of giving it my best performance possible."[17]

"Defying all odds" at the Anaheim Convention Center in the Summer Olympic Games in Los Angeles, the 240-pounder reached the finals on August 2 in the 130-kg weight gold medal match. Blatnick pinned Refik Memisevic of Yugoslavia in 5:12 in the first round, but Panayotis Pikilidis of Greece edged him, 4–3, in the second round. Memisevic subsequently pinned Pikilidis in 5:27. Blatnick edged Memisevic, 4 to 3.5, in the tiebreaker, putting him in the gold-medal round on August 2 against Sweden's Thomas Johansson. Johansson had pinned Victor Dolipschi of Romania in 4:52 in the final round of his bracket.[18]

Johansson outweighed the 248-pound Blatnick by 27 pounds. "The Swede is big," Blatnick's father warned him, "but you've come too far to let anything stop you now." Blatnick recorded two takedowns in the final 90 seconds to take the Johansson match. He triumphed, 2–0, over Johansson, marking only the second time an American had won an Olympic gold medal in Greco-Roman wrestling history. The night before, teammate and roommate Steve Fraser had triumphed over Ilie Matei of Romania in the light-heavyweight division. Americans snared two other medals in Greco-Roman wrestling. James Martinez earned a bronze medal in the lightweight division, while Gregory Gibson picked up a silver medal in the heavyweight division.[19]

Upon triumphing, "the big burly wrestler fell to his knees, kissed the mat, looked skyward, and clasped his hands together, thanking God for winning the gold medal." An ecstatic Blatnick beamed, "I've been given a lot of chances in my life, and I wasn't going to go without thanking somebody for it." He rejoiced, "Everything worked out the way it was supposed to. I couldn't believe it. All the pain and effort was worth the end result."[20]

After his match, Blatnick, "too choked with tears to talk," produced one of the most dramatic, emotional moments of the 1984 Olympic Games. "I am a happy dude!" he cried. "It wasn't enough that the super-heavyweight had won a gold medal; he had conquered Hodgkin's disease as well, believed to be a formidable opponent." Richard Hoffer of the *Los Angeles Times* wrote that the "outrageously buoyant" Blatnick "illuminated the 1984 Olympics with his own emotional fireworks, a relief of tension so mighty that grown men cried."[21] Blatnick's subsequent television interview, witnessed by viewers across the world, brought his "private struggles to the public eye." Blatnick, who did not keep his composure and wept during the television interview "spotted his parents and broke down and wept in his mother's arms." He dedicated the match to his late brother, Dave, and acknowledged, "I'd like to divide the medal into lots of pieces and give a piece to my parents and friends."[22]

On the victory stand, 27-year-old Blatnick broke into tears of joy for his remarkable comeback from Hodgkin's disease to become an Olympic champion. "The level of his emotion was stunning." "I had a lot to be thankful for," Blatnick added. "Without the help of my friends and family, I would not have made it. I might not be alive."[23] He then bear-hugged Rheingans.

Publications lauded Blatnick's remarkable comeback. *Brandweek* wrote, "Having overcome tremendous adversity with grace and strength, Blatnick reflected the Olympic spirit." "Gold medal stories are always fascinating," *Sports Illustrated* publisher Dave Long observed. "But because of the other battles he's fought, Jeff's was something special." Blatnick even realized, "I became not a famous wrestler but a famous cancer patient."[24]

The U.S. captains selected Blatnick to walk at the front of the line and carry the American flag for the closing Olympic ceremonies at Los Angeles. "Winning the gold medal was an accomplishment over my adversity," he conceded, "but an individual honor can never overtake that feeling, to be elected for something like that by your teammates. It was my biggest moment. The chill still goes up and down my spine."[25]

The American freestyle wrestling team put on an historic performance the following week. The gold medals in Greco-Roman wrestling were "a stunning development," but "a mere prelude to America's overwhelming success in the second week's freestyle competition." The United States won seven of the 10 gold medals in freestyle wrestling. Robert Weaver, Randy Lewis, Dave Schultz, Mark Schultz, Ed Banach, Lou Banach, and Bruce Baumgartner all earned gold medals in freestyle wrestling. In Greco-Roman and freestyle wrestling combined, the Americans took nine gold medals and 13 altogether. "The haul was facilitated by the absence of two world powers."[26] The Soviet Union and Bulgarian teams, which had been projected to win around 25 medals, had boycotted the Los Angeles Olympic Games.

An international hero, Blatnick received hundreds of letters from fans around the world. The correspondence largely came from individuals suffering from Hodgkin's disease or other forms of cancer. Blatnick's victory symbolized for them a triumph over the dread disease. Blatnick was named *USA Wrestling* Man of the Year in 1986, but was stripped of his amateur status because he participated in the Superstars competition. He finished seventh out of 20 and made $5,000, competing against skier Phil Mahre, trackster Greg Foster, and others.

For the next year, Blatnick often conducted wrestling clinics and spoke at banquets. He was "living happily ever after, making uplifting speeches at corporate gatherings." Although he never earned more than $15,000 a year as a wrestler, Blatnick traveled 150,000 miles that year and earned $4,500 a night on the banquet circuit delivering motivational speeches about his battle with cancer at around 25 corporate meetings.[27] He also appeared frequently on behalf of the American Cancer Society and the Leukemia Society of America.

Blatnick soon experienced stomach cramps and felt a lump in his groin. He fought a second bout with cancer in the abdominal region in 1985 and 1986. In August 1985, a biopsy disclosed a cancerous growth near his groin. Blatnick learned the tragic news about the recurrence of Hodgkin's disease via telephone at his parents' home near Schenectady. "I cried when I hung up the phone," he disclosed. The news initially depressed and enraged him. Blatnick drove 20 minutes to the residence of his sponsor, Spike Lanides, an investment counselor. "I was not a happy dude," he recalled. "I was upset and angry."[28] But his dismay did not endure very long.

Blatnick underwent 28 chemotherapy sessions from September 1985 to February 1986. He showed up in a tuxedo for his final chemotherapy injection on February 14, 1986. Chemotherapy often causes more side effects than radiation treatments. Blatnick tried working out when he could and continued delivering corporate speeches, but occasionally "overestimated his opponent." He was bedridden for three days after exercising too hard, reminding him, "Cancer still had a few respectable holds."[29]

The chemotherapy treatments forced Blatnick to quit wrestling practice in January 1986 and restrict his physical exercise to walking. Blatnick found it "frustrating" that he no longer could throw his full energy into athletics. but viewed "the whole thing as a challenge. That's all cancer is — it's just another adjustment in my life." He maintained, "You can educate the mind, and you can train your body, but you have to have spirit."[30]

In April 1986, Blatnick told the New York media about the recurrence of his cancer while attending a Leukemia Society event and reported that a CAT scan revealed the growth had shrunk. "The press conference was the equivalent of winning the gold medal for Blatnick, another happy ending." Blatnick, who had worked out for several weeks, surprised the media by announcing his intention to resume wrestling. He vowed, "I'm going right back to what I did in '82." Although realizing his vulnerability, Blatnick revealed, "I miss the mats, I miss the competition." He claimed that quitting at the top would "be like throwing the roses out the window without smelling them." He concluded, "All you can do is try."[31] Doctors pronounced Blatnick fully recovered in November 1986. After that, he did not experience any recurrence of cancer.

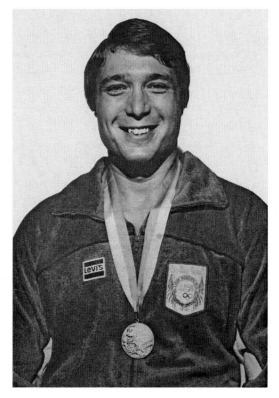

Jeff Blatnick wore his gold medal after upsetting Thomas Johannson of Sweden, 2–0, in the super-heavyweight division at the Summer Olympic Games in Los Angeles on August 2, 1984 (courtesy National Wrestling Hall of Fame and Museum).

Blatnick resumed his training in 1986 for another Olympic gold medal and competed the weekend after finishing his chemotherapy treatments. He did not perform as well as before and disliked his results, but had wanted to know if he could still wrestle. Blatnick pledged, "I'm going to try to improve myself to the point where I'm competitive again" and "let people know there's life after cancer."[32] He regained his form and lowered his wrestling weight to 255 pounds after training one year, but his endurance did not return.

Blatnick wrestled several times before the 1987 Olympic Festival in Durham, North Carolina, and was ranked third in the super-heavyweight division. He was filled with optimism entering the July 1987 Olympic Festival, but "his comeback was detoured at least temporarily." In the first round, fourth-ranked Morris Johnson of San Francisco defeated Blatnick in the best-of-three matches, 7–4, 3–0, eliminating him in the super-heavyweight division. Blatnick uncharacteristically did not try to seize the offensive when behind, 1–0, with 30 seconds left in the second match, "an obvious sign he was physically drained."[33] He did not make the U.S. Greco-Roman wrestling team for the Pan-American Games in Indianapolis that August or the 1987 World Championships in France. The disappointing outcome clouded Blatnick's status "as a world-class wrestler." Blatnick realized, "You can't worry about the Olympic team when you're No. 3 in the Olympic Festival. The odds against me to make the Olympic team and win a gold medal again are astronomical. You can't roll the dice that many times."[34]

After attending a training camp the next week in Pensacola, Blatnick continued training for the 1988 Summer Olympic Games in Seoul and the 1988 World Championships in Albany. Although finishing third in the 1987 U.S. Open, he exited after just one match at the 1988 U.S. Nationals. Blatnick's failed "comeback bid left him below the level he wanted"[35] and unable to defend his title at the 1988 Summer Olympic Games. Blatnick retired from wrestling in April 1988, having won 10 national titles and various international meets during his illustrious 16-year career. The three-time Greco-Roman national champion won eight Greco-Roman All-America awards, two World Cup medals, and two freestyle All-America honors.

Blatnick worked for a public relations firm in Albany and conducted motivational speeches, promoting amateur wrestling and helping people cope with adversities. He toured nationally as a spokesman for the American Cancer Society, the Leukemia Society of America, and United Way.

Blatnick covered the 1988 NCAA Wrestling Championships for ESPN and the 1988, 1992, and 1996 Summer Olympics as a wrestling commentator for NBC Television. Blatnick did extensive analysis of wrestling technique and strategy, commentaries, and interviews for NBC, ABC, ESPN, Bud Sports, Prime Ticket Cable, and the Madison Square Garden Network, covering the U.S. Olympic Festival, USA Wrestling National Championships, Olympic Trials, International Dual meets, and Japanese sumo wrestling, and professional wrestling.[36]

Blatnick also worked as an expert analyst for mixed martial arts from 1994 to 2001, serving as commentator for Ultimate Fighting Championships 4 to 32 and as commissioner during UFC 17. He helped modernize martial arts rules, wrote the Mixed Martial Arts Council Manual, earned a referee's license, and served as a New Jersey Commission judge.[37]

Blatnick continued championing the Olympic spirit. He served as a U.S. Olympic Committee ambassador and was on the board of directors of USA Wrestling, assisting in policy-setting, promotion, and fund-raising efforts. President Bill Clinton named him to the President's Council on Physical Fitness. Blatnick presided over the Olympians for Olympians Relief Fund, which aids needy American Olympians and sought unsuccessfully to bring the 2016 Summer Olympic and Paralympic Games to Chicago. "I'm proud to be part of the Olympic family," he affirmed. "I believe in what the Olympics stand for."[38]

Blatnick and his wife Lori Nowak had a son, Ian, and a daughter, Niki, and resided in Burnt Hills, New York. Lori often accompanied him on road trips and became "a huge fan of wrestling." According to Blatnick, "I think she screams louder than I do at times."

In 2004, Blatnick became volunteer assistant varsity wrestling coach under head coach Steve Jones at Burnt Hills-Ballston Lake High School in Burnt Hills, New York. Burnt Hills-Ballston Lake and Niskayuna High School were rivals when Blatnick wrestled. Bob McGuire, the athletic director at Burnt Hills-Ballston Lake High School, singled out Blatnick as "that special individual" who was "a role model for a lot of different children." Blatnick was also a paid coach for the local journeyman wrestling club. Blatnick also worked with youngsters at clinics and athletes in the Special Olympics. sharing his expertise on wrestling techniques. He added, "It's been fun to get back into the corner and work with kids on a daily basis."[39]

Blatnick has received numerous honors. The gymnasium at Niskayuna High School and a town park in Niskayuna are named after him. Blatnick was elected to the Niskayuna High School Hall of Fame in 1985, the NCAA Division II Wrestling Hall of Fame in 1997, and the National Wrestling Hall of Fame in 1999. He also became the youngest member of the Springfield College Athletic Hall of Fame. The U.S. Olympic Committee has nominated Blatnick four times for the U.S. Olympic Hall of Fame. Mark McGuire of the *Albany Times Union* wrote, "He may not be the best Olympic athlete ever, but you can look far and wide before finding someone who better represents the Olympic ideal." McGuire added, "He gives back as much as he's received. You can't ask for more."[40]

Blatnick survived two bouts with cancer, an airplane crash and three major automobile wrecks. His passion, sincerity, and zest for life have kept him focused on overcoming adversity. "If you can win in adversity, you can win anywhere," he affirmed. Tommy Hine of the *Hartford Courant* penned, "There is nothing — not even cancer — that can extinguish the spirit of the Olympic flame in Jeff Blatnick. And Blatnick didn't beat it once. He had to beat it twice." Blatnick reflected, "Cancer was a part of my life, a part of my life I had to deal with. But I learned that I could overcome adversity. Faith and attitude go hand in hand."[41] He explained, "I'm the white knight going after the cancer dragon. Sometimes, you just have to fight harder." He received more publicity than Fraser at the 1984 Olympic Games because of his cancer, but admitted, "I'd rather be recognized because of my athletic ability."[42]

Blatnick, who served as USA Wrestling's state director in New York, died suddenly on October 24, 2012, from the complications of heart surgery at Ellis Hospital in Schenectady, New York, at age 55. USA Wrestling National Greco-Roman coach Fraser reflected, "He has done so much for the sport as an athlete, an announcer, a leader and a spokesman." Joe DeMeo, former coach of the U.S. Greco-Roman World Team, offered, "His legacy was as a great husband and father and somebody who became a tremendous, great wrestler and willed himself into being an Olympic champion." U.S. Olympic Committee CEO Scott Blackmun reminisced, "Jeff was a legend in the sport of wrestling and a true champion." Blackmun added, "Jeff was always willing to share his story and lend his considerable talents to growing the sport of wrestling and inspiring young men and women to always do their best."[43] The spirit of the Olympic flame exemplified in his courageous story will continue to endure.

# JON LESTER

When cancer sidelined baseball player Jon Lester, he "handled it all with quiet grace, determination, and a very positive attitude." The talented young pitcher, whose compelling story resembles an art masterpiece or an Oscar-nominated movie, was diagnosed with non–Hodgkin's anaplastic large-cell lymphoma during his rookie major league season in 2006. After returning to the major leagues, Lester became a premier American League pitcher and won the clinching game of the 2007 World Series.

Lester came from a middle-class background. Jonathan Tyler Lester was born on January 7, 1984, in Tacoma, Washington, and grew up an only child in nearby Puyallup. His father, John, was a sergeant with the Pierce County Sheriff's Department in Tacoma, while his mother, Kathie, drove county snow plows and asphalt trucks.[1] Lester was a tall, powerful left-handed athlete, whose strong arm helped him in baseball and football and whose height aided him in basketball. He especially loved baseball, rooting for the Seattle Mariners and their superstar Ken Griffey Jr.

In September 1998, Lester enrolled at Bellarmine Preparatory High School, a Roman Catholic institution, in Tacoma. Baseball coach Rick Barnhart quickly inserted the freshman on the varsity squad. Lester showed great poise and competitiveness, being named league Most Valuable Player and an All-Area selection three times. In 2000, he was chosen Gatorade Player of the Year for Washington State.[2] By his senior year, the 6-foot 2-inch 190-pounder threw a fastball in the mid–'90s and attracted numerous professional scouts and college recruiters. He even hurled a no-hitter, striking out 18 of 21 batters.

The Boston Red Sox selected 18-year-old Lester in the second round of the 2002 draft as No. 57 overall. After protracted contract negotiations, Boston gave Lester the highest signing bonus among second-rounders at $1 million. Lester spent his first three seasons in the lower minor leagues with the Gulf Coast Red Sox of the Gulf Coast League in 2002, the Augusta Greenjackets of the Class A South Atlantic League in 2003, and the Sarasota Red Sox of the Class A Florida State League in 2004.[3]

Lester blossomed into the Boston organization's top prospect with the Class AA Portland Sea Dogs of the Eastern League, adding a cutter with his 92–97 mile-per-hour fast ball and occasional change-ups and curveballs. He posted an 11–6 win-loss record, leading the Eastern League with a 2.61 earned run average (ERA) and 163 strikeouts in 148 innings. His honors included Eastern League Pitcher of the Year, Red Sox Minor League Pitcher of the Year, Eastern League All-Star team, and Topps' AA All-Star squad.

When Lester struggled in spring training in 2006, the Red Sox assigned the young flamethrower to the Pawtucket Red Sox of the International League. Lester performed poorly in his first five starts, but went 3–0 with a brilliant 0.90 ERA in his next six starts. The Red Sox promoted Lester on June 10 when injuries sidelined starters David Wells, Matt Clement, and Tim Wakefield. In 11 starts with Pawtucket, Lester finished 3–4 with a 2.70 ERA.

Lester enjoyed a stellar rookie season with Boston. In his major league debut on June 10 at Fenway Park, he pitched pretty well without decision in a loss to the Texas Rangers. His parents flew to Boston to witness his debut. Lester earned his first major league victory on June 16 at Atlanta, out-dueling Tim Hudson, 4–1, limiting the Braves to one run and five hits in six innings and fanning five. The 21-year-old became the youngest Red Sox hurler to win a game since Juan Pena in 1999. His first Fenway Park victory came over the Washington Nationals, 9–3, on June 21. He not only became the first Boston moundsman that season to record 10 strikeouts, but the first Red Sox rookie to accomplish that feat in a game since Casey Fossum in 2002.[4]

Lester became the first Red Sox rookie left-handed pitcher in club history to win his first five games, handcuffing the Kansas City Royals, 1–0, on July 18. He threw eight innings, combining with Jonathan Papelbon on a one-hitter. "It was an exciting glimpse of the future for Boston fans." Mark Teahan accounted for the Royals' lone hit, a clean single to center field. Lester was the first Red Sox rookie to hurl a one-hitter since Billy Rohr blanked the New York Yankees on April 14, 1967, at Yankee Stadium.

Lester fared 5–0 with a 2.38 ERA in his first eight starts, but split four decisions with a 7.75 ERA in his next seven starts. His first major league loss came on July 28 against the Los Angeles Angels, 8–3.[5] On August 18, Lester's car was rear-ended in a minor traffic accident while he was traveling to Fenway Park to pitch against the New York Yankees. Lester pitched that day, but complained of back pain, which team officials attributed to the accident. He won his final start five days later against Los Angeles at Angel Stadium. After being staked to a 5–0 lead, he surrendered four runs before leaving the game and was awarded the decision in a 5–4 victory. Lester looked uncomfortable on the mound and took considerable time between pitches. The pressure and the back pain bothered him. "It was do or die on every pitch,"[6] he recalled. Lester had experienced back discomfort even before the accident and admitted, "Last night, it was just hard to get my back loose."[7] When the Red Sox played a three-game series against the Seattle Mariners, a doctor examined Lester in Tacoma. Lester learned that his back pain and 10-pound weight loss were warning signs of lymphoma.

Boston scratched Lester from his scheduled August 28 start against the Oakland

Athletics due to the sore back and placed him on the 15-day disabled list. Lester flew to Boston by private jet with his parents to undergo testing. He also began experiencing night sweats. The next morning, his back pain grew so intense that he could hardly walk. Lester headed for an emergency room to see leading specialists at Massachusetts General Hospital. An MRI on August 30 revealed that Lester had developed enlarged lymph nodes, and he was soon being tested for cancer. His parents were en route to the hospital in a cab when they heard the word "lymphoma" on a speaker phone. "There was dead silence,"[8] his father recalled. Cells were found in Lester's groin, lung, and collarbone.

Two days later, an oncologist diagnosed Lester with a non-fatal, treatable form of non–Hodgkin's anaplastic large cell lymphoma. The rare blood cancer, whose cause is unknown, accounts for only one to two percent of all lymph node cancers. Dr. Robert Soiffer, chief of the division of blood cancers at Dana Farber Cancer Institute in Boston, described Lester's cancer as curable with chemotherapy. "Being young is in his favor," Dr. Soiffer added.

The news stunned the injury-plagued Red Sox, who had just been swept by the New York Yankees in a five-game series at Fenway Park. "It just floored the entire organization," Boston general manager Theo Epstein said. This, he added, "really puts things in perspective."[9] Manager Terry Francona updated the Red Sox players on Lester's status before their game that night against the Toronto Blue Jays. "We met as a team before the game to make sure everyone understood what was going on," he said. Teammates were very supportive throughout Lester's ordeal. Mike Lowell, who had undergone radiation treatment for testicular cancer in 1999, noted, "The best thing is the doctor's diagnosis, that it's something treatable and curable." He advised Lester, "Take it for what it's worth, get well, and worry about baseball later." Mike Timlin observed, "This is a serious roadblock for him, but we're pulling for him." He added, "Dealing with horrible things in human life, that's a whole lot worse than losing."[10]

Lester's abbreviated stellar season ended at 7–2 with a 4.76 ERA in 15 starts. Lester finished 3–0 with a 0.90 ERA in his final six outings. Although pitching only 81 innings, he shared fourth place among American League rookies with seven victories and became the first Red Sox rookie to win 7 games since Ken Ryan and Aaron Sele in 1993.

The 22-year-old Lester remained methodical when he initially received the cancer diagnosis. "I've always associated cancer with death," said Lester, who lost both of his grandmothers to cancer.[11] He did not question why this happened, but concentrated on how to respond. Lester rationalized, "It's the hand I was dealt. I got to play the cards — and make the best of it." His father observed, "Not once did he complain. He didn't ask, 'Why me?'"[12]

During the off-season, Lester underwent six 21-day cycles of chemotherapy drug treatments in four months. He received his first chemotherapy treatment at the Dana

Farber Cancer Institute in Boston and the remainder at the Fred Hutchinson Cancer Research Center in Seattle, named after a former major league pitcher and manager who died of lung cancer at age 45 in 1964. The treatments fatigued Lester. "You're tired all the time," he acknowledged. "You want to do stuff, but you can't." Nevertheless, Lester handled the two-hour treatments well. It took him about a week to recover from each treatment. He did not work out during that period because of the side effects from chemotherapy. "When you're an elite athlete, any treatment on your body is going to take its toll," Dr. Soiffer warned.[13]

After his sixth treatment, in December, a CT scan showed the chemotherapy had removed all evidence of visible cancer and that he was in remission. Lester immediately phoned the good news to manager Francona, who had sent him inspirational text messages. Lester, who kept busy fishing, hunting, and biking, did not consider himself "any more special than any other cancer survivor or any other person who has had a sickness or a handicap."

Lester's father dropped him off at the Seattle airport in January to fly to spring training. "This is the first time I'm actually glad to see you go," his father explained. "Go have fun. Go play baseball." He added, "To be able to say goodbye was the happiest day of my life."[14]

Teammates warmly welcomed Lester at spring training in Fort Myers, Florida. Catcher Jason Varitek, who considered Lester's comeback extraordinary, remarked, "Jon treated the whole thing like he was going over a speed bump. He never wanted to be treated like a victim or for anyone to feel sorry for him." Pitcher Josh Beckett told him, "You beat cancer. This should be easy." Reliever Jonathan Papelbon said, "It's awesome to see him back, and it's amazing to think that he can come back and beat cancer." Red Sox president Larry Lucchino, who had survived both non–Hodgkin's lymphoma and prostate cancer, called Lester "an inspiration for cancer patients all over the nation."[15]

Lester worked diligently to get himself back into pitching shape. Since the treatments had caused him to lose some hair, he shaved his head completely. Lester regained his normal weight of 190 pounds by April, but needed longer to return to previous form. The cancer experience changed his pitching approach. Lester had taken pitching very seriously and was a perfectionist who insisted upon precision in his pitches and mechanics. "I'm going to lighten up and not put so much pressure on myself,"[16] he vowed. Lester wanted his dream of returning to the Red Sox to become reality, but added, "The most important thing is it's going to be fun."

Lester made 17 combined starts with the Class A Greenville Drive of the South Atlantic League and Pawtucket, increasing his velocity and regaining command of his pitches. Minor setbacks delayed his comeback. After Lester experienced cramping in his left forearm in a three-inning May 2 start with Pawtucket, Boston placed him on the 15-day disabled list and did not have him throw for several days. "Every time you knock him back a couple of days, he wants to fight you," Francona noticed. "We want this kid for years."[17] Pitching coach John Farrell advised him to temporarily stop throwing his cutter, shorten his windup, and stand more upright in the stretch. These changes improved Lester's velocity markedly.

Lester's triumphant return to the Boston Red Sox came on July 23 against the Cleveland Indians at Jacobs Field. With his parents watching from the stands, he started his first major league game in 11 months and first as a cancer survivor. The *Boston Globe* wrote, "Lester wasn't daunted by the Indians lineup" and "turned in a remarkable start in his return to the majors." The start, Tom Verducci of *Sports Illustrated* observed, signified "Lester getting his baseball career, if not his life, back to the everyday challenges and triumphs he worried about before he heard the words 'anaplastic large cell lymphoma.' He can sweat the small stuff again." Lester allowed only five hits in six innings, winning 6–2. In his emotion-packed return, he threw 96 pitches, fanned six, and walked three. The Red Sox tallied four runs in the first inning, enabling Lester to settle down against a very potent lineup. Putting Lester's comeback into perspective, Epstein said, "It's an amazing story."[18] Francona started Lester three other times on the road.

On August 14, Lester made his 2007 Fenway Park debut against the Tampa Bay Devil Rays. Fans gave him "a thunderous ovation" when he walked in from the bullpen after taking pre-game warm-ups. Lester, struggling with his emotions, walked leadoff batter Akinori Iwamura in the first inning, but then settled down and retired the next three batters. Lester dueled Scott Kazmir, allowing only two hits, striking out four, and walking just one batter in seven innings. In the fourth inning, Carl Crawford and B.J. Upton singled and Crawford scored on Carlos Pena's sacrifice fly. The *Boston Herald* wrote, "Lester pitched seven fantastic innings but was on the verge of a difficult-to-swallow defeat." The Red Sox trailed, 1–0, entering the bottom of the ninth inning, before rallying to nip Tampa Bay. Lowell clouted "a tape-measure home run on to Landsdowne Street off Tampa Bay reliever Al Reyes with one out" to tie the score. Varitek doubled to right field with two outs and scored the winning run on Coco Crisp's two-out single to right field. The rally marked the Red Sox' eighth final at-bat victory and their second in walk-off fashion. The Red Sox had been 1–41 when trailing after eight innings. "I'm glad his efforts didn't go to waste," Lowell said. "That would've been a shame."[19]

Inconsistency plagued Lester in his next start. Lester defeated Tampa Bay, 8–6, on August 21 at Tropicana Field, "thanks to generous offensive support and flawless relief from the bullpen." He allowed five runs on four hits, four walks, and a wild pitch in 5⅓ innings, and surrendered home runs to Pena and Iwamura. The Red Sox batted around in the fourth inning for the 32nd time that season. Lester "battled command problems and struggled to maintain a large lead." He said, "Luckily the bullpen picked me up and we got a win out of it, at least."[20]

Lester pitched one game for Portland in late August, allowing one run in six innings for the victory. The Red Sox recalled Lester in time to make him eligible for the post-season roster. Lester finished his abbreviated season 4–0 with a 4.57 ERA for Boston, striking out 50 batters and walking only 31 in 12 appearances. He did not pitch in the 2007 American League Division Series against the Los Angeles Angels, but relieved in the eleventh inning with one out and surrendered two runs in the 14–7, 11-inning loss in Game 2 of the 2007 AL Championship Series against the Cleveland Indians. Lester allowed an RBI double to Jhonny Peralta and a three-run homer to Franklin Gutiérrez. "We didn't do the job we came in there to do," said Lester. "I sure didn't help out. That was unacceptable."[21]

Redemption came in Game 4 at Jacobs Field in Cleveland. The Indians had broken open a scoreless duel and erupted for seven runs in the bottom of the fifth inning. Kevin Youkilis, David Ortiz, and Manny Ramirez hit consecutive homers in the top of the sixth inning. Lester relieved in the bottom of the seventh inning, with Boston trailing, 7–3, and hurled three brilliant scoreless innings.[22] The Red Sox trailed Cleveland, 3–1, in games, but made a miraculous comeback, outscoring Cleveland 30–5 in the final three games to capture the AL pennant and make their second World Series appearance in four years.

The Colorado Rockies entered the 2007 World Series on fire, but Boston easily won the first three games. Although Lester had not won since the first week in September, Francona started him in decisive Game 4 at Coors Field. In his first post-season start, Lester pitched very effectively. Kaz Matsui, Colorado's leadoff batter, popped up to Lester in front of the mound. With the tying run on second base in the third inning, Lester retired Matt Holliday, Colorado's best hitter. He shut down the Rockies until being relieved with two outs in the sixth inning. Lester pitched 5⅔ shutout innings, surrendering just three hits in a batter's ballpark, walking three, and striking out three. He held the Rockies hitless in five at-bats with runners in scoring position. Todd Helton lined a leadoff double and Brad Hawpe drew a two-out walk in the second inning, but Lester induced Yorvit Torrealba to ground out to end Colorado's only serious threat against him.[23]

Boston triumphed 4–3, capturing just its second World Series championship in 89 years. The Red Sox jumped out to a 1–0 lead in the first inning when Jacoby Ellsbury lined an opposite field double down the left field line and Ortiz singled to right field. Boston tallied in the fifth inning when Lowell lined a leadoff double to left-center field and Varitek singled to right field. Lowell homered over the left field wall in the seventh inning and pinch hitter Bobby Kielty followed suit in the eighth inning. Lester was credited with the clinching victory, becoming "the first Sox lefty ever to earn the victory in a World Series–clinching game." "It was only fitting that the storybook season had a fairy-tale ending." Only two other pitchers in World Series history had won series-clinching games in their first post-season starts. "Words cannot describe how good this feels," Lester said in the clubhouse. "It's been a whirlwind year for me." Francona added, "His ability to go out and focus on what he had to tonight, after all that he's been through and the road he has traveled, it's a storybook ending to a great year." A teary-eyed Varitek spoke emotionally about Lester's battle back from cancer. "We're talking about life, not a game," he observed. The Boston Baseball Writers Association of America in November gave him the Tony Conigliaro Award for his comeback from cancer.[24]

Lester returned to the starting rotation in 2008 and enjoyed his best major league season. On May 19, he again made headlines by hurling his first major league no-hitter and the eighteenth in Red Sox history. Boston blanked the Kansas City Royals, 7–0, at Fenway Park in Lester's career-high 130-pitch gem. Lester struck out nine, while walking two and committing an error on a pickoff throw in the second inning. Rookie center fielder Ellsbury preserved the no-hitter with a spectacular diving catch to end the fourth inning. Otherwise, Lester retired the Kansas City batters easily. After walking the leadoff hitter in the ninth inning, he induced groundouts from Tony Pena Jr. and David DeJesus and struck out Alberto Callaspo to end the game. At age 24, he became the youngest left-hander ever to pitch a no-hitter at Fenway Park.[25]

The historic 7–0 masterpiece marked Lester's first complete game in 37 starts as a major leaguer. "You don't feel tired in that situation," Lester said. "You've got so much adrenaline going that all you're thinking about is finishing the game." His gem was the first no-hitter by a Red Sox left-handed pitcher since Mel Parnell in 1956, the first no-hitter in major league baseball since teammate Clay Buchholz's masterpiece in September 2007, and the Major League Baseball–record fourth no-hitter caught by Varitek. It was only the second no-hitter pitched against the Royals. Nolan Ryan spun the other classic in 1973.[26]

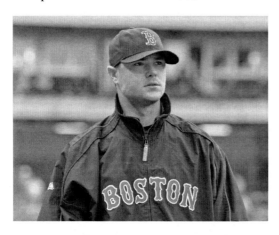

Boston Red Sox pitcher Jon Lester, shown here walking to the bullpen before facing the Cleveland Indians at Jacobs Field on July 23, 2007, allowed only five hits in six innings in a 6–2 victory in his first major league appearance since being diagnosed with non–Hodgkin's lymphoma (courtesy Andy Altenburger/Icon SMI).

In 2008, Lester posted a 16–6 mark with a 3.21 ERA in his first full major league season and led Red Sox hurlers with 210 total innings, emerging as a premier AL left-handed pitcher. He boasted a brilliant 11–1 record in 17 Fenway Park starts and shared the AL lead for most home victories. Lester hurled a complete-game, five-hit shutout in his first start against the New York Yankees at Yankee Stadium and led American League moundsmen in shutouts with two, earning AL Pitcher of the Month honors in July and September. His .771 career winning percentage (27–8 record) ranked second highest in Major League Baseball.[27]

Lester played an instrumental role

in Boston's triumph over the Los Angeles Angels in the 2008 AL Division Series, winning one decision, striking out 11 batters, and allowing no earned runs in 14 innings. He hurled seven frames in Game 1 at Angel Stadium in Anaheim on October 1, surrendering an unearned third inning run on Torii Hunter's single. The Red Sox won, 4–1, as Lester recorded the victory, allowing six hits, striking out four, and walking just one. In decisive Game 4 at Fenway Park on October 6, he blanked the Angels on four hits in seven innings, walking only two and striking out four. Boston led, 2–0, when Lester departed, but Los Angeles knotted the score, 2–2, off Red Sox relievers in the eighth frame. Boston tallied the winning run in the bottom of the ninth inning to clinch the Division Series.[28]

Lester, however, performed less effectively against the Tampa Bay Rays in the 2008 AL Championship Series. Despite striking out 15 batters in 12.2 innings, he lost Games 3 and 7 while suffering his first setbacks in consecutive starts. Although not allowing an earned run in four previous post-season outings, he gave up four earned runs on eight hits in 5.2 innings in a 9–1 loss in Game 3 at Fenway Park on October 13. Lester surrendered an unearned run on Varitek's passed ball in the second inning and allowed a three-run homer to Upton and a bases-empty homer to Evan Longoria in the third inning. Climactic Game 7 at Tropicana Field on October 19 saw Aaron Garza out-duel Lester, 3–1. Willy Aybar and Longoria homered, while Rocco Baldelli drove in the third Tampa Bay run.[29]

The Baseball Writers Association of America, nevertheless, named Lester the Red Sox Pitcher of the Year. No Boston left-hander had earned the honor since Bruce Hurst two decades earlier. Lester also received the 2008 Hutch Award for his courage in overcoming cancer, best exemplifying Hutchinson's "fighting spirit and competitive desire."[30] On January 9, 2009, he married nursing student Farrah Johnson, whom he had met two years earlier in Greenville, South Carolina. They have one son, Hudson.

On March 8, 2009, Lester signed a five-year, $30 million contract extension with a $14 million team option in 2014. After struggling in April and May, he again became a dominant, reliable pitcher. Lester struck out a career-high 12 batters in his first June start and pitched another masterpiece against the AL West–leading Texas Rangers on June 6 at Fenway Park. He did not allow a runner for 6.1 innings, striking out 10 batters on just 61 pitches through the first six frames. Michael Young lined a one-out double to left center field in the seventh inning to break up Lester's no-hit bid. Lester pitched the entire game, fanning 11 batters.[31] He struck out at least 10 batters six times in 2009, most ever by a Boston left-hander in one season.

In 32 starts in 2009, Lester posted a 15–8 record with a 3.41 ERA and broke Hurst's club record for most strikeouts by a left-hander in a single season. His 225 strikeouts ranked first among major league left-handers, third in the AL, and fifth in the major leagues. He improved after the All-Star break, limiting batters to a .224 on base percentage, second lowest in the AL and fifth best in the major leagues.[32]

In the 2009 AL Division Series, the Los Angeles Angels swept the Red Sox in three games. Lester engaged in a scoreless pitching duel with John Lackey for the first four innings of Game 1 at Angels Stadium on October 8. Hunter clouted a three-run homer off Lester in the fifth inning, leading the Angels to a 5–0 victory. Lester, saddled with the loss, allowed three runs and four hits in six innings, striking out five and walking four.[33] The game marked the first shutout ever by an Angel pitcher in post-season play and the first post-season shutout of the Red Sox since Game 2 of the 1995 AL Division Series.

Although performing inconsistently in 2010, Lester enjoyed another fine season. He struggled in his first four starts without a victory, but won his final start in April and five of his six starts in May. Lester finished May with a 5–0 mark, 1.84 ERA, and 45 strikeouts, garnering AL Pitcher of the Month honors for the third time. His fiftieth career victory came on June 16 against the Arizona Diamondbacks at Fenway Park. Lester enjoyed an 11–3 mark with a 2.78 ERA and 124 strikeouts before the All-Star break, making the AL All-Star team for the first time. In the All-Star Game, he pitched the sixth inning without allowing any base runners.[34]

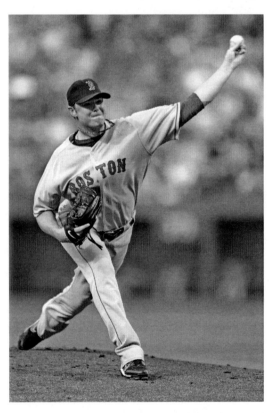

John Lester of Boston, pictured here hurling a three-hit 8–1 victory over the Toronto Blue Jays at the Rogers Center in Toronto on August 20, 2004, broke the Red Sox record for most strikeouts by a left-hander in single season and led major league left-handers with 225 strikeouts that year (courtesy Dennis Ka/Shutterstock.com).

Lester struggled after the All-Star break, losing four consecutive games for the first time in his illustrious career. He hurled a perfect game for 5.1 innings on July 24 against the Seattle Mariners at Safeco Field, striking out 10 batters. Lester's perfect game bid ended when center fielder Eric Patterson mishandled Jack Wilson's fly ball in the sixth inning. Michael Saunders clouted a two-run homer to break up Lester's no-hit bid and give Seattle a 2–1 lead. The Mariners won that game, 5–1, marking the first time Lester had lost consecutive regular-season contests in his career. Lester did not win his next two starts, but fared well in September, blanking the New York Yankees for six innings and the Texas Rangers for eight frames.

Lester finished 2010 with a 19–9 mark, 225 strikeouts in 208 innings, and two complete games in 32 starts, placing fourth in the AL Cy Young Award voting. Besides attaining a career high in victories, he ranked fourth among major league pitchers in strikeouts, shared fourth in victories, and ranked twenty-fifth in ERA in a pitcher-dominated year.[35]

In 2011, Lester compiled a 15–9 record with a 3.47 ERA and made the AL All-Star team, pacing Boston's rotation in victories (15) for the second straight year and in strikeouts (132) for the third consecutive year. He ranked among AL leaders in wins (tenth), strikeouts (eleventh), and ERA (seventeenth).[36] Lester struggled with the rest of the Red Sox in September, however, losing his final three decisions. He surrendered a career-high eight runs in one start against the New York Yankees and gave up two runs in six innings in the season finale against the Baltimore Orioles. Baltimore eliminated Boston from playoff contention when the Red Sox' bullpen blew a 3–2 lead in the ninth inning. Boston had enjoyed the best record in the major leagues through August, but won only seven of 27 games in an historic September collapse, squandering a nine-game lead over the Tampa Bay Rays and expediting the departures of Francona and Epstein.

According to the *Boston Globe*, Lester, Beckett, and Lackey, the top three pitchers in the Red Sox' rotation, drank beer, ate fast-food fried chicken, and played video games in the clubhouse during games. The trio reportedly cut back on their workouts in September, having an uncharacteristic combined 2–7 record and 6.45 ERA that month. Lester admitted that the trio occasionally drank "rally beer" in the Red Sox clubhouse during games, but countered, "Things got magnified because we lost and sources started telling people what happened."[37]

Lester experienced his first losing season as a major leaguer in 2012, finishing 9–14 with a career-high 4.82 ERA. He uncharacteristically won only three of 13 decisions with a 6.31 ERA at Fenway Park in 2012 after compiling a stellar 36–15 record and a 3.32 ERA there previously. Lester on September 21 lost his first game ever to the Baltimore Orioles, 4–2, after enjoying a 14–0 mark in 20 prior starts. In summarizing his disappointing season, he reflected, "I did what I could. I took the ball every five days and threw as many innings [205.1] as I could and the rest just didn't fall into place."[38]

Several factors contributed to Lester's struggles in 2012. Jason Varitek, who had caught Lester since the latter's rookie campaign, retired after the 2011 season. John Farrell, Lester's pitching coach from 2007 through 2010, became manager of the Toronto Blue Jays in 2011. Lester had boasted a 54–23 record and 3.41 ERA under Farrell, but had slipped to a 21–19 record and 4.23 ERA since his departure. The Red Sox left-hander, who considers Farrell an excellent communicator, observed, "He helped mold me into the pitcher I am, the player I am. My work ethic, the work I do between starts, he really helped mold all of that." The firing of player-friendly manager Francona in October 2011 also contributed to Lester's struggles. Francona had piloted the Red Sox since Lester had joined the club and had given the lefty valuable moral support when he was diagnosed with non–Hodgkin's lymphoma. Boston did not exhibit the same passion for playing under replacement manager Bobby Valentine, finishing in last place in the AL East with a 69–93 record, the club's worst performance since 1965. To Lester's delight, the Red Sox on October 21 named Farrell manager. "I'm excited to get back working with him," Lester said.[39]

Through 2012, Lester has compiled 85 wins and 48 losses with a 3.76 ERA, struck out 1,060 batters and walked only 430 in 1,163 innings, and hurled two shutouts. Lester, who ascended to the major leagues with exceptional talent, releases his pitches from a three-quarters angle with deception and throws a four-seamer, cutter, slider, curve, and change-up. "So like so many lefties, he has a motion that make his mid–'90s fastball extremely hard to hit." Although displaying occasional wildness, he often strikes out batters in clutch situations and has a great pickoff move. His enormous discipline and consistent routine, developed by former major league pitcher Bob Tewksbury, helps him average slightly over six innings per start.[40] The 28-year-old left-hander already has beaten cancer, clinched a world championship, and hurled a no-hitter.

# BABE DIDRIKSON ZAHARIAS

"Cancer was the toughest competition I'd faced yet," insisted Babe Didrikson Zaharias. "I made up my mind that I was going to lick it all the way." Zaharias, the nation's greatest female athlete, had excelled in track and field and golf when diagnosed with rectal cancer in the twilight of her illustrious athletic career. A courageous, spirited battler, she resumed playing golf just three months after undergoing a colostomy and won several more tournaments.

Zaharias grew up in an immigrant working class family. Mildred Ella "Babe" Didrikson was born on June 26, 1914, in Port Arthur, Texas, the sixth child of seven children of poor Norwegian immigrants Ole Didrikson, a seaman, furniture refinisher, and cabinetmaker, and Hannah Olson. She developed an interest in sports at an early age. Her mother enjoyed success as a skier and skater, while her father avidly followed sports and encouraged his children to participate in athletics. Didrikson moved to Beaumont at age four and graduated in 1930 from Beaumont High School, where she performed well in basketball. She became a stenographer for the Employer's Casualty Insurance Company of Dallas and starred for their Golden Cyclones basketball team, sponsored by Colonel M.J. McCombs. Besides tallying 106 points in one game, she made the Amateur Athletic Union All-America basketball team three times, and led the Golden Cyclones to national Amateur Athletic Union (AAU) Championship in 1931.[1]

Several factors contributed to Didrikson's incredible athletic success. Didrikson possessed a "natural aptitude and talent for sports," a "competitive spirit," and an "indomitable will to win." Furthermore, she demonstrated "the patience and strength of character," practicing "endless hours" to "reach the top." Didrikson's unrelenting work ethic gave her confidence and assuredness in perfecting her form. Didrikson carried the work ethic into interscholastic track and field, practicing two hours daily with her teammates and for at least two hours after supper.

The 5-foot 7-inch, 115-pound Didrikson performed well in track and field as the sole member of the Employer's Casualty Insurance Company team, winning six of the 10 events on July 16 in Evanston, Illinois, at the 1932 U.S. Women's AAU Championships. The event doubled as the Olympic Trials. "Babe staged and won a private octathlon" that day, entering eight of 10 events. She set three world records, dominating her competition in the 80-meter hurdles, baseball throw, shot put, broad jump, and javelin throw, and equaling the world record in the high jump. Didrikson was edged by Jean Shiley in the high jump, finished fourth in the discus throw, and narrowly missed the finals of the 100-meter

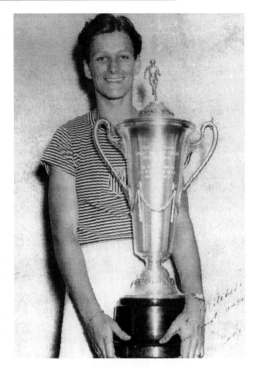

Babe Didrikson Zaharias received a trophy in 1932 as the World's Greatest Female Athlete after winning the U.S. Women's AAU Track and Field Championships (which doubled as the 1932 Olympic Trials) as a one-person team and winning three medals at the 1932 Summer Olympic Games in Los Angeles (courtesy Babe Didrikson Zaharias Foundation).

dash. She amassed 30 points to take the team title. The fully-staffed Illinois Woman's AC team finished second with 22 points.[2] No male athletes save Jim Thorpe and Jesse Owens had come close to such dominance at a track and field meet.

At the 1932 Olympic Games in Los Angeles two weeks later, Didrikson participated in only three events. She captured gold medals and set world records in the javelin throw (143 feet, four inches) and 80-meter hurdles (11.7 seconds). Didrikson tied Shiley for first place in the high jump, and both cleared the bar at 5 feet, 5 inches. The officials suddenly disqualified Didrikson for clearing the bar head first. "Babe was pretty unhappy about the whole thing since there had been nothing said about her jumping style before."[3] The Associated Press named her its Female Athlete of the Year.

Didrikson was a versatile all-around athlete. Paul Gallico of *Sports Illustrated* eulogized, "Babe excelled superlatively" in track and field, basketball, and golf, and performed "creditably" in swimming, diving, billiards, lacrosse, bowling, and tennis.

Didrikson clouted home runs in softball, proved "a crackerjack" at pool and billiards, and participated in swimming and high-diving exhibitions. She starred in baseball, setting a throwing record and hitting and pitching adeptly, threw footballs, kicked left-footed, and even contemplated boxing.

Didrikson soared to "her greatest heights" in golf. Didrikson, who married professional wrestler George Zaharias in December 1938, dominated women's golf in the 1940s. After deciding to take up the sport seriously, "she took lessons, drilled and practiced for hours on end until her hands were a mass of blisters."[4] Zaharias routinely hit 230- to 240-yard tee shots and sank 20-foot putts easily. She won 40 amateur titles before turning professional in 1947, giving the sport the flair and box-office appeal it badly needed. The Zahariases helped establish the Ladies Professional Golfers Association (LPGA) in 1946–1947, vastly improving pay for competitors.

Zaharias captured 14 consecutive golf tournaments, including the U.S. Women's Amateur, Tam O'Shanter All-American Open, North and South Women's Amateur, Augusta Titleholders, Broadmoor Ladies Invitation, and Texas Women's Open Championships, in 1946 and 1947 and became the first American woman to take the British Women's Amateur Championship at Gullane, Scotland. "She took the wind-swept, sheep-infested course by storm," persuading Scots "she was the most talented and entertaining woman the game had seen." Zaharias was named the Associated Press Female Athlete of the Year in 1945, 1946, 1947, 1950, and 1954 for her golf accomplishments and became the first woman athlete to earn over $100,000 in her career. "Babe's competitive spirit," along with "her flair for drama, her eye-popping power made her extremely popular with the galleries."[5]

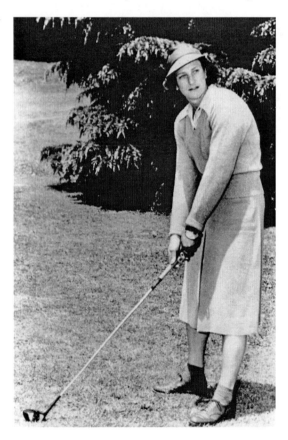

Babe Didrikson Zaharias, shown here at a promotional event in the late 1940s, captured 14 consecutive golf tournaments in 1946 and 1947, breaking Byron Nelson's record of 13 (courtesy Babe Didrikson Zaharias Foundation).

Zaharias's health remained relatively strong until the 1952 LPGA tour. Zaharias performed well in 1952, winning the Augusta Titleholders Championship and the first two legs of the Weathervane series by April. She led the Richmond Women's Open in Richmond, California, after two rounds in May when she experienced severe pain in her left side. "That evening, she was exhausted and felt pain shooting through her left hip." Zaharias noticed, "The pain and the swelling came more often" and was "more severe."[6] She competed in tournaments at Bakersfield and Fresno, California, and led the first two rounds of the Weathervane at Seattle before dropping to a career-worst eleventh place. "Those 36 holes were just agony for me," Zaharias recollected. She told George, "The pain was so bad now that I couldn't stand it any longer."[7]

After seeing her family physician, Dr. W.E. Tatum, in Beaumont, Zaharias entered Hotel Dieu Hospital. Dr. Tatum discovered Zaharias had suffered a strangulated femoral hernia on her left thigh. The protrusion at the top of her left thigh bone stopped her blood circulation. Dr. Tatum claimed that she would have died had the diagnosis been delayed a week. He postponed her surgery for three days because she was anemic and exhausted. The operation alleviated her pain considerably, but "knocked her out of some of the big tournaments." Zaharias recuperated from her hernia surgery at her Tampa Bay Country Club residence, where she designed an "ultra-modern kitchen."[8]

Zaharias pled with Dr. Tatum for several weeks to let her return to the golf circuit. Dr. Tatum finally gave his consent in August after she had undergone three months of recuperation. Zaharias tried to win her fifth consecutive World Championship at Chicago. She performed well the first two rounds, but tired on the final nine holes of the third and fourth rounds and finished third behind Betty Jameson and Patty Berg. Zaharias won the Texas Women's Open tournament in Fort Worth, Texas, that October, only her fourth victory in 20 tournaments in 1952. She did not lead the LPGA in money earned for the first time, finishing fifth, and grew fatigued after returning home in November. "No amount of rest or sleep seemed to restore her strength and energy." After golfing a round, she admitted, "I never felt like I wanted to play another nine holes."[9]

Zaharias's fortunes declined on the 1953 LPGA tour. "I wasn't winning much of anything," Zaharias complained. "Half the time I wasn't even finishing in the first five." She often tired after shooting a good round. Zaharias placed second at the Jacksonville Open in March and dropped to sixth in the Augusta Titleholders Championship. "I was feeling worse and worse," Zaharias lamented. She fared poorly in the Peach Blossom Open tournament in Spartanburg, South Carolina, barely completing the final 18 holes. George arranged a doctor's appointment for her in Spartanburg, but she declined to go. Zaharias finished second in the New Orleans Women's Open the next week, relinquishing a lead. "She barely had enough strength to eat dinner" after golfing and then slept. Zaharias "worried the fatigue was something more than a hernia," but "kept procrastinating"[10] about seeing her doctor.

Zaharias met Dr. Tatum before the inaugural Babe Zaharias Golf Tournament at the Beaumont Country Club and made arrangements for a checkup after the tournament. "I'll never know where I got the energy to play that tournament," she confessed. A nearly exhausted Zaharias led the tournament by one stroke over Louise Suggs after two rounds. "The last day it was more of an effort to play than ever," she admitted. Zaharias struggled to four over par after the fifteenth hole, but birdied the sixteenth. After bogeying the seventeenth hole, she seemed to be "crawling on [her] hands and knees."[11] Zaharias birdied the eighteenth hole, sinking a 30-foot putt to capture her tournament by one stroke over Suggs. The hometown gallery was ecstatic. "I'd never felt so completely played out," she remarked.

Dr. Tatum examined Zaharias on April 6, the day following the tournament. His face suddenly turned ashen. Zaharias feared that she had cancer. Tatum sent her to Fort Worth to see Dr. William C. Tatum, no relation, for further tests. Zaharias wanted to participate in the Phoenix Women's Open the next weekend, but saw the specialist instead. Dr. Tatum took some biopsies that night. He broke the tragic news to George the next day, "I'm afraid she has [rectal] cancer."[12] George saw three consecutive movies to try to muster enough courage to tell his wife, but still did not tell her. The Zahariases hardly slept that night.

At her 11 A.M. appointment on April 8, Dr. Tatum told her, "Babe, you've got cancer." The superbly trained athlete was just 39 years old. Zaharias explained, "That report just hit me like a thunderbolt." Deep down inside, she had suspected cancer because of her intermittent pains, diminished energy level, and exhaustion. The news proved even more devastating. Dr. Tatum confirmed Zaharias had contracted rectal cancer and needed a colostomy, requiring removal of her rectum and part of her colon. Dr. Tatum warned it would take a few months for her to recover and that she probably would never play tournament golf again. Zaharias gave her golf clubs to close friend R.L. Bowen of Fort Worth, stating, "I won't be needing them anymore." Zaharias, who was not especially religious, wondered, "What in the world have I done wrong in my life to deserve this?"[13] George, though, convinced her, "You'll play again." Zaharias soon vowed, "I feel confident that with God's help, I will be back soon to play and win."[14]

Dr. Robert Moore of the University of Texas Medical School performed the colostomy on Zaharias on April 17 at the Hotel Dieu Hospital. The media reported Zaharias was being operated on for a "serious malignancy." Her room was deluged with telegrams, letters, and flowers.[15] "It was a remarkable tribute to a woman who had made an unusual mark in our sports-loving society." Zaharias, who dreaded having the surgery, instructed George beforehand to put her golf clubs in her hospital room, vowing, "I'm going to use them again."[16] The clubs stayed in that corner for the remainder of her hospitalization.

The colostomy, "one of the most dangerous and excruciating of all operations," took four hours. Surgeons removed a malignant tumor from Zaharias' lower rectum. The doctors rerouted her intestinal tract so solid waste could pass through an incision on the left side of her abdomen. "The operation had gone well, but malignancy in the surrounding lymph node signaled doom."[17] Dr. Moore suspected the cancer would spread within a year and advised George and close friend Betty Dodd that Zaharias not be told the prognosis. He warned that she would not have much energy and added, "Babe would probably never be able to play golf again." Nevertheless, Zaharias began playing golf in her sleep. She lost considerable weight during her hospitalization and started exercising her arms and legs while still bedridden. As soon as she could, Zaharias got out of bed, grabbed one of the golf clubs in the corner, and gripped it. The surgery required an extensive "uncomfortable convalescence."[18] She spent slightly over one month in the hospital and recuperated at the home of her brother, Louie, and his wife, Thelma.

Zaharias returned to Tampa in early June. She never felt well again, but did not complain and showed enormous courage. In hopes of inspiring others, she wanted her health problems made public. The operation had given her renewed hope, as she tried to live each day to the fullest. Zaharias yearned to show others with colostomies that life could proceed as before.

Drs. Moore and Tatum permitted Zaharias to start practicing golf. Zaharias pledged "to come back and win golf championships just the same as before."[19] She gradually practiced more each day at the Tampa Golf Club, increasing the number of holes played, and even shot a 37 over nine holes. "I'll beat it," Zaharias insisted. She won the Babe Didrikson Zaharias Open Tournament the last week of June at the Beaumont Country Club, donating the proceeds to the Damon Runyon Cancer Fund. "Babe had become a leading spokesperson for cancer fund-raising and education."[20]

Fourteen weeks after the surgery, Zaharias competed in the All-American Open Championship for Women at the Tam O'Shanter Country Club in Niles, Illinois. Gallico observed, "This incredibly brave and unquenchable girl was back on a golf course again," competing in torrid temperatures. Zaharias needed to know if she could still play tournament golf. She was paired with Dodd. According to Zaharias, Dodd "could step in and help if I had any trouble."[21] George wondered whether she could walk 18 holes.

Before a gallery of nearly 5,000 people, Zaharias hit the first ball 250 yards straight down the middle. According to Gallico, "Her presence on that first tee was an act of heroism that should have been rewarded with the Congressional Medal of Honor." Her example inspired others of "less courage and steadfastness." Jameson, who was amazed with Zaharias's determination, observed, "What grit."[22] But Zaharias could not control her shots on the short green and recorded discouraging rounds of 82 and 85 the first two days. "I couldn't do anything right," Zaharias lamented. She broke down emotionally during the third round. "I was beginning to think that I'd never play championship golf again," Zaharias recalled. After three-putting the fourth green, she missed a little chip shot, and took another three putts on the fifth hole.

Zaharias walked to the sixth tee and sat down. "I put my face in my hand and just bawled," she recalled. George and Dodd suggested that Zaharias return to the clubhouse if she did not want to golf anymore that afternoon. But Zaharias retorted, "I don't want to quit. I'm not a quitter!" She three-putted again on the sixth green, terming it "the blackest of moments," and prayed to God to give her strength. Zaharias pulled her game together and shot the last nine holes in 34, two under par, to finish with a 78 for the third round and shot an 84 on the final round to tie for fifteenth out of thirty. "The power in her tee was gone," and she feared "what might happen."[23]

A few days later, Zaharias played in the World Championship at Tam O'Shanter and led after three and one-half rounds. She tired on the final nine holes, shooting a 43. "My back was killing me," Zaharias revealed. Berg won the tournament, while Zaharias finished third. Zaharias was pleased about being able to "stay up as long as I did that soon after the operation," but "a third-place finish hardly lived up to Babe's own standards."[24] Zaharias, who was accustomed to winning, received many inspirational letters encouraging her to continue golfing. "The Babe is back," *Time* magazine declared. Doctors marveled at her "recuperative power."[25] Zaharias competed in the Texas Women's Open that October. Despite missing numerous tournaments that year, she won two events and miraculously ranked sixth in money earned with $6,345 prize money. She edged baseball slugger Ted Williams of the Boston Red Sox for the Ben Hogan Comeback Player of the Year Trophy.

Although tiring easily, Zaharias returned to the LPGA tour in January 1954 and gradually regained championship form. After placing seventh in the Tampa Women's Open, she tied Beverly Hanson after four rounds of the St. Petersburg Open before losing on the third playoff hole. Zaharias pondered "whether I'd ever be capable of winning tournaments again." "I'm starting to feel myself on the golf course," she wrote, but "I just miss silly easy shots."[26]

Zaharias battled Berg for first place in the Serbin Women's Open in Miami Beach in February, sharing the lead at two strokes under par 220 for the first three rounds. They were still tied after nine holes in the final round. Despite fatiguing on the back nine, Zaharias needed just a par-four on the 430-yard final hole to defeat Berg. She drove the ball, however, into a spot among the palm trees and clouted the next ball over them to within 100 yards of the green. Zaharias blasted the next ball onto the green and sank her par putt for her first tournament victory since the cancer operation. "After so many losses, Babe's spirit soared." She beamed, "I'll have to call this the biggest thrill of my life. I didn't think I would ever win another one."[27]

After capturing the Serbin Women's Open, Zaharias ranked among the top three golfers in nearly every 1954 tournament. "In one of sport's all-time dazzling ascents after adversity," Zaharias captured four more tournaments that year.[28] President Dwight D. Eisenhower and his wife, Mamie, hosted her at the White House in Washington, D.C., where she opened an American Cancer Society crusade drive.

After taking the National Capital Women's Open in Washington, D.C. in May,

Zaharias resoundingly captured the U.S. Women's Open in July at the challenging Salem Country Club in Peabody, Massachusetts, competing in that event for the first time in three years. Sportswriter Jack Newcombe termed her triumph on the long 6,393- yard course "Babe's finest golf victory." Zaharias seized the lead with a par-72 the first day, never exceeding five on any hole. She widened the margin with a 71 on the second round and a 73 on the third round. She tired on the last five holes of the final round, bogeying each and ending with 75 for the round. "Heroically, she had played thirty six holes on the final day." She routed Betty Hicks by a tournament-record 12 strokes and Suggs by 16 strokes, recording a 291 for the tournament, "as impressive as the best male professional of the day."[29]

Following Zaharias's clinching putt, the roaring crowd applauded her "master-piece" for nearly five minutes. Zaharias celebrated with George and Dodd. Although experiencing some fatigue, She was ecstatic "over the way I'd come back to win the biggest title in women's golf." Zaharias, who had received over 15,000 letters from cancer victims, said, "I can tell people not to be afraid of cancer." She added her victory would "show a lot of people that they need not be afraid of an operation and can go on and have a normal life."[30] Zaharias even predicted, "I'll go on golfing for another 20 years." The triumph marked her third U.S. Women's Open victory in just five attempts. USGA president Isaac Grainger gave her a silver cup and $13,000 check, pronouncing her "the greatest woman athlete in the world" and praising her "wonderful attitude in fighting against what many consider an insurmountable handicap." Sports columnist Jim Murray of the *Los Angeles Times* lauded her triumph as "probably the most incredible athletic feat of all time, given her condition."[31]

Zaharias dominated the Tam O'Shanter All-American Open Championship for Women by eight strokes with a 294 score, one stroke off the women's 72-hole record she set for that course for her final major triumph. She finished fourth in the Tam O'Shanter World Championship, lacking the endurance to compete in consecutive tournaments. Zaharias acknowledged, "I didn't have quite as much stamina as I used to." She struggled in subsequent tournaments at Wichita, Kansas, and Ardmore, Oklahoma, but still finished second in earnings with $14,452 on the 1954 LPGA tour. Zaharias won the Vare Trophy for lowest scoring average and the Serbin Trophy for highest cumulative finishes in tournaments. The Associated Press named her Female Athlete of the Year for the sixth time. "No other athlete, male or female, has won the award six times."[32]

Zaharias volunteered her time to help in cancer-related organizations, becoming "America's all-star trailblazer against cancer." She had pledged, "I'd do everything in my power when I got out to help the fight against cancer." Besides opening a Babe Didrikson Zaharias chapter of the American Cancer Society in Seattle, she made personal appearances and recorded television and radio advertisements for the American Cancer Society and Damon Runyon Cancer Fund, sponsored several golf tournaments to benefit cancer treatment and research, and visited children's cancer wards. "She gave people hope," Berg recollected. Fatigue and illness eventually forced her to reduce those appearances. Zaharias and George built a new dream house, Rainbow Manor, near the Tampa Golf and Country Club and moved there in March 1955. Zaharias spent considerable time designing the home while traveling to tournaments. "She planned every inch of it,"[33] George recalled.

Zaharias had rejoined the golf tour after her 1954 surgery for several reasons. Her comeback inspired other cancer victims, especially those having colostomy operations. "She wanted so desperately to get well and to help relieve tension and fear in others of this dreaded disease." Zaharias also desired to help the LPGA continue to grow. The LPGA tournament had nearly quadrupled to 25 events and offered higher purses. Tournaments drew larger crowds, Zaharias acknowledged, "when all of us are in there." She also aspired to convince skeptics that she could still triumph and "prove all over again I'm still a championship golfer."[34]

Zaharias won the Tampa Women's Open by one stroke over Suggs in January 1955, but did not prevail in her next two tournaments. She withdrew following the first round of the Sarasota Open in February and shared sixth place in the Augusta Titleholders Championship in March. "Slowed, often in great pain, Babe kept playing."[35] A two-year checkup revealed no signs of a relapse. Doctors found her anemic and prescribed a vacation.

In mid–April, Zaharias struggled to thirteenth place in the Babe Zaharias Open at Beaumont. Her back ached, which she attributed to fatigue. Zaharias ruptured a disk in her spinal column getting a car out of sand when it got stuck in Port Arthur on the Texas coast. She writhed with back pain and could not sleep. Zaharias took Vitamin B-1 injections before finishing sixth the next week in the Carrollton Women's Open in Georgia. She won the Peach Blossom Open tournament in late April in Spartanburg, South Carolina, with a 293, two strokes ahead of Marilynn Smith. Zaharias "shifted into high gear" and "started smashing those long drives off the tee." The tournament proved an ordeal, however, because her back problems worsened. Zaharias sadly never played another tournament. "Isn't it kind of fitting," Betsy Rawls observed, "that Babe would win the last tournament she ever played?"[36]

Doctors at Hotel Dieu Hospital in Beaumont searched in vain for the cause of Zaharias's back pain. Zaharias collapsed after returning to Tampa, suffering unbearable pains in her right leg and numbness in her right foot. Zaharias returned to John Sealy Hospital in Galveston, Texas, in late May. Dr. Robert Moore diagnosed her with a herniated slipped disk in the spinal column. Dr. S.R. Snodgrass operated on her ruptured disk on June 22. Doctors wanted to "relieve Babe's intense back pain," but her suffering persisted. In late July, doctors discovered a new cancer on the right side of the rear of her pelvis. "Both Babe and George knew the score." She welcomed the stream of hospital visitors, "many of whom were moved to tears by her bright courage."[37]

Zaharias kept unswerving optimism in the face of the physical pain because of "her belief in her own invincibility and denial of her mortality." She told doctors, "There was no doubt about my coming back again." Zaharias also yearned to return to competition, "her life's blood."[38] Doctors told her that she could not return to the LPGA circuit for three to six months. After leaving the hospital in September 1955, she vowed to continue competing in golf tournaments. "My autobiography isn't finished yet."

Harry T. Paxton, a ghost writer, helped Zaharias pen her autobiography. Zaharias signed a contract with A.S. Barnes and Company and told her story from the late spring to midsummer to Paxton, who tape-recorded her recollections. Paxton wrote, "Perhaps her most important golf triumphs ... were the titles she came back to win after undergoing major cancer surgery in 1953."[39]

Zaharias, unable to bear the pain in her left leg and foot, returned to John Sealy Hospital in Galveston from December 1955 through late January 1956 and from March 1956 until her death. Despite the ordeal, "her fiery spirit remained undimmed." When looking at the clubs in her room, she could "play mentally over old courses" and "plan to correct old mistakes."[40] The pain, though, frustrated her, and prevented any further comebacks. According to close friends, "Her final days were agonizing."

Cancer ultimately was "one challenge she couldn't conquer." No one knew what kept her alive, as her weight dwindled to 62 pounds. Zaharias battled for six more months, succumbing at age 45 on September 27, 1956. George told reporters, "It's been a long battle and Babe fought it the way she knew how to fight — giving ground reluctantly, an inch at a time." Upon her death, "Babe achieved a level of public approval, purposefulness, and valor that transcended all of her athletic honors. Her earthly achievements were stupendous, but her dying, despite and beyond all her emaciated physique, had been magnificent."[41]

Eloquent tributes came from the media. The Associated Press called her "the greatest woman athlete the world has ever known" and noted "her stubborn battle with the one competitor she couldn't beat — cancer." The *New York Times* eulogized, "Babe Didrikson has finally lost the big one. It was the greatest and most gallant struggle of her great and gallant career."[42]

Zaharias garnered three Olympic medals in track and field, earned All-America honors in AAU basketball, held hundreds of sports records, and won 82 golf tournaments, including seven after her 1953 colostomy, in her 18-year dominance of women's golf. She was inducted into the LPGA Hall of Fame in 1951, World Golf Hall of Fame in 1974, the National Track and Field Hall of Fame in 1974, PGA Hall of Fame in 1976, the International Women's Sports Hall of Fame in 1980, and the U.S. Olympic Hall of Fame in 1983. Her other honors included being named top Female Athlete of the Twentieth Century by the Associated Press and ESPN.[43] The Babe Didrikson Zaharias Museum in Beaumont, opened on November 27, 1976, celebrates her life.

Zaharias revolutionized the way the media and American public viewed women athletes. "A star athlete," Jack Newcombe wrote, "Babe began as a muscular phenom who mastered all sports and ended as a brilliant, beloved golfer." Gallico eulogized that Americans watched her "become the greatest woman golfer that ever lived, a champion of champions, and then thrill a nation with the courage and gallantry of her battle against cancer." Although her track and field and Olympic records (except for the baseball throw) were later broken, no woman "has matched her record of events won in a diversity of sports" nor "even approached her in the number and caliber of golf championships captured, some of them played while suffering from pain, illness and physical handicaps." Gallico boasted, "She carved herself an imperishable niche in the great American world of sports,"[44] and claimed, "She was probably the most talented athlete, male or female, ever developed in our country." Zaharias also helped spark the growth of the LPGA, with nearly $200,000 in tournament money and 35 tour participants by 1956.[45]

Zaharias won the Academy Awards of Sports Courage in 1987 for "overcoming tremendous physical hardships." Since 1985, the American Sport Art Museum and Archives, which is dedicated to the preservation of sports art, history and literature, has given the Mildred "Babe" Didrikson Zaharias Courage Award to an individual who demonstrated courageous action in overcoming adversity to excel in sport. The recipients have exhibited courage, perseverance, grace, and strength in sports achievement. The award honors Zaharias's spirit and zest for life, along with her courage, strength, and achievement. Her fight to overcome life-threatening cancer and return to the winner's circle has withstood the test of time. Rocky Bleier, Jim Abbott, Gail Devers, and Scott Hamilton, four subjects in this book, have received this prestigious award.

Zaharias distinguished herself as a medical humanitarian involved in cancer education and fund-raising. Through her foundation, she increased cancer awareness and vowed "to emerge victorious over any foe, including cancer." But she "offered instead a conqueror's independent stoicism faced with denial, courage, good humor, and distorted hope."[46]

# *Diabetes*

## GARY HALL JR.

"I live every day as if it's going to be my last"[1] was the motto of Gary Hall Jr., who battled back from Type 1 diabetes to return to swimming excellence. Hall already had won four Olympic medals before being diagnosed with Type 1 diabetes. He learned to cope with that debilitating disease to regain Olympic form, earn six more Olympic medals, and set several world freestyle records.

Hall was reared in an elite setting. Gary Wayne Hall Jr., the oldest of six children, was born on September 26, 1974, in Cincinnati, and grew up in a swimming environment. His father, Gary Sr., an ophthalmologist, swam at Indiana University under legendary coach "Doc" Counsilman. A very intense competitor, Gary Sr. held 11 world records, including the 200-meter butterfly, competed in three Olympics, and won a silver medal in the 200-meter butterfly at the 1972 Munich, Germany, Summer Olympic Games. He was the American flag bearer at the opening ceremonies at the 1976 Montreal, Canada, Summer Olympic Games, the last swimmer so honored. After winning a bronze medal in the 100-meter butterfly there, Gary Sr. took his two-year-old son from his wife, Mary Keating, and walked him around the pool to a standing ovation. To his dismay, however, he never won a gold medal in three Olympic Games. He later moved to Paradise Valley, Arizona, and operated the Gary Hall Eye Surgery Institute in Phoenix.

Gary Jr. possessed innate swimming ability and was considered "the most talented U.S. swimmer since [seven-time Olympic gold medalist] Mark Spitz." He exhibited less passion than his father for swimming and felt being pushed by his father to swim. The pair clashed over what his father termed a lack of commitment. "I resisted the whole talent thing,"[2] Gary Jr. recalled. Hall started swimming at a very young age at the Phoenix Swim Club and spent considerable time around the pool, but did not take the sport seriously until age 16.

Hall enjoyed an extremely close relationship with Charles Keating, his maternal grandfather, often visiting the latter's financial office in Phoenix and traveling abroad with him. As a teenager, Hall rebelled when Keating, a 1946 NCAA Champion swimmer in the 200-yard butterfly, was convicted in 1991 of fraud, racketeering, and conspiracy in the Lincoln Savings & Loan scandal and sentenced to prison. Hall, who called Keating's imprisonment "the greatest tragedy of my life,"[3] started struggling academically and "battling his parents." Hall and a few friends were caught blowing up mailboxes and doing donuts in a station wagon on the ninth green at a Phoenix golf course. Hall tried "to block out everything that was happening then" and admitted, "I just felt helpless." Swimming helped Hall deal with Keating's imprisonment. Hall tried reviving America's slumping swimming program, which had not performed well since the 1976 Olympics, and dedicated his efforts to Keating. He found swimming "a way to release that frustration" and "to give him some joy."[4]

Hall's first swimming success came in 1992, when he won the Junior National Championships. Hall graduated from Brophy College Preparatory High School, a Jesuit institution, in 1993. He attended the University of Texas, noted for its swimming program, from 1993 to 1994 and Arizona State University from 1995 to 1996. At the 1994 Long Course World Championships in Rome, Hall won a gold medal in the 4×100-meter medley and silver medals in the 50-meter freestyle and 100-meter freestyle. In 1995, he began training with Mike Bottom, co-head swimming coach of the University of California, Berkeley. Under Bottom's leadership, Hall and his teammates worked out twice daily, mixing long slow swims with high intensity sprints, weight lifting, running, jumping, and speed bag punching. The speed bag punching helped Hall improve his hand-eye coordination. The free-spirited Hall exhibited antics before competitions, frequently strutting onto the pool deck in motorcycle pants listening to the Grateful Dead on a Discman or donning boxing shorts and robe, shadow boxing and flexing for the audience. At the 1995 Pan-American Games in Mar del Plata, Argentina, he won the gold medal in the 4x100-meter freestyle. The 1995 Pan-Pacific Championships in Atlanta saw him take gold medals in the 50-meter freestyle, 100-meter freestyle, 4×100-meter freestyle, and 4×100-meter medley.

The 6-foot 6-inch, 187-pound Hall possessed "the prototypical build for a sprinter," whose smooth stroke "creates an optical illusion." Hall often did not appear to swim as fast as he actually did and usually gained considerable momentum on his turns. "He gets so much propulsion," his coach Tim Dalbey observed. "It's like God gave him a set of fins." Hall's inconsistency, however, sometimes baffled Dalbey. At the U.S. National Championships in February 1996 in Orlando, Hall perplexed Dalbey by stopping to kick on the final turn in the 100-meter freestyle.

At the Olympic Trials in Indianapolis in March, Hall easily made the 1996 U.S. Olympic team by winning the 50-meter freestyle race and placing second in the 100-meter freestyle. He "shoots down his lane like a torpedo when the big meets arrive, slicing off yards with a stroke that has been called biomechanically perfect by every coach he had ever had."[5]

Hall, noted for his blithe spirit, lacked his father's legendary training zeal and took a "low thermostat approach to the Olympics." He described his training as "quality over quantity." Despite his relaxed approach to training, Hall swam well in the major meets. "I just think I can do it," he maintained. "The speed has just always been there" when he needed it. His father concurred, "Every time he's had to swim fast in his life, he has."[6] Gary Jr. seemed confident about his prospects at the Atlanta 1996 Summer Olympic Games and even asked Coach Dalbey for a three-day training break instead of the traditional two.

Hall's self-confidence was warranted. At the 1996 Olympic Games, Hall won silver medals in the 50-meter freestyle and 100-meter freestyle and gold medals in two relay events. "The best head-to-head duel of the entire Olympics was the matchup of Alexander Popov and Gary Hall." Popov of Russia, who had swum an estimated 1,000 miles in seven months of training, entered the 1996 Olympic Games as the most dominant sprinter of all time, world record holder in the 100-meter freestyle, and winner of gold medals in the 50-meter freestyle and 100-meter freestyle in the 1992 Barcelona Summer Olympic Games. The 100-meter freestyle on July 22 was almost a dead heat from the start, with Hall leading by 0.11 seconds after the first 50 meters. The 6-foot 7-inch Popov used his reach to nose Hall at the wall by about six inches for the gold medal, his 48.74 seconds clocking besting Hall by 0.07 seconds. Hall, meanwhile, recorded a personal best 48.81 seconds, starting out very quickly and "just holding on at the end," Hall stated. "I think I did a lot better than anybody expected me to."[7]

In the shorter 50-meter freestyle on July 25, Popov won the gold medal in 22.13 seconds, edging Hall by 0.13 seconds. Popov accelerated his pace about halfway through the race and pulled ahead in the final 10 meters. "I think anybody could have won it," Hall contended. "It was the fastest field in Olympic history." Hall "exacted a measure of revenge," earning gold medals in the 4×100-meter freestyle and 4×100-meter medley. He swam the anchor leg of the 4×400-meter freestyle relay in "a sizzling 47.45 seconds," recording the fastest split in the event's history to give the U.S. team an Olympic record of three minutes, 15.41 seconds. Hall also anchored the 4×100-meter medley relay to a world record three-minute, 34.84-second-time, boasting another very fast split in defeating a Russian team that included two world-record holders. The Americans were underdogs entering the race, but Hall pointed out, "This is a perfect example of how a team can come together."[8]

Hall then took an extended break in 1997. He injured his shoulder in the weeks before the U.S. National Championships, the qualifying meet for the Pan-Pacific and World Championships. "I had a bad meet,"[9] he admitted. The 1998 season started and ended well for Hall. He won a gold medal in the 4×100-meter freestyle and a silver medal in the 4×100-meter medley at the Long Course World Championships in Perth, Australia, and captured his second and third U.S. National titles in April.

Hall's swimming career, however, suffered two major setbacks. Hall possessed a free spirit and a 1960s-style irreverence, delighting fans, but often frustrating swimming authorities. He was known "as a flake, a hey-dude character, with his headphones sending Grateful Dead music through his ears." In May 1998, FINA, swimming's international body, suspended him for testing positive for marijuana, his second violation in three years. The marijuana charge caused his sponsor, Speedo, to drop him. "It stripped me of all credibility," he lamented. "I became delusional, delirious and crazy. I'd totally lost myself."[10]

The marijuana problems forced Hall to clean up his lifestyle. Hall had smoked marijuana since his grandfather was imprisoned. Pot enabled him to maintain a pleasant facade. Elizabeth Peterson, his girlfriend and future wife, said, "When he quit smoking pot, he came in touch with his feelings" and learned how "to stay in control." By December 1998, he had recovered sufficiently to win the 50-meter freestyle at the World Cup meet in Texas.

In 1999, Hall confronted even more devastating problems. He constantly felt fatigued and experienced an unquenchable thirst and blurry vision. After collapsing at a party, Hall visited an internist in Phoenix in March just one week before the U.S. Nationals and learned that he had contracted Type 1 diabetes. The doctor's words crashed down on the Olympic gold medal-winning swimmer like a tidal wave. The internist told Hall, "You'll need to give yourself insulin by injection, several times a day, for the rest of your life. If you don't, you'll die." His body did not produce enough insulin, necessary for the body to use sugar. Sugar is the basic fuel for the cells in the body, and insulin takes the sugar from the blood into the cells. The endocrinologist predicted Hall's diabetes would terminate his competitive swimming career and warned, "You'll never swim at the world-class level again."[11]

The devastating news of his having diabetes was extremely difficult for a disbelieving Hall to handle. "I immediately felt the urge to defy him," Hall admitted. He took a brief hiatus from swimming, struggling with the possible impacts he knew the medical condition would have on his life. "I was extremely upset, shocked and discouraged," he recalled. Hall had believed that older, overweight, and under-active people contracted diabetes. "I had spent my entire life eating right, exercising, minding my health, etc.," he explained. Hall, who also found no history of diabetes within his family, asked, "Why me?"

Hall encountered difficulty accepting diabetes. He tried to learn as much as he could about the disease, but did not know if he could resume his swimming career. "It was frightening," he confessed, "because I had gone through so much."[12] Hall had faced the suspension for drug use and suffered through his toughest season since the Atlanta Olympics.

Peterson supported Hall throughout his ordeal. Four days after the diagnosis, Hall and Peterson flew to Costa Rica. Hall spent around two months in Costa Rica soul-searching and visited Peterson's uncle, David Butterfield, a Presbyterian minister who owned a nut farm overlooking a lake. Over the next three weeks, he was very depressed and contemplated suicide. "Right after we arrived," Peterson recalled, "he told me that he wasn't going to be going home with me. I pounded on his chest, bawling my eyes out and begging, 'Don't do it!' But Gary kept saying, 'Let's make this a nice farewell.'" Hall even swam a considerable distance into the Pacific Ocean, with Peterson waiting frantically on the beach for him to return. Hall admitted, "I'd swim until I couldn't see land, then I'd swim further. I thought, 'This is it. This is more than I can handle.' My life was total darkness."

But the trip ultimately rejuvenated Hall, who hiked with Peterson down to Lake Arenal and trekked up Mount Arenal. "We spent the larger percentage of our time porch sitting, overlooking the lake with a view of the spectacular natural beauty and tranquility," Peterson recalled. Hall observed, "I needed to know that a place this beautiful existed. I regained my hope, optimism, and a sense of well being." Hall said, "I found the will to continue on."[13]

The athletically powerful Hall became emotionally strong and celebrated a new dawn. He decided to prove to himself and over 120 million diabetics worldwide that the limitations of the disease are self-imposed. The disease forced the free-spirited Hall to discipline his life. As his father recalled, the diabetes "made him worry about how he was going to function as a person." The experience also changed his priorities, as he became a spokesman for diabetics "to show how a person can live a full life."[14] Hall managed his disease like a scientist, injecting himself with insulin up to eight times daily and trying to maintain high energy while monitoring his sugar levels at least 10 times a day by pricking his finger. He also reduced his aerobic work in the pool, attacked his dry-land training, including weightlifting, running, boxing, and circuit training, and adopted a high-protein, low-carbohydrate diet.

Upon returning from Costa Rica, Hall visited several doctors. Three doctors told him that he should not resume swimming. Hall, however, learned about Anne Peters, an endocrinologist at the University of Southern California School of Medicine in Los Angeles. Peters encouraged Hall to resume swimming and continue competitive swimming. She accompanied him to practices, the Olympic Trials, and Olympic Games. Peters also talked with him over the phone, monitored his health, answered his questions, and allayed his fears. She regarded Hall's case as exceptional, stating that among diabetics, "nobody's competing in the Olympics, nobody's trying to become the world's fastest swimmer, and nobody's doing anything anywhere near this intense."[15]

Peters explained how the battle with diabetes helped Hall. "Initially, Gary flipped out," she recalled, but he learned to cope with it. "He had had all of those hard knocks in his life, which helped him grow up." Peters added, "Gary has dealt with this disease with more grace and maturity than I've ever seen. His determination, strength and readiness to absorb information makes him stand out, separate from his swimming." Other diabetics were by awed Hall. "His Olympic quest means everything to them," Peters stated. "He's such an inspiration." Hall, who considered Peters his "godsend," found his way back into life and into the sport. Hall's attitude toward life changed dramatically. "I definitely don't take anything for granted," he said. "I live every single day as if it's going to be my last."[16]

Hall trained seriously with Coach Bottom at the Phoenix Swim Club, recording the fastest times of his career. He practiced with the Sprint Team 2000, consisting of a dozen sprinters from various countries preparing for the Olympics. Hall and 6-foot 3-inch, 165-pound, 19-year-old Anthony Ervin, a confident University of California at Berkeley sophomore and his chief competitor, followed the same program and ate Platinum Performance vitamins. "They listened to the same sports psychologists. They hit the same speed bags for coordination."[17]

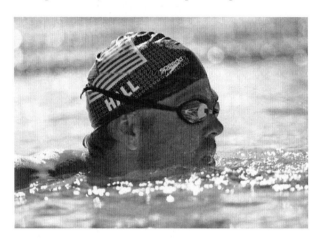

Gary Hall Jr., pictured swimming circa 2000, set an American record in the 50-meter freestyle at 21.76 seconds at the U.S. Olympic Trials at Indianapolis (photograph by Guillaume Deutsch, International Swimming Hall of Fame).

A few days after having influenza, Hall won the 50-meter freestyle with a personal best time at the 2000 U.S. National Championships for his fourth title and placed second in the 50-meter freestyle at the Pan-Pacific Championships. He also made the 1999–2000 All-America team, the national A team, and the national All-Star team, comprising the highest-ranking Americans in each event in the FINA World Rankings.

At the 2000 U.S. Olympic Trials in Indianapolis in August, Hall defied the doctor who had diagnosed his diabetes. He won the 50-meter freestyle by edging Ervin, the first swimmer of African American descent to make the U.S. Olympic team. His 50-meter freestyle time of 21.76 seconds broke Tom Jager's decade-old American record and was the second fastest in history. "No matter how tough, no matter what kind of outside pressure, no matter how many bad breaks along the way, I must keep my eye on the final goal — to win, win, win,"[18] Hall said in a voice choked with emotion. Hall placed second to Neil Walker in 48.24 seconds in the 100-meter freestyle and also qualified for the Olympic team in the 4×100-meter freestyle relay and the 4×100-meter medley relay.

Hall completed his incredible comeback at the 2000 Sydney Summer Olympic Games. On the opening night at the International Aquatics Center, he won a silver medal in the 4×100-meter freestyle relay. Before that September 17 race, Hall predicted an American victory. He called the American team "untouchable" and vowed to "smash" the Australians like "guitars," having taken "every Olympics in which the event had been contested."[19] The Australians moved ahead at the outset and maintained the lead entering the final leg.

Hall swam last against Australian ace Ian Thorpe, a 50-meter specialist, who jumped into the pool first and held the lead. He passed Thorpe midway through their 100-meter leg. "But Thorpe refused to fold. As both men churned to the finish, Thorpe methodically reeled Hall in, giant stroke by giant stroke." He regained the lead, finishing a body length ahead of Hall. Hall had cut slightly into Thorpe's margin by six-hundredths of a second, outpacing the Australian 48.24 seconds to 48.30 seconds on the final leg. But the Australian team set a world record with a three-minute, 13.67 seconds clocking to edge the American team by .21 seconds, the latter's first ever Olympic defeat in the event. Thousands of delirious Australians shouted joyously. After the race, the Australian team played air guitars on the pool deck. Hall admitted later, "I don't even know how to play the guitar." He considered that competition "the best relay race I've ever been part of. I doff my cap to the great Ian Thorpe. He swum better than I did."[20]

Five nights later, Hall won a bronze medal in the 100-meter freestyle. Twenty-two-year-old Peter van den Hoogenband of the Netherlands won the gold medal in that event and became the first man since Mark Spitz to triumph in the 100-meter freestyle and 200-meter freestyle in the same Olympics, setting world records in both events. Popov, two-time defending champion, finished second.

Two nights later, however, Hall denied van den Hoogenband a third gold medal in the 50-meter freestyle. The momentum shifted toward the American swimmers. Hall posted the best qualifying time, with van den Hoogenband second, Ervin third, and world record-holder Popov fourth. During the introductions, Hall flexed his muscles and threw imaginary uppercuts. The race featured "the usual explosion of froth and flailing." No swimmer conserved energy. "The only strategy was to go as fast as you could."[21] Hall started the quickest, but Ervin soon caught him with van den Hoogenband and Popov very close behind. The crowd of 19,500 roared throughout the race.

For the first time in an Olympic sprint race, Hall and Ervin tied for the gold medal, churning to victory in 21.98 seconds. They reached the wall at the same time "in one of the most dramatic sprints in Olympic history" for "yet another stunning upset by U.S. swimmers." Van den Hoogenband finished third in 22.03 seconds, while Popov fell to sixth place. Leigh Montville of *Sports Illustrated* poignantly described the photo finish: "They all reached the finish as if they were carried by one large wave." Hall and Ervin were perplexed when they looked at the wall at the far end of the pool and noticed that both were clocked at 21.98 seconds. "It took me a while to figure out what had happened," Hall acknowledged. He initially thought that van den Hoogenband had tied him, but then realized that it was Ervin. "If I had to share the gold with anyone," Hall reflected, "I'm glad it was him." Hall, who had never dreamed of finishing in a tie with Ervin, queried, "Who ever could have predicted such a long journey could end at the same time and the same place?"[22]

On September 23, Hall helped the U.S. team earn a gold medal in the 400-meter medley relay. He swam the last leg in 47.92 seconds to vault the Americans to a world record of three minutes, 33.73 seconds. Lenny Krayzelburg, Ed Moses, and Ian Crocker swam the first three legs. Australia finished second, while Germany placed third.

Hall's performances highlighted an unexpected display of dominance by the U.S. swimming team, which earned 33 medals, including 14 golds, eight silvers, and 11 bronzes in eight days. During the Olympic Trials, the Australians had set five world records. By contrast, no records were set at the American Olympic Trials. The Australians battled the Americans valiantly at the Olympic Games, but the latter ultimately prevailed. "This was the fastest meet in history, and we dominated it,"[23] U.S. team coach Dave Marsh boasted.

In August, 2001, Hall won the 50-meter freestyle at the U.S. National Championships and qualified in the 50-meter freestyle for the Goodwill Games in Brisbane, Australia. His blood sugar level, however, fluctuated erratically because he was required to compete several races in one day.

Hall also competed in the 50-meter freestyle at the 2002 U.S. National Championships and the 2003 Pan-American Championships in Santo Domingo, Dominican Republic. Although training substantially less than usual, he took the bronze medal in 22.43 seconds, just three-one-hundredths of a second behind victorious Fernando Sherer of Brazil.

At the 2004 Olympic Trials in July, Hall qualified for the 4×100-meter freestyle relay and the 50-meter freestyle. His appearance at the 2004 Summer Olympic Games in Athens made him and Gary Sr. the only father-son combination in the event's history to each compete in three Olympics. At age 29, he became the oldest American Olympic male swimmer since Duke Kahanamoku had vied in the 1924 Games.

The 2004 Olympics, however, did not begin well for Hall, who swam the anchor leg in the preliminaries of the 4×100-meter freestyle relay. Neil Walker swam more than a half-second quicker than Hall in the preliminaries and was selected instead to participate in the finals. Sprinters Jason Lezak and Crocker were reserved spots on the relay team by virtue of their one-two finish in the 100-meter freestyle at the Olympic Trials. Michael Phelps, who was attempting to surpass Mark Spitz's record seven Olympic medals in an individual games, was the fourth relay member selected for the finals.

The U.S. team of Crocker, Phelps, Walker, and Lezak placed a disappointing third, the worst American finish ever, in the 4×100-meter freestyle relay. South Africa set a world record at three minutes, 13.17 seconds, followed by the Netherlands at three minutes, 14.36 seconds. Hall, who still received a bronze medal for having competed in the preliminary heats of the relay, criticized coach Eddie Reese for bypassing him in the relay. He lamented, "I was bitter. I took it personally."[24] Hall added, "I very much wanted to be part of the relay that reclaimed that medal." He claimed, "The team would have had a better chance at gold if I had swum the final."[25] Hall also questioned Reese's decision to include "the ailing Crocker" and "the inexperienced

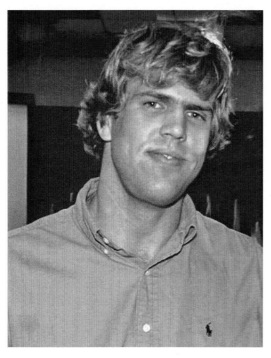

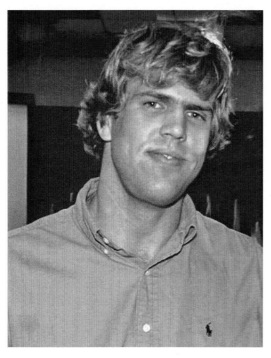

Gary Hall Jr., shown here at the International Swimming Hall of Fame induction ceremonies in 2011, was elected to the U.S. Olympic Hall of Fame in 2012 (courtesy International Swimming Hall of Fame).

Phelps" in the final. Crocker was ill and finished a second off his personal best, while Phelps had not done any relay exchanges with the team. The relay exchange with Phelps took half a second, "the difference between gold and the bronze" and "the slowest relay exchange out of anybody."[26] Reese assured Hall that "his relay selections were made strictly according to times"[27] and tried to convince him that he was not showing favoritism toward Phelps.

Hall's week ended, however, on a brighter note in the 50-meter freestyle. In the year preceding the Olympics, Hall had swum the fastest 50-meter freestyle. He walked to the starting line for the final dressed in a stars-and-stripes boxing robe and trunks, a code violation that cost him a $5,000 fine from USA Swimming. Although rated a long shot in the 50-meter freestyle finals, Hall surpassed the American record for most medals won over an Olympic career in any sport by garnering a gold medal. He covered the 50 meters in 21.93 seconds, two one-hundredths of a second ahead of Duje Draganja of Croatia, five one-hundredths of a second better than his 2000 Olympics time, and just .02 of a second off the Olympic record. Hall traveled "the most important inches of a race faster" than his competitors. Roland Schoeman of South Africa won the bronze medal, recording 22.02 seconds. "Very few people have been able to defend their Olympic title,"[28] Hall pointed out. He celebrated his victory by climbing out of the pool and bowing to the fans. His triumph did not surprise Coach Bottom. After the race, Schoeman remarked, "People may not like him for it, but I love him for what he is. He is a guy with a lot of heart. He's special!"

Although nearly 34 years old by the 2008 Summer Olympic Games, Hall hoped to defy the odds to become the first four-time American Olympic swimmer. He explained, "They told me it couldn't be done in '96 because I was too premature and then they said in 2000 it couldn't be done because I had diabetes, and this time they said that I was too old. So why not? Defiance is fun."[29] He failed to qualify for the 2008 U.S. Olympic Team, however, finishing fourth in the 50-meter freestyle at the Olympic Trials.

Hall serves as a national spokesperson for the American Diabetes Association and gives motivational speeches for those with diabetes, encouraging them to live full lives. He travels globally, sharing his love for swimming and his experiences as a diabetic with children, parents, coaches, doctors, and executives. He was on the regional board of directors of the Diabetes Research Institute and has been a consultant for medical device, pharmaceutical, and health companies.

Hall also handles television commentary for sporting events and hosts swim competitions. He and his father in 2003 founded The Race Club, an academy for those swimmers ranked among the top 20 in the world for three years or the top three of their national events in the past year. The club, coached by Bottom and based at the Islamorada, Florida, training center, offers swimming camps and clinics year around for young swimmers.

Hall, who possessed "a sprinter's here and now attitude," battled immaturity, drug problems, and especially diabetes to become one of the world's elite swimmers. He medaled in all ten of his Olympic races spanning three Olympic Games, earning five gold medals, three silver medals, and two bronze medals, and winning the 50-meter freestyle two consecutive Olympics. In 2012, Hall was elected to the U.S. Olympic Hall of Fame. Reese, who had observed Hall for nearly 15 years, summed up, "He had that killer instinct and he always tried to win."[30]

# RON SANTO

"I was very fortunate to be at the right place at the right time," recalled Ron Santo, who endured a debilitating disease to fulfill his dream of becoming a major league baseball player. Doctors diagnosed Santo with Type 1 diabetes shortly before he pursued a professional baseball career. Santo did not let that disease deter him from becoming the premier third baseman of his era.

Santo came from a lower-middle class background. Ronald Edward Santo was born on February 25, 1940, in Seattle and grew up in an ethnic working-class neighborhood known as Garlic Gulch. His alcoholic father, Louis, a bartender, and his mother, Vivian Danielsen, divorced when he was only seven years old. His mother sent the mischievous Santo to parochial school to learn more discipline. Santo participated in competitive school athletics and Little League baseball. "Sports saved me," Santo wrote. To support Ron and his older sister, his mother worked extremely hard as a waitress and drugstore clerk for several years. In 1954, she married John Constantino, a dry cleaner. The tempestuous Santo experienced difficulty adjusting to the masculine discipline and "fought all the time, especially in sports."[1] His family moved near Sick's Stadium, where he worked for the Seattle Rainiers (Pacific Coast League) baseball team.

Santo graduated in 1959 from Franklin High School in Seattle, having made All-City three years as a third baseman-catcher in baseball, quarterbacked in football, and played basketball. Although offered three college football scholarships, he explained, "I just loved baseball."[2] Santo made two hits in the Hearst 1958 All-Star Game, featuring the nation's premier high school baseball players at the Polo Grounds in New York. He married classmate Judy Scott in January 1960. They had three children, Ron Jr., Jeff, and Linda, before their 1982 divorce.

In 1959, the Chicago Cubs signed Santo for $20,000, promising him "a quick promotion to the major leagues." Although the other major league clubs offered him at least $50,000, Santo signed for much less with the Cubs because he had enjoyed watching them, especially Ernie Banks, on television. "The incredibly long dry spell" of the Cubs "since their last championship" in 1908 also intrigued him. His stepfather asked him whether making more money while performing in the minor leagues or playing in the major leagues sooner with the less-talented Cubs was more important. Santo replied, "I want to get to the big leagues."[3]

The 18-year-old Santo scheduled his annual physical examination with Dr. Mark Tupper, the family physician, before leaving Seattle for his initial minor league training camp. After finding sugar in Santo's urine, Dr. Tupper ordered him to have a glucose tolerance test at Providence Hospital to determine if he had Type 1 juvenile diabetes. Santo's blood sugar exceeded 400, confirming his juvenile diabetes, the most serious and insulin-dependent form of the disease. The devastating news startled Santo, who recalled, "I woke up that morning a happy, healthy teenager, and suddenly I had a disease I had never heard of." When Santo asked if he could still play baseball, Dr. Tupper replied, "I don't know."[4]

After conversing with Dr. Tupper, Santo's mother assured him that he still could pursue his baseball career. But she warned him about possible side effects and complications. Santo, who was diagnosed before measuring blood sugar was possible, read numerous diabetes books and articles at the public library. He learned that diabetics had just a 25-year life expectancy after being first diagnosed and wondered if that meant if he was supposed to live only to age 43.[5] Santo found the disease was a leading cause of blindness, hardened arteries, kidney failure, and gangrene. "I stopped reading," he admitted. "I couldn't absorb the horror."

Although prevalent theory regarded diabetes as strictly hereditary, Santo found no genetic link to his disease. He later discovered that "a traumatic event in one's life can trigger the disease"[6] and suspected his father's desertion of the family perhaps caused it. He had not yet experienced the fatigue, frequent erections, weight loss, and constant thirst associated with diabetes.

Santo attended a three-week course for newly diagnosed diabetics at a Seattle clinic that gave individual assessments for patient treatment. One doctor told him that he needed to take insulin daily for survival and exercise regularly to help lower his blood sugar. Despite the doctor's warning, Santo insisted that professional baseball players should not take insulin and believed that he could control his condition through diet and exercise. "The younger you are, the stronger the denial," he realized.

A woman sitting adjacent to him at one course session suddenly collapsed into a coma. Santo wondered if that could happen to him during a professional baseball game. The doctor urged that Santo learn the various symptoms of Type 1 diabetes. He told Santo, "You are a juvenile diabetic," and insisted, "You *will* go on insulin." Santo, who admitted being "just as scared as ever," shifted his focus to playing major league baseball. He vowed, "I wasn't going to let this thing beat me."[7]

Santo possessed the personal qualities to battle adversity. Pitcher-author Jim Brosnan termed him a "physically rugged" and "always doggedly fierce competitor." Santo combined a fiery personality with an intense desire to win, God-given talent, and blue-collar work ethic. Future teammate Banks called him "a hard worker and a leader. He had intensity. He was determined and ambitious. He wanted to win more than anybody I've ever known."[8]

Santo could not check his blood sugar easily and initially gauged his blood sugar levels on his moods. "I had to go by how I felt," he said. Santo quickly recognized the symptoms of hypoglycemia, including starting a cold sweat, being very hungry, feeling numbness in his nose and lips, and starting to weaken. If he felt his blood sugar was low, he snacked on a candy bar in the clubhouse.

Santo, meanwhile, spent three weeks catching at the Cubs' rookie camp in Mesa, Arizona, homering in his initial plate appearance. Legendary hitter Rogers Hornsby, who instructed Santo in batting, assured him, "Kid, you can hit in the big leagues, TODAY." The Cubs shifted Santo to third base at their full-scale spring training camp and nicknamed him "the Cheerleader" because he "yelled so much."[9]

Santo ascended through the Cubs' farm system, batting .327 with 11 home runs and 87 runs batted in (RBI) for Class AA San Antonio of the Texas League in 1959. "I felt great," he beamed. Santo thought he could keep his diabetes under control by exercising and eating properly. He trained with Chicago in 1960 at Mesa, primed to replace Alvin Dark. After acquiring Don Zimmer on April 8, the Cubs, however, assigned Santo to Houston of the American Association. The acquisition infuriated Santo, who had been promised the third base job by manager Charlie Grimm. "I quit," Santo told Grimm. "I stormed back to my room and started packing my bags."[10] Chicago general manager John Holland dissuaded him, giving him a major league contract to play for Houston.

The 6-foot, 190-pound Santo, who threw and batted right-handed, spent two months with Houston and joined the Cubs at age 20 on June 26, becoming the second Little Leaguer to make the major leagues. Santo debuted in a doubleheader that day against the Pittsburgh Pirates at Forbes Field with two hits and three RBI off Bob Friend in Game 1 and two hits and two RBI off Vernon Law in Game 2. Chicago swept the twin bill, ending its nine-game losing streak. "I was so nervous," Santo recollected. "There were 40,000 people in the stands." He quickly became the Cubs' regular third baseman.

Santo refused to take insulin until 1962. The Cubs conducted routine physicals, but did not check Santo's urine. During that winter in Chicago, "Santo's condition reached the life-or-death point of needing insulin."[11] His pancreas stopped working and his right leg began hurting. He suddenly lost 22 pounds and urinated frequently, and he recognized the source of those problems. His son's pediatrician urged him to see a doctor immediately. "I knew I was in trouble," Santo realized. The doctor told him to start taking insulin. "If you don't start taking it now, you will lose that leg," he warned.[12]

Two months before the 1962 season, the doctor ordered 15 units of insulin and instructed Santo to visit his office every other day. The doctor told Santo about the warning signs of diabetes, the symptoms of collapsing from low blood sugar, and how to take the daily insulin. "After years as a begrudging student," Santo understood, "I had to become his willing pupil." Teammates erroneously thought he was deliberately losing weight to increase his speed. One week before spring training, the doctor increased his insulin dosage to 30 units. Santo displayed diabetes symptoms while playing basketball with a friend. After 45 minutes, he felt a cold sweat, experienced blurriness and dizziness, turned ashen, and began slurring words. When Santo took insulin and drank orange juice, his body gradually returned to normal.

Santo told his doctor what had happened. The doctor ordered him to regulate his insulin, urging him to recognize his symptoms and always carry a candy bar in the dugout. He advised, "When you feel that very first symptom, take that candy." With Santo's busy schedule, he added, "It's going to be very important to regulate that insulin."[13]

At spring training in 1962, Santo notified Cubs physician Dr. Jacob Suker that he had taken insulin for two months to treat diabetes. Each morning, he took insulin shots in his legs and drank some orange juice. Santo concealed his condition from his teammates and swore Dr. Suker to secrecy. Since a teammate roomed with him on the road, he recalled secretly taking his insulin injection in the bathroom early each morning. Santo worried, "If the Cubs found out and I slumped badly, they would attribute it to the diabetes." He feared that they might send him back to the minor leagues or release him.

Santo wondered what teammates might do if he slipped into a diabetic coma. "The following season, my anxiety increased," he noted. Santo befriended rookie catcher Cuno Barragan, his new roommate. He informed Barragan about his condition, "swearing him to secrecy."[14] Barragan pledged not to tell teammates or the media. No other Cub knew for three seasons. "I lockered right beside him for years," Banks wrote, "and I never knew he had the disease."

Glenn Beckert, Santo's 1965 roommate, accidentally learned about the diabetes when mired in a batting slump. Beckert noticed that Santo was taking shots. At dinner one night, he whispered to Santo, "I hate needles, but I want it." "You want what?" Santo queried. Beckert had seen Santo giving himself a shot and explained, "You're hitting .320 and I'm hitting .220. Whatever it is, I want it."[15] Santo told Beckert about his diabetes and that the shots were insulin. Beckert looked dumbfounded and initially doubted Santo's explanation, but soon realized that his roommate was telling the truth.

Santo, Banks, and Billy Williams provided Chicago with offensive firepower from 1961 through 1966, but the leaderless Cubs languished in the second division. Chicago lost 90 games in 1961, although Santo batted .284 and clouted 23 home runs with 84 RBI. Santo, the National League (NL) Sophomore of the Year, wondered how he did it amidst all the mental turmoil, admitting he "had one helluva year." He estimated having lost 20 base hits by just a step in 1961 and vowed to increase his speed by losing 15 pounds to 175 pounds. In his first season while taking insulin (1962), Santo's batting average dropped to .227, home run production declined to 17, and errors rose to 24.

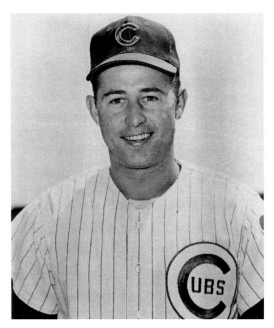

Ron Santo provided the Chicago Cubs with offensive firepower from 1960 to 1972, batting over .300, clouting at least 30 home runs, and knocking in over 100 runs four different seasons (courtesy National Baseball Hall of Fame Library, Cooperstown, N.Y.).

Since Santo had bypassed college, Chicago eventually became "the campus for Santo's million-dollar education." Gen Pullano, wealthy Old Heritage Life Insurance Company executive, met Santo when he was mired in a batting slump in 1962. The third baseman "needed someone who would help take his mind off his horrible season." The brash, self-confident Pullano helped him become assistant president of Nova Oil Company, giving him "an education in good common sense," Santo acknowledged. "He's given me a lot of responsibility and I've had to make decisions."[16] Pullano taught Santo responsibility and decision-making. Santo opened a pizzeria in Park Ridge, invested in four Chicago-area Kentucky Fried Chicken franchises, organized a baseball school for youngsters, and started Interpoint Corporation, which eventually operated 76 truck stops in seven states.

By 1963, Santo's lofty goals were to bat .300, clout 30 home runs, and knock in 100 runs each year for ten consecutive years. "A latter-day flannel-uniformed Man of La Mancha, Santo set himself an impossible dream." Furthermore, he aspired to become "the best all-round third-baseman in the game."[17] For the next five years, he "nearly matched his grandiose ambitions," averaging 30 home runs and 100 RBIs and winning five consecutive Gold Gloves as the NL's best defensive third baseman.

In 1963, Santo was named the NL Player of the Month in June and made his first All-Star Game appearance. Besides batting .297 with 187 hits, 25 home runs, and 99 RBI, he set a major league record for a third baseman with 373 assists. Santo had become the "spiritual and physical leader among Cub players."[18]

Santo hit a career-high .313 with 30 home runs in 1964, finishing second to Willie Mays with a .564 slugging percentage and second to Ken Boyer with 114 RBI. In 1965, he batted .285 with a career-high 33 home runs and 101 RBI. The Cubs, "a rag-tag bunch of leaderless losers 'managed' by a committee of coaches," made 25-year-old Santo the youngest team captain in franchise history. Head coach Bob Kennedy wanted Santo to unify the team. The Cubs still languished in the second division, dropping 90 games. According to Santo, "There was 'too much animosity' among the players" that boiled in 1965. Kennedy observed, Santo "took every defeat as if it were a personal disaster."[19]

Upon becoming team captain in 1965, Santo informed teammates about his diabetes at a hasty pre-game meeting. The third baseman disclosed how he needed candy or juice between innings following a dizzy spell in the field and discussed blood samples, urine tests, insulin injections and diet adjustments. Teammates pledged to keep the information confidential. Santo concluded, "I expect you to judge me by what I do on the field."[20]

Leo Durocher, who became the Cubs' manager in 1966, boasted, "Santo's my kind of ballplayer." Santo broke Hack Wilson's club record, hitting safely in 28 consecutive games. On June 26, he singled off Jack Fisher of the New York Mets to extend his streak to 26 games. In his next at bat, he stepped into the pitch, which "was higher and tighter than he calculated."[21] He turned his head, and the pitch hit him on the cheek. Santo realized his left cheekbone was broken and feared becoming blind, an affliction affecting diabetics. "I went down like a fighter," he recalled. Santo told Durocher, "I can't see out of my left eye." Durocher countered, "You're not blind. Your eyelid is completely shut."[22] An ambulance rushed Santo to nearby Northwestern Memorial Hospital, where doctors operated on his cheekbone. His clean break knit quickly.

Santo's hospitalization lasted only three days. Upon returning to the Cubs, Santo became the first major league player to wear a batting helmet with protective ear flaps. He rejoined the lineup on July 4 at Wrigley Field, making three hits off Law of Pittsburgh in Game 1. Don Cardwell held Santo hitless for most of Game 2. When Santo batted the next time, umpire Jocko Conlon told him that would be his last opportunity to extend his hitting streak because he planned to call Game 2 after that inning due to darkness. Cardwell threw Santo a fast ball down the heart of the plate that the latter lined to right field for a single, breaking Wilson's record. "The record was all mine,"[23] Santo beamed.

In 1966, Santo batted .312 with 30 home runs and 94 RBI. Defensively, he led NL third basemen in chances for the fifth consecutive year, tying Pie Traynor's record.

Fred Katz termed Santo "a winner playing for a loser." Although Chicago finished last and tied a franchise record with 103 losses, Durocher's arrival made Santo's season worthwhile. Typifying Durocher's competitiveness, Santo aspired "to win as badly as anybody, under any circumstances."[24] Durocher admired Santo's courage, declaring, "If I had eight more like him, we'd win the pennant every year." According to Santo, "1966 was the last year of the dark ages for the Chicago Cubs. 1967 was the beginning of the Renaissance."[25]

Santo excelled again in 1967, hitting .300, pacing Chicago with 31 home runs and 98 RBI, and finishing fourth in the NL Most Valuable Player (MVP) balloting. The Cubs exhibited more confidence and talent, vaulting to third place behind the St. Louis Cardinals and San Francisco Giants. Chicago, led offensively by Santo, Banks, Williams, and Beckert, recorded its best winning percentage since 1945 with 87 victories. Santo rejoiced at "playing on a winning team for the first time."[26]

At Wrigley Field on September 25, 1968, Santo's diabetes problem resurfaced against the Los Angeles Dodgers. Before the game, Santo ate his usual candy bar and drank a Coca-Cola. Bill Singer blanked the Cubs on one hit through eight innings and still led, 1–0, with Williams at bat, two men on base, and two outs in the ninth frame. Santo, who sensed an oncoming diabetic reaction while in the on-deck circle, recalled suddenly getting dizzy. His head began spinning because his blood sugar level plummeted. He recollected, "I looked up to centerfield and I saw three scoreboards out there."[27] Williams fouled off several pitches. Santo hoped that Williams would strike out so that he could return to the dugout for a much-needed candy bar. Williams walked instead.

Upon reaching home plate, Santo barely could swing the bat. He vowed to swing at Singer's first pitch regardless of where it was thrown. The first pitch looked "like it was attached to a slinky," Santo recalled. He remembered seeing "three balls instead of one." He clouted a grand slam home run over the left field wall, giving the Cubs a 4–1 victory. According to Santo, "The place went nuts."[28] Santo, who belted six career grand slam home runs, wanted to circle the bases quickly, but Williams sauntered ahead of him. "I thought for sure I would pass out and not make it to home plate," he noted. His face was ashen, his body numb. Santo lamented, "All of the warning signals the doctors had warned me about for years were there."[29] After struggling to the Cubs' dugout on the third base side, Santo quickly ate a candy bar and sat for about five minutes. He then trekked to the Cubs' clubhouse and talked to the media, who were unaware of his diabetic reaction.

In 1968, Chicago battled St. Louis for first place before finishing third again with 84 victories. Banks, Williams, and Santo combined for 88 home runs and 279 RBI. Although batting only .248, Santo contributed 26 home runs and 98 RBI and again led the NL in walks. During Santo's prolonged batting slump, the Cubs broke a record with 48 consecutive scoreless innings. "I didn't even have a good week,"[30] he recalled.

The Cubs came closest to winning NL pennants in 1969 and 1970, featuring Santo, Banks, Williams, pitcher Ferguson Jenkins, Beckert, and shortstop Don Kessinger. The 1969 season proved Santo's most frustrating. "Every time I went out there I thought we would win," he recollected. The opposing team or pitcher made little difference. Chicago finished April atop the senior circuit with a 15–6 record. "The Cubs set a blistering pennant pace,"[31] winning 22 of 30 games from May 11 through June 15 and holding first place for 155 consecutive days.

On June 19, Jim Hickman clouted a towering, walk-off home run with two men out in the ninth inning to give the Cubs a 7–6 come-from-behind victory over the Montreal Expos at Wrigley Field. The Expos had led 6–3 entering the final frame. "There may have been a time in my career when I was more excited, but if so, I can't remember it," Santo said. Santo led the reception when Hickman crossed home plate, "pounding on his helmet, hugging, slugging, yelling and screaming like a Little Leaguer." He ran down the left field line, watching the boisterous crowd. "I jumped into the air and kicked [*sic*] my heels" three times, he recalled. WGN featured his acrobatics as the headline story the next morning. To motivate the team, Durocher wanted him to make the heel-clicking demonstration the Cubs' victory signal. Chicago triumphed again the next day. Santo raced down the left field line at the end of the game and clicked his heels three times. "A tradition was born," Santo reminisced.

Cubs' fans adored Santo's antic, but critics associated the routine with overconfidence. "We were a close-knit group," Santo acknowledged. Chicagoans conversed mainly about the Cubs rather than politics, economics, or foreign policy that summer. "We were treated like rock stars," Santo claimed. Chicagoans really believed "we could win."[32] Santo repeated the heel-click routine after every home triumph until September 2, the last time the Cubs held first place.

Chicago led the New York Mets by seven games in July and derided the prospects of the Mets, their only East Division challengers. When the Cubs visited New York, sportswriter Dick Young asked Santo, "What do you think of the Mets?"[33] Santo replied, "How can they beat us? They ought to take a look at our club and give up." His comments infuriated the Mets and may have sparked their late season resurgence.

Chicago lost that crucial series to New York. Santo was involved in a controversial incident on July 8. "Suddenly, the tide turned"[34] against the Cubs. Durocher criticized Cubs rookie center fielder Don Young for dropping routine fly balls by Ken Boswell and Don Clendennon at Shea Stadium in a 4–3 setback. Young ripped off his uniform and left without meeting the media or waiting for the team bus. Santo was quoted by the media as saying of Young, "When he hits, it's a dividend, but when he fails on defense, he's lost — and today he took us with him." Within hours, Santo retracted his comments, admitting, "It was very wrong of me" to "jump all over him."[35]

Some columnists vilified Santo. The *Chicago Sun-Times* headlined the July 9 issue, "Santo Says Young Loses Game." Young questioned how Santo could blame him for losing the game. Santo denied he had said that and apologized to the team for anything the reporter misconstrued. Fans loudly booed Santo when he returned to Wrigley Field on July 11. "It was traumatic. My heart sank."[36] Vindictive hate mail and letters arrived, threatening him, his wife, and his children. Police protected the Santos for about a year.

Chicago led New York by eight games when Ken Holtzman no-hit the Atlanta Braves on August 19, but lost seven of its next nine games. The biggest setback came on September 6. Jenkins blanked Pittsburgh, 1–0, until the ninth inning, when Willie Stargell homered. The Pirates triumphed, 4–1, in 11 innings in "the pivotal game of the 1969 season." Santo claimed, "You could hear a pin drop as we walked into the clubhouse." The Cubs lost 17 of their final 25 games and finished eight games behind the Mets, who won 35 of their final 49 games and upset the Baltimore Orioles in the World Series. Santo still insisted, "We were the best team in the National League,"[37] and labeled the final three weeks "a nightmare." Chicago still recorded 92 wins, the most since its 1945 pennant club tallied 98. Besides batting .289, Santo finished second to Willie McCovey with a career-high 123 RBI, led the Cubs with 29 home runs, fielded superbly, and finished fifth in the National League MVP balloting.

Santo batted .267 and drove in 114 runs with 26 home runs in 1970, as Chicago finished second, five games behind the Pittsburgh Pirates. "It may have been our last great chance with the club we had to go all the way,"[38] he acknowledged. Santo slumped offensively until July 6, when he enjoyed the best day of his major league career. His two-run homer off Carl Morton of the Montreal Expos won the first game, 3–2. In the second contest, Santo belted a grand-slam home run in the third inning, walked with the bases loaded in the fourth frame, and slammed a three-run homer off Claude Raymond in the seventh inning. His offensive assault included three hits and 10 RBI, eight in the finale.

The Cub management held Ron Santo Day at Wrigley Field on August 28, 1971, when the third baseman disclosed his diabetes publicly for the first time. At the ceremonies, Santo told the nearly 35,000 fans about his courageous battle with diabetes. According to Brosnan, Santo "found a way to drum up support and understanding for other diabetics."[39] Proceeds from the sale of Santo buttons were donated to the Juvenile Diabetes Association of Greater Chicago. He devoted more time to visiting diabetic children in hospital pediatric units.

Santo again batted .267 in 1971, but his power production declined, with only 21 home runs and 88 RBI. The following year, he hit over .300 for the first time in five years and clouted 17 home runs with 74 RBI. The 1973 season saw him hit .267 with 20 home runs and 77 RBI. The Cubs traded him to the crosstown Chicago White Sox in December 1973. Santo spent his final major league season there, struggling as a designated hitter.[40]

Santo, the only diabetic playing a full major league career as a field position player, demonstrated enormous fortitude. "No one had ever played the game on a daily basis as an insulin-dependent diabetic." To survive, he injected himself with insulin every morning for 15 seasons. An optimistic attitude helped him. "I've got to do my best and be very positive about it,"[41] Santo insisted. His personal qualities, especially his "unusual capacity to learn and mature," made him a success. In addition, Santo kept "his boyish enthusiasm, his total unpretentiousness, his full-throttle approach, his sensitivity, and his fresh outlook."[42]

The nine-time All-Star often carried the Cubs defensively and offensively. "Santo was the National League's premier third baseman in the 1960s," demonstrating consistency and durability. He missed just 25 games from 1961 to 1971.[43] The third baseman led the NL nine times, including eight consecutive

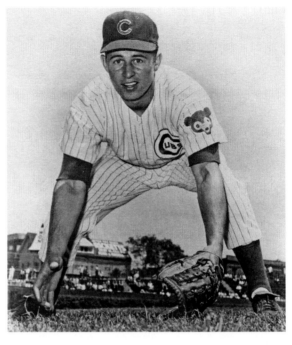

Nine-time All-Star Ron Santo, pictured here fielding, consistently led National League third basemen in several defensive categories and won five Gold Glove Awards (courtesy National Baseball Hall of Fame Library, Cooperstown, N.Y.).

(1961–1968), in total chances, and shares the record for most seasons topping the league in games, putouts, and assists with seven and double plays with six. Santo, who established a NL mark by playing 364 consecutive games at third base (April 19, 1964-May 31, 1966), also led the senior circuit in games played twice and fielding percentage once. His 164 games at third base in 1965 remain the major league record. Santo compiled a .954 fielding percentage as a third baseman, ranking sixth in career games (2,130), fifth in assists (4,581) and total chances (6,853), and seventh in double plays (395). He held NL records for career assists, total chances, and double plays, all later broken by Mike Schmidt. His 2,102 games at third base fell just 52 short of Eddie Mathews's NL record. Only four major leaguers participated in more games or belted more career home runs without making the playoffs.

In 15 major league seasons, Santo batted .277 with 365 doubles, 67 triples, 342 home runs, 1,331 RBI, and 1,108 walks in 2,243 major league games. He batted over .300, clouted at least 30 home runs, and plated over 100 runs four seasons, and ranked consistently among the top five in RBI, home runs, total bases, and slugging average. Only three Cubs belted more career home runs. His 337 home runs ranked eighth among NL right-handed batters. Santo was just the second third baseman to record at least 300 career homers and win five Gold Gloves, since joined by Schmidt. He ranked second among third basemen in slugging percentage (.464) and third in RBI, total bases (3,779), and walks. A patient hitter, Santo paced the NL in triples in 1964 with 13, in walks four times (1964, 1966–1968), and in on-base percentage twice (1964, 1966). The Cubs retired his uniform number 10 on September 28, 2003, before 40,000 fans at Wrigley Field. In April 2004, he was inducted into the inaugural class of the Washington Interscholastic Activities Association Hall of Fame.

During his 15 times on the Baseball Writers Association of America ballot, Santo never came close to the 75 percent figure required for election to the National Baseball Hall of Fame. He peaked at 43.1 percent in 1998, his final year of eligibility. His only opportunity for selection, thereafter, rested with the Veterans Committee. In February 2007, Santo missed selection by just five percent. Some baseball observers rated Santo "the best player not in the Hall."[44] Several factors initially hurt his Hall of Fame candidacy. Santo hit .296 at home, but only .257 on the road. He never played in a World Series and fell far short of the traditional 2,500 hit and 500 home run standards. Yet, upon Santo's retirement, only Brooks Robinson and Lave Cross had attained 2,500 hits and only Mathews had slugged 500 home runs among third basemen.

During the early 1980s, Santo met Vicki Tenace at the stable where he kept his horse. They married in 1983. She had a daughter, Kelly, from a previous marriage.

Santo joined the Cubs as a WGN radio color commentator in 1990, exhibiting unabashed enthusiasm and impassioned commentating. ESPN noted, "Nobody rooted harder for the Cubs and nobody took it harder when they lost." Santo, "beloved by the home crowd for the way he eagerly cheered for his favorite team on the air, hollering 'Yes! Yes!' or 'All right!' after good plays and groaning 'Oh, no!' or 'It's bad!' when things went wrong." In August 2009, Santo told the Associated Press, "The emotion for me is strictly the love I have for this team. I want them to win so bad."[45] In 1993, he coauthored with Randy Minkoff an autobiography, *For Love of Ivy*, describing how he developed diabetes and affirming that the disease did not interfere with his baseball career.

Santo, meanwhile, suffered myriad serious medical problems related to his blood sugar fluctuations. He underwent laser eye surgeries on both retinas in the 1980s, suffered a heart attack requiring quadruple-bypass surgery in June 1999, and endured 15 operations from 2000 to 2003. In June 2001, he experienced sharp pain while walking in St. Louis and discovered a penny-sized sore that never healed on his right foot. Doctors amputated his right leg below the knee in December 2001 because of circulation problems. In December 2002, his left leg was amputated below the knee. Blue vacuum-sealed prostheses replaced parts of both legs. Santo underwent surgery for bladder cancer in 2003, was hospitalized for an irregular heartbeat in 2007, and contracted pneumonia several times. Despite these setbacks, he rarely missed any broadcasting assignments. Steve Stone, Chicago White Sox analyst, remarked, "He's truly the strongest man I know and has the greatest attitude of any man I've met.

The competitive thing that drove him to be a star baseball player is the same thing that drives him now."[46]

Santo, whose spirits never dampened, remained a wonderful role model for diabetics, working tirelessly to raise money for diabetes research. He embarked on a special mission to raise diabetes awareness and began serving on the board of directors of the Juvenile Diabetes Foundation in 1976, raising badly needed funds to fight the disease. Santo sponsored the Juvenile Diabetes Research Foundation's annual Ron Santo Walk to Cure Diabetes in Chicago from 1974 to 2010, raising over $60 million for diabetes research. He also secured donations through golf outings, personal appearances, and royalties. At Santo's inspiration, Bill Holden walked 2,100 miles from Arizona to Chicago to raise $250,000 for diabetes research.

Santo visited various diabetics in Chicago hospitals and wrote inspirational letters to diabetics detailing his personal struggles. He phoned many diabetic children, trying to alleviate their fears and encouraging them to learn more about the disease. Santo gave inspirational talks to diabetic children, encouraging them to use "their own God-given gifts."[47] He added, "The only difference between me and any other ballplayer is the ten seconds a day I spend taking insulin." His life priorities changed. Santo previously believed he had made his biggest impact as a baseball player, but discovered it was "after I started speaking up about diabetes that I really made a difference."[48]

Santo's storied battle against diabetes was featured in the 2004 documentary film, *This Old Cub*, directed by his son, Jeff. Santo considered his family his biggest inspiration. "They just kept me fighting." Despite his myriad problems, he noted, "I'm so happy, so lucky, so blessed. I really have everything that any 61-year-old person could want." Santo also believed that his Cubs connection prolonged his life. In September 2003, he claimed, "If I hadn't had this when my troubles started, I don't know if I would have survived."[49]

Santo truly became an inspirational figure. *Chicago Sun-Times* sportswriter Toni Ginnetti eulogized, "Santo's career was as remarkable as it was miraculous." Banks wrote, "He is the most courageous person I've ever been around. I'm inspired by him and by his spirit. He is one of my idols, one of my heroes."[50] Santo died December 3, 2010, at a Phoenix, Arizona, hospital of complications from bladder cancer. The Cubs in August 2011 unveiled a statue of Santo south of Wrigley Field, depicting him ready to throw.[51]

Although the Cubs did not win a World Series during his lifetime, Santo posthumously fulfilled another dream almost exactly one year after his death. On December 4, 2011, the Golden Era Committee resoundingly selected him to the National Baseball Hall of Fame. He was named on 15 of 16 ballots by the committee considering players who made their mark from 1947 to 1972, becoming just the twelfth third baseman so honored. The committee broadened its perspective about what Santo meant to baseball, discussing his struggles with diabetes and work with juvenile diabetes research as well as his contributions to baseball. "Everybody saw the numbers — the home runs, the Gold Gloves," committee member and former teammate Williams reported, "but I think they looked at [him] with a different view."[52]

The posthumous Hall of Fame selection would have thrilled Santo. "It is a place he wanted to be," Williams stressed.[53] Vicki, Santo's widow, visualized, "He'd be pumping his fist in the air, saying, 'Yes! yes!,' like he did with so much enthusiasm as he did as a player and when he was broadcasting." She believes "he was meant to be in the Hall of Fame," and philosophized, "It just shows you can't give up."[54]

The baseball community, including several Hall of Famers and executives, welcomed Santo's selection. Pitcher Juan Marichal remembered, "He gave 100 percent on the field," while baseball commissioner Bud Selig wrote, "Ron was a staple of the Cubs' experience every single day for decades. I always admired Ron's courage and loyalty."[55] Cubs team chairman Tom Ricketts called him "the beating heart of Cubs' fans. As an athlete, he was our All-Star. As a radio analyst, he carried our passion. For those battling illness or disease, he remains an inspiration."[56]

# Other Debilitating Diseases

## GAIL DEVERS

"If you have faith and never give up your dream or goal, anything is possible," reflected Gail Devers, who conquered a crippling disease to mount one of the most inspirational comebacks in track and field history. Doctors diagnosed Devers with Graves' disease after the 1988 Olympic Games. Strong religious faith enabled her to cope with the disorder and return to track and field competition, becoming the greatest female sprinter-hurdler in history and even winning three Olympic gold medals.

Devers grew up in a middle-class family. Yolanda Gail Devers was born on November 19, 1966, in Seattle, the second of two children, and spent her childhood in National City, California, near San Diego. Her father, Larry, served as associate minister of the Mount Erie Baptist Church, while her mother, Alabe, worked as an elementary school teacher's aide. Devers excelled academically and especially enjoyed reading. She dreamed of becoming an elementary school teacher, following her mother's example. Her very strict, close-knit family especially enjoyed picnicking and recreational activities. She recalled watching *I Love Lucy* and stated, "We were a *Leave It to Beaver* family."[1]

Devers did not intend to participate in track. Before her sophomore year at Sweetwater High School in National City, her older brother, Parenthesis, persuaded her to run with him and teased her until she ultimately defeated him.

As a Sweetwater High School sophomore in 1982, Devers competed in middle-distance events and established a California Interscholastic Federation (CIF) record of two minutes, 11.07 seconds in the 800 meters. Henceforth, "Running was all that mattered," she recalled. Devers trained without a track coach, often competing as the sole Sweetwater entrant. "It was the loneliest feeling in the world," she recalled. "Slowly, however, Gail began to realize that she had real speed."[2] She switched to the sprints as a junior in 1983, running the 100 meters in a personal best 11.69 seconds and competing in the more challenging 100-meter hurdles.

During her senior year in 1984, Devers excelled in the 100 meters and rapidly improved her hurdling and long jumping skills. "She won the San Diego sectional team title for Sweetwater High all by herself!" Devers captured both the 100 meters and 100-meter hurdles and placed second in the long jump at the 1984 California State High School Championships. She faced the nation's best interscholastic competition, finishing second in the 100 meters at the Track Athletic Congress (TAC) Junior Championship. Devers won the bronze medal in the 100 meters and participated on the gold-medal winning U.S. 4×100-meter relay team at the Pan-American Junior Games. Her resume included three state championships, four Southern California regional crowns, and 12 San Diego intramural titles. Devers, who advised classmates, "Follow your dreams,"[3] graduated in 1984 from Sweetwater High School.

The naive, sheltered Devers, talented athletically and academically, entered the University of California at Los Angeles (UCLA) on an athletic scholarship in September 1984. She majored in sociology and maintained good grades. Upon entering UCLA, her personal best times were 11.51 seconds in the 100-meter dash and 14.32 seconds in the 100-meter hurdles. Under intense, renowned Bruins coach Bobby Kersee, she blossomed into a world-class sprinter and hurdler. Kersee, a physical fitness expert, realized her enormous track potential and wanted to make her "a world-class competitor." He envisioned her setting an American 100-meter hurdles record, making the 1988 Olympic team, and winning a gold medal in 1992, and he sought to motivate her. Devers realized that he "believed in me more than I believed in myself." Kersee learned, once "she sees what she can do, she's unstoppable."[4] Under Kersee, Devers's sprint and hurdle times improved dramatically. As a freshman, Devers finished sixth in the 100 meters, 200 meters, and 100-meter hurdles at the 1985 NCAA Track and Field Championships. Her times of 11.19 seconds, 23.12 seconds, and 13.16 seconds in these events approached world-class levels.

As a sophomore, Devers ranked seventh nationally in the 100 meters and 100-meter hurdles. She also participated in the long jump, and ran on relay teams. At the 1986 NCAA Championships, she placed fourth in the 100-meter hurdles and second in the long jump. Devers won six events, including the 100 meters, 200 meters, and 100-meter hurdles, at the 1987 Pacific 10 Championships. The 1987 NCAA Championships saw her finish second in the 100 meters in 10.98 seconds and run the 200 meters in 22.71 seconds. She captured the 100 meters at the 1987 U.S. Olympic Festival and Pan-American Games and was ranked second nationally and seventh globally.

Skeptics, however, questioned whether Devers would become a 100-meter hurdles champion because her 5-foot 4-inch, 115-pound frame made it difficult for her to clear the hurdles without breaking stride. According to Kersee, however, "her tremendous lower-body strength, her speed, and Her long arms" destined her for success. As a UCLA senior, Devers fulfilled Kersee's prediction by lowering the American record for the 100-meter hurdles to 12.71 seconds on April 19. But Jackie Joyner-Kersee, who trained with Devers and specialized in the heptathlon and long jump, broke the 100-meter hurdle mark on May 7 with a 12.70 finish. At the 1988 Pacific Ten Championship in late May, Devers reclaimed the American standard negotiating the 100-meter hurdles in "a blazing 12.61."[5] She also won the long jump and 100 meters, registering the world's second best time.

UCLA, meanwhile, was heavily favored to win the 1988 NCAA Championship. Despite her "illustrious" UCLA career, she still lacked an individual NCAA crown. In the long jump, Nena Gage of George Mason University edged her, 21 feet, eight inches to 21 feet, six inches. Devers captured her first individual NCAA title, winning the 100 meters. Never trailing, she built a substantial lead in the latter half. "I figured I must be going pretty fast," Devers admitted. Her 10.86-second clocking lowered Diane Williams's 1983 record by .06 seconds, but the wind exceeded the allowable limits for the mark to stand.

Devers started well in the 100-meter hurdles an hour

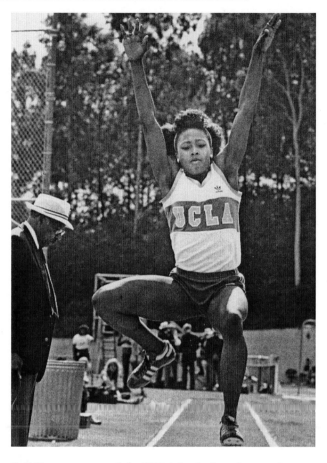

Gail Devers competed for UCLA in the long jump, winning the 1988 Pacific-Ten Championship and finishing second at the NCAA Championships (courtesy ASUCLA).

later, with Lynda Tolbert of Arizona State University close behind. LaVonna Martin of the University of Tennessee made a move at midpoint. Devers touched the eighth hurdle and knocked over the ninth, as Tolbert darted past to triumph in 12.82 seconds, nosing Martin. Devers finished a disappointing third with a 12.9-second clocking, costing UCLA anticipated points. UCLA trailed Louisiana State University, 53 to 48, entering the final 4×400-meter relay. Devers' "strong 51.4 second leg"[6] helped UCLA win that relay, but LSU still upset UCLA, 61 to 58, for the NCAA team title.

After marrying UCLA miler Ron Roberts in May 1988, Devers qualified for the U.S. Olympic team by faring second in the 100-meter hurdles at the 1988 U.S. Olympic Trials, fulfilling another Kersee prediction. "She was very excited. Things couldn't have been better."[7]

Devers, however, sensed something was wrong with her health before the 1988 Summer Olympic Games in Seoul, South Korea. "I lost weight, strength, and memory," she lamented. "I had terrible migraine headaches. I had involuntary shakes, convulsions, and I lost a lot of blood." At Seoul, her health deteriorated further. She

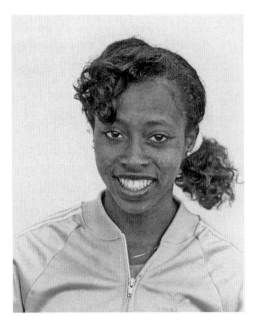

Gail Devers entered UCLA in 1984 and earned a bachelor's degree in sociology in 1988 (courtesy ASUCLA).

finished last in the 100-meter hurdles semifinals. Devers's 13.51-second clocking marked her slowest since high school. She found her non-medal performance "extremely disappointing." Devers initially attributed her lackluster performance to the rigorous training and intense pressure. Kersee blamed himself and wondered what mistake he had made in her training, but "a mysterious illness"[8] diminished her performance. Her problems "had nothing to do with Bobby Kersee's coaching, Gail's willingness to work, or the pressure of the Olympics." Devers admitted, "I was scared to death that my life as an athlete was over." She continued suffering "vision loss, wild weight fluctuations, fits of shaking and nearly perpetual menstrual bleeding."[9]

After returning to California, Devers consulted 13 doctors over 30 months to determine the cause of her illness. Physicians initially attributed her symptoms to physical exhaustion and emotional stress and prescribed rest. Repeated misdiagnoses compounded her illness. Devers realized that her illness was serious and began thinking it was "God's will that she stop running." She resumed training in December, but health problems sapped her physical strength and slowed her practice times. Doctors told her, "Just take some time off."[10] Physicians speculated that she might have bronchitis or diabetes, but tests ruled otherwise. Others attributed her problem to exhaustion. She had graduated with a bachelor's degree in sociology in 1988.

The fatigued Devers, suffering from the mysterious illness, did not compete in 1989 or 1990. Her skin began peeling off in layers, making it difficult for her to look into a mirror. She nicknamed herself "the alligator woman."[11] Her eyes began bulging and her left eye became blurry.

A UCLA physical therapist noticed a bulging cyst "the size of a child's fist" on Devers's thyroid gland. In September 1990, tests confirmed that Devers had contracted incurable Graves' disease, an enlarged thyroid gland. The gland, located toward the side of the neck, secreted a hormone that regulated growth and the rate at which the body cells produced energy. Her body's immune system malfunctioned. Devers's overactive thyroid was twice the normal size and needed to be reduced. Devers was heartbroken and shocked. "I left his office and sat in my car for a long time trying to absorb the devastating news."[12]

Since Graves' disease usually can be controlled with medication, doctors prescribed a beta-blocker for her. Her husband, Ron, wanted her to drop coach Kersee and take a beta-blocker. Devers, however, considered Kersee the nation's best track coach. Kersee did not want her to take a beta-blocker because the International Olympic Committee banned it. Devers declined to take the drug, not wanting to surrender her dream of competing in the 1992 Barcelona Summer Olympic Games.[13]

Homebound, Devers instead chose radiation therapy to destroy a cyst and the bad part of her thyroid gland. "The radiation treatment was a disaster," destroying her whole gland. The side effects made her even sicker, eroding other body tissue and causing her feet to swell, blister, crack, ooze, and bleed. "My feet were swollen," she revealed. "I had little holes all over my skin."[14] Devers recollected, "My face was constantly peeling." She found the pain "so excruciating that she sometimes crawled because it hurt too much to walk."[15]

The Robertses' marriage ended in divorce in 1991. Roberts seemed unable "to deal with Gail's illness or understand her desire to run again." Podiatrists ordered Devers completely off her feet. Devers's parents moved into her duplex in Van Nuys, California, because she could virtually do nothing by herself. "Her father had to carry her around her apartment, while her mother bathed her."[16] Neither Devers nor her doctors knew what triggered her skin problems. One podiatrist diagnosed her with athlete's foot. Her condition had deteriorated so much by March 1991 that one doctor told her, "If she had walked on her feet for two more days, they would have had to be amputated." Preserving her life and restoring her good health were paramount. Devers, who believed her track career had ended, admitted being "scared" and said, "I was just hoping God would save my foot so I would be able to walk again."[17]

An internist fortunately realized the radiation treatments caused her foot problems and changed her therapy immediately, prescribing an antibiotic instead to treat her sores. Although the antibiotic caused her to develop skin rashes, Devers's health gradually improved. Within a month, Devers began walking again and riding a stationary bicycle. The medication steadied her system and dramatically healed her feet. According to *Sports Illustrated*, "It was the start of the greatest comeback in track history."[18]

Under Kersee's guidance, Devers resumed her track and field training in late March 1991. She initially found the pain unbearable, recollecting, "I felt like my feet were falling off." Kersee, however, encouraged her to battle through adversity, "urging her forward step by step." He put her through a strenuous physical training regimen. Within 30 days, she began walking gingerly around the UCLA track in socks.[19] Devers survived her first workout in over two years and soon donned track shoes. She jogged lightly, strode, and then miraculously sprinted within two weeks. Devers regained her strength through "lots of hard work, determination, perseverance, and faith in God."[20]

Kersee insisted that Devers return to hurdling in May. Much of her former speed returned. Miraculously, Devers clocked 13.28 seconds in the 100-meter hurdles at Modesto, California, on May 11, 1991, finishing slightly faster than her first year at UCLA. She worked "harder than ever to get back to her old form." Devers dreamt again of participating in the 1992 Olympics at Barcelona. Despite her ordeal, she insisted, "The word quit has never been part of my vocabulary."[21] Kersee resumed training his star hurdler for an Olympic gold medal. At the 1991 USA/Mobil Championships in June, Devers captured the 100-meter hurdles in 12.83 seconds, displaying excellent form and regaining some speed and strength.

Devers exhibited renewed enthusiasm. "She once again saw the chance to become the best, and she went after it."[22] In the 1991 outdoor season, Devers concentrated on the 100-meter hurdles. In August, she finished second to Russia's Lyudmila Narozhilenko in the 100-meter hurdles at the World Championships in Tokyo. "I was the happiest silver medalist in Tokyo," she exulted. "Six months ago, I had no idea I would be here," Devers revealed. "It was just a matter of believing in myself." In September in Berlin, she established a personal best with an American record of 12.48 seconds in the 100-meter hurdles. Others lauded her for recording "the greatest comeback in modern track history."[23] In 1991, the American Sport Art Museum and Archives gave Devers, who aspired for an Olympic gold medal, the Mildred "Babe" Didrikson Zaharias Courage Award for demonstrating courage, perseverance, grace, and strength in overcoming adversity to excel in sport.

Devers originally planned to compete only in the 100-meter hurdles at the 1992 Barcelona Summer Olympic Games. During that spring, however, her times improved markedly in the 100-meter dash. "I'm starting to feel like a sprinter again," she explained. Although the favored Gwen Torrence won the 100 meters in a dazzling 10.97 seconds at the Olympic Trials in New Orleans, Devers qualified for the U.S. Olympic team by finishing second in that event in 11.02 seconds and winning the 100-meter hurdles in 12.55 seconds. She was just elated to qualify after having battled Graves' disease. "My goal was simply to finish both races,"[24] she disclosed.

Pundits favored Devers in the 100-meter hurdles and considered her a long shot to medal in the 100 meters at the 1992 Summer Olympic Games. The 100 meters on August 1 was rated a tossup between Torrence, Juliet Cuthbert of Jamaica, Irina Privalova of the Commonwealth of Independent States, and Merlene Ottey of Jamaica. The "pale, powerful" Privalova and the "short, quick" Devers led the first portion of the race. At 50 meters, Cuthbert and Ottey surged. Torrence closed fast, too. The race was too close to call with five meters remaining. The crowd had stopped cheering. All five runners crossed the finish line together, leaning or lunging simultaneously for the tape, "to exhalations of disbelief" and "stunned muttering." "Even the blurry, warped finish photo on the scoreboard, freezing the sprinters in the throes of their final efforts was of no immediate help." The race had decided the world's fastest woman. "But no one could tell who she was. She herself didn't know." Devers stuck her head forward and seemed to cross the finish line barely ahead of the others. Cuthbert told Devers, "You got it," but the latter was uncertain. Judges scrutinized replays before declaring Devers victorious. Photographers and sportswriters rushed toward her. "Only then did she know." She hurried over to Kersee, who yelled, "You wanted it. You got it."[25]

Devers captured the gold medal in the 100 meters in 10.82 seconds, edging Cuthbert by .01 seconds. She had lowered her previous best time "by 13 hundredths of a second, a whopping deduction." Only world-record holder Florence Griffith Joyner (10.49 seconds) had ever run that distance quicker. The race marked history's closest 100-meter Olympic final, as the first five runners finished within .06 of a second of one another. Privalova came in third at 10.84 seconds, Torrence fourth at 10.86 seconds, and Ottey fifth at 10.88 seconds. No sixth-place finisher had ever run that fast. "You couldn't ask for anything closer, anything better,"[26] Devers observed. "In one of the closest and fastest races ever run," she had won an Olympic gold medal and had authored "one of the most amazing comebacks from illness in sports history." During her victory lap, she reflected, "A year ago, you couldn't walk. Now, you're running. You've just won gold." Devers was ecstatic. "This was a long time in coming," she sighed. "I'm back where I wanted to be."[27] The triumph made her the "World's Fastest Woman." "I'm a better person for having gone through this," Devers concluded. "I'm happier. I'm stronger. I'm more determined."[28]

Devers shifted attention to the 100-meter hurdles, hoping to become the only woman besides Fanny Blankers-Koen of the Netherlands in 1948 to win Olympic gold medals in both the 100 meters and 100-meter hurdles. She quickly seized the lead and "was blowing the field away" at 50 meters. "That's the fastest I've ever gone through the hurdles," she noted. Devers held "a huge lead" and seemed "a sure winner." She controlled the race approaching the final hurdle, 10 meters from the finish line. "But then what happened is every hurdler's nightmare." Devers could not "force her all-out sprint stride to change to a controlled hurdle stride."[29] Upon reaching the hurdle, her lead leg lacked the height to clear the 33-inch barrier. Devers' right toe struck the final hurdle on the way up, causing her to stumble. "She toppled forward, staggering, falling, driving toward the line," while the competitors "shot by." Devers finished the race, resembling "Pete Rose diving for the bag." Paraskevi Patoulidou of Greece triumphed in 12.64 seconds for Greece's first track medal since 1896, nosing LaVonna Martin by .05 seconds. Devers came in fifth, suffering "a devastating loss," with "her sure gold suddenly transformed into an abrasion on her left shoulder."[30] She could not believe her sudden fate and concluded, "It just wasn't meant to be." Although "terribly disappointed," Devers noted, "I still had my 100-meter gold."[31] Kersee blamed himself for not reminding her to shorten her stride for the final three hurdles.

Nevertheless, the 1992 Summer Olympic Games marked a significant comeback for Devers, who had defeated the world's best in the 100-meter race. "Gail had won the most impressive victory of her life. She had hauled back from a debilitating disease to win the greatest prize in sports — an Olympic gold medal." Devers summoned the spiritual and physical resources for the requisite focus, determination, perseverance, and support to triumph. "Seldom has the grand stage of the Olympics produced a winner who has won so much more than the medal she wore around her neck and the flowers she held on the victory podium. She stood as a beacon of hope, an example of fortitude to others who have suffered with some kind of illness."[32] Global rankings still listed her first in the 100-meter hurdles and third in the 100 meters.

During the winter 1993 indoor season, Devers competed in shorter 60-meter races. She aspired to be both the best sprinter and hurdler in the world. Devers ran seven indoor meets, winning the 60 meters six times. Her only setback came on February 11 at Madrid, where Privalova set a world record of 6.92 seconds. Devers finished second with an American record 7.05 seconds time. In March, she established an American mark while taking the 60 meters in 6.99 seconds at the USA/Mobil Indoor Championships.

Before the 1993 World Indoor Championships in March in Toronto, Kersee warned Devers that it was harder to defend the major title and reminded her, "It takes determination, willpower, and mental toughness."[33] Kersee uncharacteristically challenged her to control her emotions and concentrate completely on the 60-meter race. Devers surged from the outset and "blew away from world-record older Irina Privalova," lowering the American record to 6.97 seconds. Her time ranked the second fastest in history, barely missing the world record by .03 seconds. After having battled Graves' disease, she denied that "there's anything in my life that will come up that I can't get over."[34]

During the 1993 outdoor season, Devers concentrated on the 100-meter hurdles. Her speed represented her biggest asset as a hurdler. Devers, who intimidated other hurdlers, viewed herself "as a sprinter who happened to have to go over obstacles." "Remove the hurdles," Kersee claimed, "and there's no way they can outsprint her."[35] Devers captured the 100 meters in 10.82 seconds at the USA/Mobil Outdoor Championships in June and the 100-meter hurdles in 12.76 seconds at the U.S. Olympic Festival in San Antonio.

Devers entered the 1993 World Championships in Stuttgart, Germany, in top condition. She prevailed in both the 100 meters and 100-meter hurdles, accomplishing the first double since Blankers-Koen's 1948 Olympic feat. In the 100 meters, Devers and Ottey of Jamaica "raced stride for stride to the finish line" and "crossed at almost the same time." Devers edged Ottey with a 10.82-second clocking. Her shoulder barely crossed the finish line before Ottey's chest. Judges spent three minutes examining the photo finish, which showed Devers winning by inches. Devers observed, "This was just my time."[36] In the 100-meter hurdles, Devers demonstrated unmatched speed, controlled her stride, and handled each hurdle cleanly. Her winning time of 12.46 seconds lowered her own American record. Devers anchored the silver-medalist 4×100- meter relay team to an American record of 41.49 seconds. Although disappointed over the photo-finish relay loss to the Russians, she maintained, "We got an American record."

During 1993, Devers lost only twice. *Track & Field News* recognized her as its 1993 U.S. Female Athlete of the Year, marking "the crowning glory to her comeback, one of the greatest in all of sports."[37] The U.S. Olympic Committee named the trackster its Sportswoman of the Year.

Nagging hamstring and back injuries kept Devers from competing in the hurdles in 1994, but she repeated as the 100-meter titlist at the USA Outdoor Championships in Knoxville, Tennessee. Another injury, however, prevented her from competing against Torrence at the 1995 Millrose Games in New York City. Devers won the 100-meter hurdles in 12.77 seconds at the USA Outdoor Championships in Sacramento, and she retained the 100-meter hurdles crown at the World Championships at Gothenburg, Sweden, preserving her top global ranking.

At the 1996 U.S. Olympic Trials, Devers qualified for the U.S. team with a victory in the 100-meter hurdles in 12.6 seconds and a second-place finish to Torrence in the 100 meters. In June, the Showtime network featured *Run for the Dream: The Gail Devers Story*. The film chronicled Devers's battle with Graves' disease and her remarkable comeback to a stirring victory in the 100 meters at the 1992 Summer Olympic Games. Devers, who served as film producer, became "a national celebrity"[38] and was deluged with offers to endorse commercial products.

The centennial Atlanta 1996 Summer Olympic Games brought special meaning for Devers, as she joined Wyomia Tyus as the only women in Olympic history to repeat as the 100-meter gold medalist. Her strongest challengers were Ottey, four-time Olympic bronze medalist, and Torrence, the 1995 world champion. Devers quickly darted to the lead. Ottey and Torrence then closed the gap. Near the tape, "Devers twisted her left shoulder forward and ducked her head. Ottey kept her head higher and her chest forward." Kenny Moore of *Sports Illustrated* wrote, "No one knew who had won. For long minutes they waited, watching slow-motion replays on the scoreboard of races that were too close to call." Judges ruled Devers the victor after reviewing photos. In an extremely close finish, Devers and Ottey both crossed the finish line in 10.94 seconds. Torrence placed third in 10.96 seconds. "Devers clearly got her head across the line before Ottey." Kersee, caught up in the celebratory moment, flung Devers "wildly."[39] The Jamaican Federation protested the decision on Ottey's behalf, but its complaint was disallowed.

Although Kersee had helped Devers improve her hurdle stride since 1992, Devers ended a disappointing fourth, one-hundredth of a second from a bronze medal in the 100-meter hurdles. She cleared all the hurdles this time, but Ludmila Enquist of Sweden won the gold medal and two other competitors outraced her. Devers reflected,

"It just was not to be." Her fourth-place finish was better than her Barcelona outcome mainly because she had not stumbled. Devers lamented, however, "I never found my speed. I never got into the rhythm of my mechanics."[40] She also ran the second leg on the U.S. gold medalist 4×100-meter relay team. Kenny Harrison, who lived and trained with Devers, won the gold medal in the triple jump, setting an Olympic and American record with a leap of 59 feet, 4¼ inches.

In February 1997, Devers captured the 60 meters in 7.07 seconds at the Mobil Invitational Championships, edging Torrence by .05 seconds. She clocked an incredible 7.0 seconds in defeating Torrence again at the U.S. Indoor Championships and won the 60-meter title at the World Indoor Championships. During the outdoor season, Devers concentrated on sprinting and anchored the U.S. 4×100-meter relay team to victory at the World Championships, setting an American record. The Women's Sports Foundation named soccer star Mia Hamm and Devers their 1997 Sportswomen of the Year. Persistent injuries and medication problems sidelined her the 1998 and early 1999 seasons. She returned to form, however, triumphing in the 100-meter hurdles at both the 1999 USA Championships and World Championships in Seville, Spain. Her 12.37 seconds time for the 100-meter hurdles established an American record.

The 2000 season bode well for Devers until the Sydney Summer Olympic Games. Devers finished second in the 100 meters and 100-meter hurdles at the IAAF Grand Prix in Croatia and won the 100-meter hurdles in 12.50 seconds at the Athletissima Tournament in Lausanne, Switzerland, in July. She lowered her 100-meter hurdles record again to 12.33 seconds and claimed her sixth 100-meter hurdles U.S. Outdoor title at the Olympic Trials. She injured her right Achilles tendon and left hamstring while training for the 2000 Summer Olympic Games. Devers led halfway through the semifinals of the 100-meter hurdles at Sydney, but stopped abruptly before reaching the fifth hurdle with a torn hamstring. "Today, it was someone else's turn to shine," she explained. "This does not mean that Gail Devers's Olympic dream is over."[41]

Although dismissing Kersee as coach in 2001, Devers still enjoyed considerable track success. She won the 2001 USA Outdoor crown in the 100-meter hurdles and finished second at the World Championships, trailing teammate Anjanette Kirkland. Devers dominated the 100-meter hurdles in 2002, winning the USA Outdoor Championships at Palo Alto, California, in June and the IAAF Grand Prix Final at Paris in September. She ranked second in the 2002 Grand Prix Season Standings and ended Marion Jones's five-year reign as the female track and field ESPY award recipient. In 2003, Devers set the American indoor record for the 60-meter hurdles, clocking 7.78 seconds at the Verizon Millrose Games. She won the 60-meter hurdles at the USA and World Indoor Track and Field Championships, breaking her own American indoor record in the semifinals at the USA Indoors. Devers dominated the 100-meter hurdles on the outdoor track circuit until being eliminated in the semi-finals of the 2003 World Championships at Saint-Denis, France, in August.

In 2004, Devers became the first athlete to capture both the 60 meters and 60-meter hurdles at the USA Indoor Championships, clocking 7.06 seconds in the dash and 7.81 seconds in the hurdles. She garnered a gold medal in the 60 meters and a silver in the 60-meter hurdles at the 2004 World Indoor Championships. Although qualifying for the 2004 Athens Summer Olympic Games, she failed to reach the finals in the 100 meters and was eliminated in the 100-meter hurdles when she aggravated an injured calf muscle.

Devers, now married to businessman Mike Philips, did not compete in 2005 and gave birth to a daughter, Karsen, that June. She has another daughter, Legacy, born in 2007. At age 40 in February 2007, Devers "burst back into the track spotlight," unexpectedly edging 2004 Olympic champion Joanna Hayes in the 60-meter hurdles at the Millrose Games in New York. "I always knew I could come back,"[42] she affirmed. Her 7.86-second clocking temporarily set the standard for the best in the world that indoor season, but was surpassed the next night by Susanna Kallur of Sweden.

Devers eventually plans to open a day care center, hoping "to intervene in their [children's] lives" earlier. The avid reader originally aspired to teach elementary school, "but now I think that by then it's almost too late to start. I really want to go after kids in the earliest years."[43] Devers has represented Your Thyroid Gland Central, spreading thyroid disease awareness in communities nationally since 1996. The Gail Devers Foundation, established in 1999, funds education, health, and community development projects to help youngsters fulfill their potential. "I've encountered many challenges and had to reach inside myself for powerful spiritual and physical forces to make it through," Devers stressed. "Now it's time for me to give back."[44] The Gail Force enforcement center offers educational programs, sports training, mentoring and career development, affording all young people the same opportunities to advance their lives. The foundation helps offer college scholarships and provides needy families with food and clothing, helping spread her dreams and values.

Graves' disease taught Devers valuable lessons. "I'm a stronger, more determined person because of it," she said, explaining, "There's no hurdle I can't get over." Devers combined "a strong spiritual foundation with a solid work ethic, drive, and determination to be the best," soaring "to the top of her field" and sustaining her during the battle with Graves' disease. "Her courage, belief in God, and confidence in herself brought Gail back" both "as an Olympic star and, more important, as a person."[45]

Devers combatted Graves' disease to attain track and field stardom. She reigned as history's fastest combination sprinter-hurdler, having been ranked first globally by *Track & Field News* twice in the 100 meters and eight times in the 100-meter hurdles. Devers triumphed in three Olympic races, winning gold medals in the 100 meters in 1992 and the 100 meters and the 4×100 meters in 1996. At the World Outdoor Championships, she won three gold medals in the 100-meter hurdles (1993, 1995, 1999) and gold medals in the 100 meters in 1993 and the 4×100 meters in 1997. Devers also

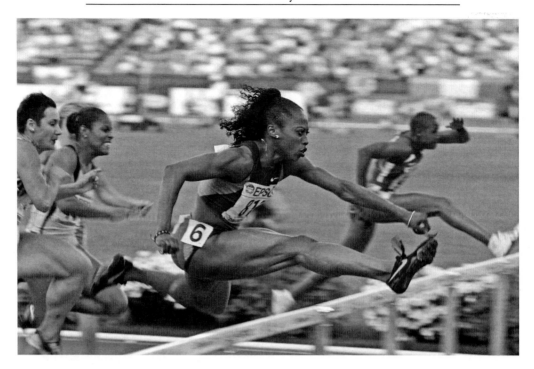

**Gail Devers finished second to Anjanette Kirkland in the women's 100-meter hurdles during the IAFF World Championships on Athletics at Commonwealth Stadium in Edmonton, Alberta, Canada, on August 10, 2001 (courtesy Philippe Millereau/DPPI/Icon SMI).**

excelled at the World Indoor Championships, winning gold medals in the 60 meters in 1993, 1997, and 2004 and the 60-meter hurdles in 2003.

Devers has received considerable recognition for her achievements. In 1999, the American Sports Art Museum and Archives gave Devers the Mildred "Babe" Didrikson Zaharias Courage Award for demonstrating courage, perseverance, grace, and strength in overcoming adversity to excel in sport. The 10-time USA Outdoor 100-meter hurdles champion received ESPY awards for being Women's Track and Field Athlete of the Year in 2003 and 2004. She was inducted into the National Track and Field Hall of Fame in 2011 and the U.S. Olympic Hall of Fame in 2012. USA Track & Field described her career as "one of perseverance" and lauded her recovery from Graves' disease "to become one of the most dominant sprinters and hurdlers of her time."[46]

# ALICE MARBLE

"Everyone is endowed with the qualities of a champion and can succeed in spite of handicaps in the most important game of all — the game of life"[1] sums up the stellar career of tennis player Alice Marble. Marble collapsed while playing several tennis matches in extreme heat at age 21 and was diagnosed with tuberculosis and anemia. After Marble spent several agonizing months recuperating, her extraordinary courage, enormous spirit, and resourcefulness enabled her to become one of the world's best tennis players.

Alice Marble was born on September 28, 1913, in Beckwith, California, the fourth of five siblings, and grew up in a working-class environment. Her father, Harry, worked as a high-climbing lumberjack in the logging industry in the Sierra Nevadas and owned a farm and cattle ranch near Beckwith. He labored for a lumber company after the Marbles moved to San Francisco in 1920, but died of pneumonia when Alice was just seven years old. Her mother, Jessie, a nurse, and two older brothers held jobs to support the family.

Marble, "a tomboy," loved athletics and constantly played baseball with her younger brother, Tim. Her uncle, Woodie, a former semi-professional baseball player, had taught her how to play. By age 13, Marble saw the San Francisco Seals, a New York Yankee farm club, play baseball daily and impressed them with her tremendous throwing arm. She served as team warm-up player and mascot, being dubbed the "Little Queen of Swat."[2] She graduated in 1931 from Polytechnic High School in San Francisco, where she participated in girls' basketball, track and field, and baseball.

When Marble was 15 years old, her brother, Dan, an accomplished handball player, bought her a tennis racket so she could play "a more ladylike sport." Dan wanted her to cease acting like a tomboy and encouraged her to play tennis. Marble retorted, "I won't play that sissy game." The next day she played tennis with her friend, Mary, on the public courts at Golden Gate Park. Mary taught her the tennis rules and promptly defeated her. Although still preferring baseball, Marble rapidly became "hooked on tennis."[3] She played at Golden Gate Park daily after school and spent the entire weekend there. Blessed with "natural athletic ability,"[4] she soon triumphed in local tournaments.

Although a tennis novice, Marble quickly ranked among the premier northern California players. California tennis associations and an anonymous donor funded her participation in the 1931 Northwest and Canadian Championships. At age 18, Marble represented Northern California as junior champion in the U.S. Nationals at the West Side Tennis Club at Forest Hills, New York, and the under-18 National Junior Championships at the Philadelphia Cricket Club. After taking the train to New York, she was trounced in the first round of the U.S. Nationals. Former national champion Mary K. Browne told her, "You have worlds of natural ability but no strokes or strategy."[5] She advised Marble to take tennis lessons "to improve her game and make it more adaptable to the eastern grass courts." Marble reached the finals of the National Junior Championships before losing to Ruby Bishop in two sets. She performed well on hard courts in California, but needed a coach to instruct her about playing on grass.[6] Bonnie Miller teamed with her to take the doubles tournament in three sets.

In 1932, Marble successfully defended her California State singles title and traveled east to the U.S. Nationals. After upsetting American Sarah Palfrey in the first round, she lost to Joan Ridley of Great Britain in the next round. Marble and fellow American Midge Morrill finished second in the doubles. "Her excellent hand-eye coordination, natural athletic ability, quick foot speed, and years of practice pitching had given her an aggressive game and a powerful serve." But the stocky, 5-foot 7-inch, 150-pounder's ground strokes were not proficient. "I had gone as far as I could on my own,"[7] she realized.

Eleanor Tennant, renowned American tennis coach, became Marble's instructor in 1932 and remained her mentor for the next 13 years. Tennant profoundly influenced Marble's career. Marble spent several months that year with Tennant in Los Angeles, defraying her lesson expenses by helping her with the other students and doing secretarial work at Wilson Sporting Goods. The very slow progress frustrated her. "I expected miracles," she confessed, "but they didn't happen."[8]

With Tennant's help, Marble changed her grip, improved her ground strokes, and started using "her athleticism to play an attacking game at the net." Unlike other contemporary women players, she gradually combined her powerful service and attack and volley game to dominate opponents. Marble excelled at doubles due to "her ability to get to every shot, and her ferocious net game." Marble "pioneered an aggressive style of power tennis for women,"[9] a strategy later employed by champions Billie Jean King of the United States and Martina Navratilova of Czechoslovakia.

Marble's game lacked proper technique until she received instruction from Harwood White at his mountaintop home near Santa Barbara, California. After watching Marble play for 10 minutes, White remarked, "That's the worst tennis game I've ever seen."[10] He taught her the theory and execution of stroke production, starting with the Eastern grip, while Tennant taught her strategy and honed her competitive edge. Her strokes featured more power and became more controlled. Marble lost in the semifinals of the Southern California Championship and won the California State Championship at Berkeley, employing the new techniques. By 1933, her national ranking surged from seventh to third.

Marble experienced her initial health crisis in 1933 in a three-day qualifying tournament for selection of the Wightman Cup team at the Maidstone Club in East Hampton, Long Island. "Ill health caused by overexertion nearly brought Marble's tennis career to a halt." The tournament revealed Marble's "great spirit, courage, and fortitude."[11] Marble was appalled at being placed in both singles and doubles in the short tournament and protested to Julian Myrick, tournament chair, that it was impossible to compete in both events. She only wanted to compete in the doubles and preserve her strength for the singles in the Wightman Cup the following week, but was forced to participate in both events to make the team. Myrick replied, "You will have to prove your worth by making a good showing here." Marble countered, "I've won two tournaments to Sarah Palfrey's one, and neither she nor Carolin Babcock is scheduled to play both events." Myrick responded that he would determine the schedule. Several California players advised her to skip the qualifying tournament and take a chance that she would still be chosen for the singles position, but she played both events anyway. "I was nineteen, ambitious, and stubborn,"[12] Marble recollected.

Marble fared well the first two days and competed in the semifinals of both events the final day. Marble's first singles match against fellow American Midge Van Ryn started at 10 A.M. Marble defeated Van Ryn in three sets. "The pounding in my temples reverberated through my body, painfully in my joints and turning my stomach into a queasy knot," she recalled. Marble and American Helen Wills Moody played a lengthy doubles contest against Betty Nuthall and Mary Heeley of Great Britain immediately after the Van Ryn match. Marble remarked, "We played three long sets," triumphing "by a small margin."[13] Moody's back hurt her, forcing Marble to compensate. "I took every overhand shot, compounding the match's toll on me."[14] The match finished at 1 P.M., an hour before she played Nuthall in the singles final. Marble, who trembled from heat and fatigue, ate very little.

By 2 P.M., the temperature at center court had soared to 104 degrees with high humidity. Marble won the first set over Nuthall, 7–5, taking "everything I had," she admitted. Nuthall triumphed easily in the second set. Marble reflected, "My body simply would not do what I asked." Her muscles stiffened during the two-minute rest period. Nuthall won that deciding set in just 10 minutes. "I was completely exhausted,"[15] Marble explained.

Marble had just a few minutes to change into her fourth outfit that day for the doubles final. Committee members and players warned her, "It was suicide to try and play another match." But she countered, "I was too tired to care." Myrick reminded Marble the attendees wanted to see Mrs. Moody perform. The ultimate decision about playing was left to Marble, who "never quit at anything." In that match, she lamented, "Neither my muscles nor my brain cared to function."[16] Marble and Moody were defeated in straight sets, with the former largely responsible for losing the match. "I had lost fourteen pounds in nine hours,"[17] she disclosed. Tournament officials had asked Marble to play 11 sets and 108 games in nine hours on the year's warmest day. Marble, who could not eat after the match, lay down on a sofa and collapsed from sunstroke and anemia.

Marble made the Wightman Cup team anyway and played at Forest Hills the next week. The team doctor, however, forbade her from performing in the singles competition because she had not recuperated sufficiently. "I was heartbroken," Marble recalled, "for I had worked so hard for the chance." American Babcock replaced her in the singles. The U.S. won four of the five matches, but Marble and Van Ryn lost soundly in the doubles. "I felt weak and tired all the time,"[18] Marble confessed.

Marble reached the quarter-finals of the 1933 U.S. Nationals at the West Side Club and lost to Nuthall, squandering a 5–1 lead and 40–15 advantage in the next game. "It was a bitter blow," she observed. In the doubles, Marble partnered with American Elizabeth Ryan against Nuthall and Freda James of Great Britain. Nuthall lined a fast volley that struck Marble in the eye, suspending the match.[19] During 1933, her national rankings had risen from seventh to third.

Although competing the following summer, Marble still experienced fatigue. She easily defeated Dorothy Round, the best British player, in two sets at the Northern California Championships, but then was bedridden with anemia. Marble played no tennis for several months and worked that winter for the Wilson Sporting Goods Company. Marble sailed to Paris to compete in the 1934 French Open, but wanted to stay in her hotel room and be left alone. "My muscles ached and I couldn't sleep,"[20] she recalled. When her blood count dropped dramatically, the French doctor diagnosed her affliction as anemia.

On a very hot June 1934 afternoon, Marble tried to compete against Sylvia Henrotin, number two French player, at Roland Garros Stadium in Paris. "I felt more dizzy and more nervous than at any other time on a tennis court," she revealed. Henrotin, who forced Marble to run all over the court, built a 5–1 lead and led 15-love in the next game. "It was hopeless," Marble recalled. "I felt my knees buckling, the racquet slipping from my hand."[21] After collapsing, Marble was carried off the court and rushed to the American Hospital at Neuilly. "I was in agonizing pain,"[22] she disclosed. Doctors told her she could not accompany the Whiteman Cup team to England, but did not know what ailed her.

Although Marble really suffered from sunstroke, anemia, and pleurisy, Dr. Dax, who misdiagnosed her affliction as tuberculosis, bluntly told her, "You will never be strong enough to play tennis again." Marble, shocked and dismayed, noted, "I couldn't believe what I had heard." Teammates vainly tried to cheer her up, but she felt "morose and bitter," had no appetite, and was depressed. "It was all like a terrible dream,"[23] Marble recollected. "My life was over. Tennis was my life."

After being hospitalized six weeks, Marble persuaded Dr. Dax to let her return to the United States to recuperate. Tennant, teary-eyed, met her in New York City. Marble rested one week at the Roosevelt Hotel. A doctor who examined her at the hotel concluded, "This girl will never play tennis again." Tennant blamed Myrick for Marble's illness, since he had forced her to play too many matches in one day. But Marble countered, "I could have defaulted had I wanted, at the risk of losing my place on the team."[24] The U.S. Lawn Tennis Association refused to foot her medical bills.

Marble returned to her San Francisco home in June to convalesce. Marble's family doctor prescribed rest and quiet and confined her to bed. Her medical care burdened "her economically precarious family."[25] Her mother Jessie, who suffered from cancer and weight loss, already was overworked trying to care for other family members. She and Dan, though, did not want to leave Marble in an outsider's care.

Tennant offered to let Marble recuperate at her Beverly Hills home so she could improve more rapidly in a warmer, quieter atmosphere. She ultimately assumed responsibility for Marble's care, arranging and paying for her to stay several weeks at Pottinger's Sanitarium in Monrovia near Los Angeles. Tennant's financial and moral support enabled Marble to launch a rehabilitation program to resume her tennis career. Tennant persuaded Marble to rest several weeks at the sanatorium under Dr. Pottinger's supervision. Although Tennant visited her daily, Marble despised staying at the sanatorium. "Every day was a slice of hell," she recalled, "and the nights were worse — sleepless desolate hours of staring into darkness."[26]

Upon Marble's insistence, Tennant disobeyed doctor's orders and snuck her out of the sanatorium after twelve weeks. "I'm never going to get well here," Marble convinced Tennant. Before reaching Tennant's car, Marble nearly fainted. After leaving the sanitarium, she gradually fought back from being a semi-invalid. Dr. Commons from Los Angeles permitted Marble to play tennis again if she recovered from the anemia and reduced her weight substantially. "Your lungs are scarred," Dr. Commons said, "but I see no reason why you can't play tennis."[27]

Marble and Tennant planned the former's return to tennis. Tennant furnished financial support, while Marble restored her health and honed her tennis skills. Commons let Marble resume tennis when she lost 14 pounds. "I was immediately swept up in the game I loved, illness forgotten," she recollected. Tennant, who became manager and teacher at the Racquet Club in Palm Springs in September 1934, instructed Marble 15 minutes daily. Marble had lost some of her stamina and quickness. Few athletes from that era had come back from anemia. Marble, however, soon noticed her health and tennis improved "by leaps and bounds."[28]

Tennant showed considerable patience with Marble and predicted that she would become "the world's best woman player." Marble eventually played two sets of doubles daily and easily defeated Babcock, the third-ranked women's player, 6–2, 6–2, for her first single's triumph in nearly two years. "I had won a far more important victory — victory over illness," she boasted. "Through philosophy, hard work and faith I had completed the crossword puzzle, which a year before had seemed impossible to complete." Few people believed that Marble could play competitive tennis again. But she countered, "I had beaten a devastating disease." She added, "Nothing was going to stop me."[29]

Dr. Commons wanted Marble to compete in two West Coast tournaments before joining the eastern tournament circuit. Marble decisively defeated American Margaret Osborne for the California State Championship and also won the doubles crown at Golden Gate Park in San Francisco. "I was happier than I had been in two years," Marble beamed. Commons, though, refused to let her travel east because her blood count dropped 15 points. Marble rested as much as possible and continued improving her tennis, stamina, and health through tennis lessons with Tennant and afternoon practice at the Los Angeles Club. When Marble won the Southern California Championship, Commons gave her a clean bill of health and let her play in all the Eastern grass court and Forest Hills tournaments. "No trophy ever was so gratifying as that,"[30] Marble recalled.

Marble dominated women's tennis from 1936 to 1940. U.S. Lawn Tennis Association (USLTA) officials initially refused to let Marble enter any of the 1936 Eastern tournaments because of her anemic health. The USLTA tested Marble's readiness to return to tennis competition by forcing her to play exhibition matches against several male players. When these players could not match Marble's relentless power and endurance, USLTA officials narrowly permitted her to compete by a 3–2 margin. In 1936, Marble won the women's singles at the Seabright Invitation and the Longwood Cricket Club near Boston and with American Gene Mako upset Palfrey and American Don Budge, 6–3, 6–2, in the mixed doubles at the U.S. Nationals.[31]

Marble returned to championship form, upsetting fellow American Helen Jacobs, four-time U.S. National champion and 1936 Wimbledon titlist, 4–6, 6–3, 6–2, for her first U.S. Women's Singles crown. The cheering crowd energized her in the second set. "I just couldn't believe it when the second set ended and I had won it ... quite easily," she recollected. As the third set commenced, she realized, "I had nothing to lose and everything to gain." Marble swept the first four games in record time, surprising even herself. After Jacobs took the next two games, Marble took a 5–2 lead and seized a 40–15 advantage in the next game. She then smashed a ball hard into Jacobs' backhand side to take the game, set, and match. "I never thought I could do it right up to the last point,"[32] she said in disbelief.

Marble realized the significance of her triumph. "I had won much more than just the championship," she reflected. "I had won a fight for health against odds." Marble added, "I had been counted down and out, but I didn't stay down, and I surely wasn't out." She teamed with Mako to best Palfrey and Budge, 6–3, 6–2, for the 1936 U.S. Mixed Doubles crown. Marble had fought back to become the premier American female tennis player. "The story of my comeback," she detected, "had transcended the sports pages and become an inspiration for everyone who had a debilitating disease."[33] The USLTA ranked Marble the number one American women's tennis player from 1936 to 1940. Marble's "tennis skills, determination, and winning spirit," along with courage, brought her numerous titles. In 1937, Marble combined with Budge to conquer Simone Mathieu and Yvon Petra of France, 6–4, 6–1, for the Wimbledon Mixed Doubles crown, and with Palfrey to edge Van Ryn and Babcock, 7–5, 6–4, for the U.S. Women's Doubles title.[34]

Marble hoped to win the 1938 Wimbledon Women's Singles Championship, but Jacobs eliminated her, 6–4, 6–4, in the semifinals. She teamed with Palfrey to defeat Mathieu and Billie Yorke of India, 6–3, 6–3, in the Wimbledon Women's Doubles and with Budge to win their second consecutive Wimbledon Mixed Doubles title over Palfrey and Henner Henkel of Germany, 6–1, 6–4. Budge became the only player in Wimbledon history to win all three championships in his first attempt. Marble had captured two of three Wimbledon titles, "reason to be proud."[35]

The year 1938 marked Marble's first Triple Crown. Marble captured her second U.S. Women's Singles title at Forest Hills, surviving a spirited semifinal match with Palfrey. After Marble led 5–1 in the first set, Palfrey became more intense and recovered to win, 7–5. "I couldn't touch her," Marble recollected. In the second set, Palfrey seized a 5–2 advantage. She needed just two points to win the set, when Marble staged an incredible comeback. "By some miracle," Marble recalled, she made a backhand volley on an almost certain match point that Palfrey could not return. "I'll never understand what makes a player's game suddenly start to click," she said. Palfrey took only four points in the last four games of that set.

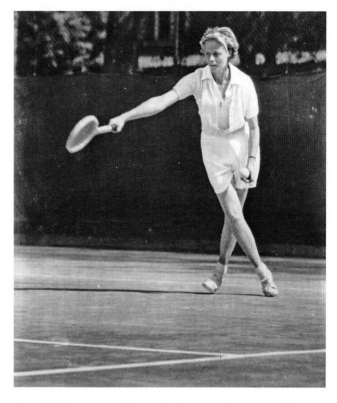

Alice Marble, pictured here returning a volley, circa 1940, dominated women's tennis from 1936 to 1940, sweeping the U.S. women's singles and doubles titles and the U.S. mixed doubles crown from 1938 to 1940 (courtesy International Tennis Hall of Fame & Museum).

Marble won both that set and the third set by identical 7–5 scores to take the match, noting, "I had to fight for every point in the third set."[36] The spirited match saw both players score 122 points.

In the U.S. Women's Singles final, Marble trounced Nancy Wynne of Australia, 6–0, 6–3, in just 20 minutes. She combined with Palfrey to win the U.S. Women's Doubles title over Mathieu and Jadwiga Jedrzejowska of Poland, 6–8, 6–4, 6–3, and with Budge to capture the U.S. Mixed Doubles championship over John Bromwich and Thelma Coyne of Australia, 6–1, 6–2, to complete the rare triple crown in the same year.[37]

Marble reached her pinnacle at Wimbledon in 1939. "I was at the peak of my game," she maintained. Marble easily ousted Hilda Sperling of Germany, 6–1, 6–1, in under 20 minutes in the Wimbledon Women's Singles semifinals. In the Women's Singles championship, she overwhelmed Kay Stammers of Great Britain, 6–2, 6–0, for her first Wimbledon title. "Everything about my game was working," she beamed. The Britishers were shocked to witness their very popular contender exit so quickly.

Marble exulted, "I had done it! I was champion of the world!" Her victory marked "the culmination of a life time of striving." She hugged her racquet to her chest, "prouder than I'd ever been in my life."[38]

Marble, playing on "sheer adrenaline," dominated her other Wimbledon matches, combining with Palfrey to trounce Jacobs and Yorke, 6–1, 6–0, in the Women's Doubles finals, and with fellow American Bobby Riggs to defeat Nina Brown and Frank Wilde of Great Britain, 9–7, 6–1, in the Mixed Doubles. "This is my day!" she beamed. Marble had attained her primary objective of being the first twentieth-century female to win the Wimbledon singles, doubles, and mixed doubles championships in the same year, while Riggs became the only player to take the Wimbledon Singles, Doubles, and Mixed Doubles titles in his first attempt. "The day had become a magnificent day, and I never wanted it to end,"[39] Marble declared.

Marble met Jacobs again in the 1939 U.S. Women's Singles finals. She admitted, "The 1939 Nationals final was as fierce a match as the two of us ever played." Marble blanked Jacobs, 6–0, in the first set, but the latter rallied from a 5–3 deficit to take the second set, 10–8. After Jacobs seized a 3–1 lead in that set, Marble regained the momentum to win the set, 6–4, and the match. Jacobs twice fought back from match point before capitulating. "The match could have gone either way,"[40] Marble conceded.

Marble then teamed with Harry Hopman of Australia to defeat Palfrey and American Elwood Cooke, 9–7, 6–1, to win the 1939 U.S. National Mixed Doubles championship and with Palfrey to overcome Stammers and Freda Hammersley of Great Britain, 7–5, 8–6, for the U.S. Women's Doubles title at Chestnut Hill, Massachusetts. Months later, "I still had trouble believing that I was the world champion,"[41] Marble noted.

The 1940 U.S. Nationals tournament likewise was dominated by Marble. After besting Jacobs 6–2, 6–3, for the U.S. Women's Singles crown, Marble paired with Palfrey to defeat American Dorothy Bundy and Van Ryn, 6–4, 6–3, for the U.S. Women's Doubles title and with Riggs to overcome Bundy and fellow American Jack Kramer, 9–7, 6–1, to capture the U.S. Mixed Doubles titles. Her Triple Crown in the U.S. Singles, Doubles, and Mixed Doubles championships between 1938 and 1940 matched a record shared by American Hazel Hotchkiss Wightman from 1909 to 1911 and Browne from 1912 to 1914. She destroyed competitors "with her well-executed ground strokes, strong serves, and crisp volleys, enhanced by speed and agility around the court."[42]

Marble also represented the United States in the Wightman Cup matches against the best English women players between 1937 and 1939. She was selected the outstanding Amateur Athlete of the Year by the Helms Foundation. The Associated Press named her Woman Athlete of the Year in 1939 and 1940.

Marble's personal financial obligations and desire to contribute to the World War II effort caused her to turn professional in 1940. In 1941, Marble toured the

United States playing exhibition tennis matches with Mary Hardwick of Great Britain. Her other activities included directing physical training for women in the Office of Civilian Defense, entertaining the military with tennis exhibitions, visiting military hospitals, selling war bonds across the United States, singing in New York City nightclubs, and designing tennis clothes.

After secretly marrying Army Captain Joseph Crowley, an army intelligence officer, in 1941, Marble experienced personal tragedy. She "plunged into despair" after suffering a miscarriage, and especially after Crowley was killed in a 1944 plane crash in Germany. Army intelligence recruited Marble as a spy. During a tennis tour in Switzerland, Marble retrieved

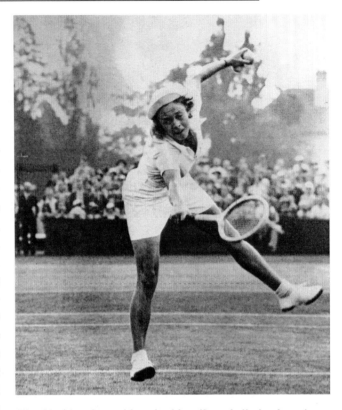

Alice Marble, pictured here backhanding a ball, dominated the U.S. National Tournament at Forest Hills, New York, in 1940, defeating Helen Jacobs for the women's singles title, combining with Sarah Palfrey to win the women's doubles crown and with Bobby Riggs to take the mixed doubles title (courtesy International Tennis Hall of Fame and Museum).

information about Nazi financial accounts. She was shot in the back while escaping a counter-agent but was rescued. Marble reflected, "I have been a loser before and have had to learn through hard work, patience and faith just a bit of the way to overcome defeat."[43]

Marble remained involved with tennis after World War II. "She lectured, played exhibition matches, and taught, particularly after she moved back to California from New York City in 1951." Marble contributed columns for *American Lawn Tennis* magazine, influencing the careers of Doris Hart and Althea Gibson of the United States. She commended Hart for overcoming adversity and inspired her to achieve championship potential. Marble berated the USLTA for denying Gibson, an African American star, the opportunity to participate in tennis tournaments and thus demonstrate her court skills. Her criticism "sparked an outcry that forced the organization to change its rules and allow Althea Gibson to play in USLTA tournaments."[44] The author of *The Road to Wimbledon* (1947) and *Courting Danger* (1991, with Dale

Leatherman), Marble coached tennis champions Americans Darlene Hard, Maureen Connolly, and King.

Colon cancer and the loss of a lung to pneumonia later slowed Marble. In 1964, Marble was inducted into the International Lawn Tennis Hall of Fame. She taught tennis at the Palm Desert Country Club in Palm Desert, California, from the mid–1960s until her death there from pernicious anemia on December 13, 1990.[45]

Marble suffered from health problems throughout her life, but "nothing seemed to stop her." She overcame enormous adversity to become "one of the great players of women's tennis" and "utilized her natural athletic talents to develop a powerful, all-court game. She played tennis with the same verve, style, and daring sense of adventure that she brought to all aspects of her life." Marble, "a woman of extraordinary courage, resourcefulness, and spirit,"[46] was blessed with exceptional athletic skills and a profound love for sports.

# ALONZO MOURNING

"Resilience, faith, focus and triumph" inspired basketball star Alonzo Mourning's rebound from kidney failure. After having played eight National Basketball Association (NBA) seasons, Mourning learned in October 2000 that he had developed a life-threatening kidney disease. The tragic news sent shock waves through the NBA. Mourning launched a miraculous comeback after receiving a kidney transplant in 2003, helping the Miami Heat win an NBA Championship.

Mourning was reared in unsettled circumstances. Alonzo Mourning was born in Chesapeake, Virginia, on February 8, 1970. His father, Alonzo Sr., who worked as a machinist in the Portsmouth, Virginia, shipyards, divorced his wife, Julia, when Alonzo was 11 years old. Mourning moved in with Fannie Threet, a family friend and retired teacher who ran a foster home. Up to nine children lived in Threet's four-bedroom house. Mourning did not adjust well to his parents' divorce and "began getting into trouble."[1]

To keep Mourning occupied, friends and teachers encouraged him to participate in basketball. Mourning, who grew to six feet, three inches by seventh grade, began playing basketball. He witnessed the 1982 NCAA Championship game between Georgetown University and the University of North Carolina on television and idolized the Hoyas's center Patrick Ewing.[2] "I was very awkward, very clumsy," Mourning admitted. "People were laughing at me, but that made me work harder."

Mourning improved his basketball skills markedly under coach Bill Lassiter at Indian River High School in Chesapeake, becoming a dominant presence. In summer 1986, he impressed college scouts at the prestigious Five-Star Camp near Pittsburgh. His undefeated Indian River High School team won the 1987 Virginia State Class

AAA Championship, and he was named Virginia High School Player of the Year. As a senior, Mourning led Indian River in scoring and rebounding and was rated the nation's premier scholastic basketball player. "It was kind of exciting at first. But it was tough keeping things in perspective,"[3] he realized. In 1988, Mourning made McDonald's All-American. Gatorade and *USA Today* selected him as National High School Player of the Year.

Georgetown University, coached by John Thompson, recruited Mourning as a center to follow in the giant footsteps of Ewing and Dikembe Mutombo. "Mourning picked up Ewing's torch, ignoring entreaties to show his good-guy side and his intelligence." As a freshman in 1988–1989, Mourning averaged 13.2 points, 7.3 rebounds, and 4.9 blocks and led the nation with 169 blocked shots. His 11 blocks in one game broke Ewing's record. In 1989, Mourning was selected the Big East Conference (BEC) Defensive Player of the Year and to the All-BEC Second Team and BEC All-Rookie Team. He proved a ferocious interior player, constantly battling. Mourning, who averaged 16.5 points and 8.5 rebounds in 1989–1990, was named BEC Co-Defensive Player of the Year, First Team All-BEC, and Associated Press Second Team All-America.[4] A serious foot injury sidelined him for nine games as a junior.

In the summer of 1991, Mourning worked out with NBA stars Ewing and Mutombo. He gained greater control over his personal life and "showed a new level of maturity." Mourning returned to center in 1991–1992 and led Georgetown to the BEC Co-Championship, averaging 21.7 points, 10.7 rebounds, and five blocks. He became the Hoyas' team leader, blocking shots, feeding the ball to teammates when double-teamed, and converting foul shots. Mourning joined Ewing as the only players in Georgetown history to amass over 2,000 career points and 1,000 rebounds. His career average of 3.78 blocked shots per game ranked second only to Mutombo. Mourning was named the BEC Tournament's Most Valuable Player (MVP), becoming the first player chosen BEC Player of the Year and BEC Defensive Player of the Year in the same year. He garnered AP First Team All-America honors and the Henry Iba Defensive Player of the Year Award, and earned a bachelor's degree in sociology in 1992.[5]

In 1992, Mourning joined the Charlotte Hornets, a struggling NBA expansion team in its fifth year. Charlotte made Mourning the second overall selection after Shaquille O'Neal of the Orlando Magic. Mourning made an immediate impact, becoming the Hornets' all-time leading shot blocker in his forty-ninth game and compiling the highest scoring average of any rookie in Charlotte franchise history. He averaged 21 points, 10 rebounds, and 3.5 blocks per game in 1992–1993 while earning runner-up honors for NBA Rookie of the Year and making the NBA All-Rookie First Team. Mourning helped the Hornets make their first playoff with a 44–38 record in 1992–1993 and a first-round playoff victory on May 5 over the Boston Celtics. He drained the clinching shot, a 20-footer at the buzzer, to send Charlotte into the NBA Eastern Conference semifinals against the New York Knicks.[6]

Although plagued by injuries in 1993–1994, Mourning played for the "Dream Team II" U.S. squad that won the 1994 World Basketball Championship in Canada and made the NBA Eastern Conference All-Star team for the first of four consecutive seasons and seven times altogether. In his third season with Charlotte in 1994–1995, he became one of four players to lead an NBA team in four categories, including

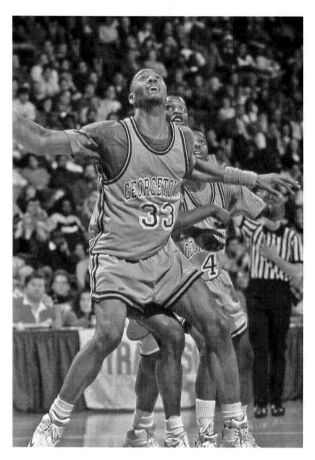

scoring, rebounding, blocked shots, and field-goal percentage. Mourning played in his initial NBA All-Star Game and helped the Hornets achieve 50 victories for the first time.[7] He also joined Mutombo and Ewing in conducting basketball clinics for children in South Africa.

Mourning established an enviable reputation as an industrious player with a feisty persona, declining the Hornets' $11.2 million per year salary offer. *Sports Illustrated* writer Jack McCallum pictured Mourning as "a joyless, brooding man." In November 1995, Charlotte traded Mourning to the Miami Heat for Glen Rice. Heat head coach Pat Riley, impressed with Mourning's skills, said, "Zo, come to Miami, and let's go to work."[8]

Mourning starred for Miami from 1995 to 2003, missing much of the 1997–1998 season with injuries. The 6-foot 10-inch, 261-pounder resembled other small pivot men Willis Reed, Dave Cowens, and Wes Unseld.

**Alonzo Mourning prepares to rebound a shot during a Georgetown University game circa 1990. He amassed over 2,000 career points and 1,000 career rebounds, winning the Henry Iba Defensive Player of the Year Award (courtesy Georgetown Sports Information).**

Mourning employed "a unique, intimidating style" and began controlling "his intense moodiness." Riley, who lauded Mourning's work ethic, raved, "Alonzo is a whirling dervish, a cyclone of a player. He embodies everything we want this team to be — passionate, committed, aggressive, tireless."[9]

Miami relied primarily on Mourning both offensively and defensively. Mourning paced the Heat in points (career-best 23.2 average), rebounds (10.4 average), and blocked shots and led them to the 1995–1996 playoffs with a 42–40 record. He set a personal and team record with 22 rebounds in a January game. In 1996–1997, the Heat won a record 61 games and captured the Atlantic Division. He helped the Heat to the NBA Eastern Conference Finals, where they lost to the Chicago Bulls.

Mourning married Tracy Wilson in August 1997 in the Caribbean and has one son, Alonzo Jr. and a daughter, Myka.[10]

A knee injury and broken cheekbone sidelined Mourning for 22 games in the 1997–1998 season. In 1998–1999, Mourning averaged 20.1 points, 11 rebounds, and 3.9 blocks, finishing second to Karl Malone in the NBA MVP balloting and making the All-NBA First Team. He was named NBA Defensive Player of the Year, made the NBA All-Defensive First Team, and led the NBA in blocks in both 1999 and 2000, bettering O'Neal and Ewing.[11]

In the 1999–2000 season, Mourning played a career-high 79 games, averaged 21.7 points, 9.5 rebounds, and 3.7 blocks, made the All-NBA Second Team, and finished third in the NBA MVP voting. He played a physical series in the NBA Eastern Conference semifinals against the New York Knicks.[12]

Mourning helped the USA men's basketball team win a gold medal at the 2000 Sydney Summer Olympic Games. During the games, he flew home to witness the birth of his daughter, Myka. "A lot of people would have loved to have traded places with me at that particular point," Mourning reflected. "Things were just great."[13]

Although normally having abundant energy and stamina, Mourning grew increasingly fatigued and weak. "I was tired all the time and was not able to even complete everyday tasks," he lamented. His kidneys began to fail. Mourning attributed his lethargy to unhealthy eating habits and to "being tired after participating in the Summer Olympics."[14]

At the annual, pre-season team physical, a doctor diagnosed Mourning with a chronic kidney disease called focal segmental glomerulosclerosis (FSGS). FSGS attacks small filters in the kidney that remove waste from the blood, causing protein to spill into the urine and scar the kidney. It inhibits the kidney from filtering toxins out of the body, causing kidney failure and anemia. The rare, sometimes fatal, and incurable disease was considered untreatable until the mid–1990s. It tends to affect younger men, especially African Americans. The doctor warned him that he would need dialysis for 10 to 12 months and require a transplant shortly hereafter.[15] Two other doctors gave Mourning a more optimistic assessment, prescribing an oral medication regimen. Mourning, who never went on dialysis, began taking Procrit, a drug that stimulates red blood cell production to fight anemia. "That gave me my energy and my life back,"[16] he recollected.

The news about the kidney disease shocked the young, athletic, and seemingly healthy Mourning, who had enjoyed one of his best seasons. Some nights soon afterward, Mourning lay awake "wondering if he would die." He admitted, "It was very, very tough to digest, I was totally in denial, and I felt like that, like all the other injuries I had in my life, I could beat it."[17] The disease taught Mourning to become a more active participant in his own health. Mourning stressed, "When you're dealing with an obstacle of that magnitude, you've got to start with having faith, with believing, and staying positive." He also needed to learn everything he could about the disease and then make proper adjustments in his life to cope with it.[18]

At an October 2000 press conference, Mourning announced that he would miss part of the 2000–2001 season to undergo treatment for kidney disease. He missed the first five months of that campaign and began medication treatments. Others discussed possible dialysis or a transplant and his likely retirement, but the Heat center insisted upon returning to the NBA. "Quit isn't in my vocabulary," he explained. "I love the game too much."[19] The competition and friendships meant everything to him.

Upon returning to the Heat in March 2001, Mourning played limited minutes. His offensive production dropped to 13.6 points and 7.80 rebounds per contest in 13 games. He explained, "The medication that I am on affects my endurance," which reduced his normal playing time. He was selected to the Eastern Conference team for the 2001 NBA All-Star Game, but his illness sidelined him.[20]

Mourning possessed the requisite qualities for defying the odds. McCallum claimed that only an athlete "with a lot of steel inside, could do what Mourning is doing now." Indiana Pacers coach Isiah Thomas lauded Mourning's standards and work ethic. Although the average American with Mourning's wealth likely would have retired already, the Heat's center continued to play. Mutombo of the Philadelphia 76ers observed that to witness him courageously "compete again almost at the same level as he used to is amazing." Fatigue, however, posed the biggest challenge for the determined Mourning. Both on and off the court, Mourning often felt physically exhausted. The doctors did not know whether the disease, the medication, or a combination thereof caused his fatigue. But Dr. Gerald Appel, kidney specialist at Columbia University Medical Center, stressed, "We simply don't have another 6'10", 260-pound world-class athlete expending this kind of energy and battling this."[21]

Mourning played nearly the entire 2001–2002 NBA campaign, which McCallum termed "a season full of fight." He worked diligently to keep his body healthy and added, "Thankfully we saw my body respond to the medications." His blood tests returned to a level allowing him to compete. Mourning drank plenty of water, did not play too long at one time, and continued to consult his doctors regularly. He struggled initially, missing five games due to food poisoning and a virus, as the Heat won just five of 23 games.[22]

Mourning inspired a dramatic Heat turnaround, suddenly becoming "electric" with his drives to the basket and dunks. Miami defeated premier teams and won 11 consecutive second halves of back-to-back games over a three-month stretch. Teammate Brian Grant claimed, "Zo was the catalyst," recalling what Mourning had endured during rehabilitation. By late March, Mourning already had recorded 20 double doubles and again competed "at a high level." In an 89–79 loss at the San Antonio Spurs on March 23, Mourning battled David Robinson and Tim Duncan for 32 minutes. Although Mourning tallied 16 points and 11 rebounds, his "inestimable efforts had gone for naught."[23]

During 2001–2002, Mourning averaged 15.7 points and 8.4 rebounds in 75 games and participated in the NBA All-Star Game for the seventh time in his career. Besides leading the Heat in rebounding, he ranked sixth in the NBA in field-goal percentage (51.6), third in the NBA in blocked shots (2.48 average), and second on the team in scoring. Despite Mourning's yeoman efforts, the Heat finished next to last in the Atlantic Division with a 36–46 record and missed the playoffs.[24]

Several factors sparked Mourning's resurgence. Drs. Appel and Victor Richards of New York changed his daily eight-pill regimen in late December. Mourning's hard work and conditioning exercises started paying dividends. Riley attributed Mourning's performance to positive mental attitude. Mourning also trained diligently off the court. His agent Jeffrey Wechsler often found him working out with weights in his garage after a hard practice. Mourning still needed to build his leg strength.

Mourning's point and rebound averages, however, had declined. NBA scouts observed, "Mourning can be his old self only in spurts."[25] His average playing time dropped from at least 40 minutes to 32 minutes, as his stamina declined in consecutive games. The reduced minutes, however, did not diminish his effectiveness, he insisted.

A roadblock stymied Mourning's miraculous comeback. In September 2002, doctors persuaded Mourning to skip the 2002–2003 season because test results indicated his condition had worsened. Since that was the final year of his seven-year, $105 million deal with Miami, the Heat did not renew his contract. Mourning even realized he had concentrated too much on basketball and not enough on his health. "Like so many athletes," he admitted, "I thought about our sport before I thought about my health, not realizing that your health is the driving force behind all the things you want to do in life. If you don't have your health, you don't have anything."[26]

The New Jersey Nets signed Mourning to a four-year, $22 million contract in July 2003, but the seven-time All-Star played only 12 games from October 29 through November 22. Mourning averaged eight points and 2.3 rebounds in 215 minutes for the two-time defending Eastern Conference champions, who struggled with a 5–7 mark. He saved his best game for last with a season-high 15 points in 16 minutes in an 81–80 loss to the Toronto Raptors, but looked exhausted when he left the court for a fourth-quarter breather. Mourning still epitomized determination and a strong work ethic. Teammate Jason Kidd observed, "For him to come out and almost kill himself to just play the game that he loves, it just shows the kind of person Zo is." Nets coach Byron Scott noted, "He played every game like it was his last game."[27]

By November 2003, Mourning's illness worsened so he could no longer compete on the court. His team and personal doctors considered him medically unfit to play.

As the Nets embarked on a West Coast trip, Dr. Appel told Mourning that his kidney function had deteriorated rapidly and advised him to retire. "It is no longer medically safe for him to play basketball," Dr. Appel warned. "The medical imbalances in his blood make it dangerous for him to play." He feared that Mourning might have a heart attack if he continued playing basketball. "No, doc, no," Mourning retorted. "Why?" Appel replied, "Your potassium has gotten to a level where if you play, then you put yourself into a position for heart palpitations and cardiac arrest." Mourning found it difficult accepting Dr. Appel's advice. He told TNT NBA analyst John Thompson, "I still feel there's an emptiness in my career that just wasn't filled."[28]

On November 25, 2003, Mourning left the NBA because of the kidney disease complications. Nets general manager Rod Thorn announced Mourning's retirement, stating, "Alonzo is a true champion and a very courageous athlete who attempted to defy the odds with his comeback to the NBA. Unfortunately, his medical condition will not allow him to continue his basketball career." Riley reflected, "It's a sad day in anyone's life when they can no longer do what they love, especially when they have no control over their situation." But Kidd reminded Mourning, "The game of basketball is just a game."[29]

Mourning immediately began seeking a donor for a kidney transplant. Although the average wait in America for a kidney transplant is two to four years, many people offered Mourning one of their own kidneys. Mourning luckily found a family donor. The same day, Jason Cooper, his estranged cousin whom he had not seen in 25 years, was visiting their gravely ill grandmother in the hospital. Mourning's father informed Cooper about the kidney transplant need. Cooper was tested for compatibility, along with other family friends, relatives, and Ewing. During his grandmother's funeral, Mourning learned that Cooper was a good match. Cooper agreed to donate his left kidney to his cousin. On December 19, Mourning underwent a three-hour kidney transplant surgery. The disease drew the cousins closer together. "We have established a brotherly type of relationship,"[30] Mourning revealed.

Mourning sobbed uncontrollably right after the surgery, shedding tears for the first during the entire ordeal. His tension, built up over three years, burst forth. "I felt helpless," he told Ian Thomsen of *Sports Illustrated*. Mourning suffered "horrible pain" that night and earnestly prayed, "God, if you ever get me back on my feet to where I am able to work out, I'll do everything I can to take care of myself."[31] Mourning's hospital visitors believed that his NBA playing career was finished.

Defying the odds, the physically weak Mourning began planning his return to the NBA the next day. Doctors released Mourning from the hospital on December 23. For several months, the self-conscious, frail Mourning seldom left his Miami home. He began his recovery in February 2004, walking on a treadmill and pressing 20-pound dumbbells. The exercise initially made him "sick and dizzy," but he vowed to continue the workouts until his physical strength was restored.[32]

Doctors were amazed how well Mourning recovered from such a radical procedure. Mourning's physical fitness foundation expedited his recovery. Mourning knew that it would be a tough road, but never doubted his ability to come back. He promised "to touch other people's lives through the pain that I had to go through" and provided hope and support to others battling kidney disease, cancer, diabetes, and other diseases. "Being back on the court," he added, "has helped lift other people's lives."[33]

Mourning made the Nets' roster for the 2004–2005 season. Doctors assured him that playing would not jeopardize his long-term health if he followed his physical regimen. While Kidd was recovering from off-season knee surgery, Mourning helped the Nets keep afloat in the first six games, averaging 11.8 points, 7.2 rebounds, and 2.7 blocked shots in 26.2 minutes. Mourning wore a small plastic shield with foam to protect his new kidney during games, looking "as strong as ever." In mid–November, he even played 77 minutes in consecutive games. "I've been nothing but amazed," observed Nets coach Lawrence Frank. "Everything he does, he does hard."[34]

In mid–November 2004, however, Mourning told the media that he wanted to be traded to a contender and asked the Nets to buy out $14 million of the $18 million on the remaining three years of his contract. He was disheartened upon hearing rumors that Nets owner Bruce Ratner wanted him to retire for salary cap reasons. Mourning also protested the Nets' cost-cutting trades that summer of forward Kenyon Martin and Kerry Kittles, claiming those transactions removed the Nets from title contention and would make his comeback "a waste of time."[35]

Since Mourning's contract was uninsured, no team offered equal value to the Nets. Thorn, therefore, initially kept his second best scorer and rebounder. In December 2004, Mourning did not accompany the Nets on a road trip. A week later, the Toronto Raptors acquired Mourning and four other players for Vince Carter. Mourning never reported to Toronto and bought out the remaining $9 million of his contract.

NBA fans and team executives criticized Mourning's stance, but he replied that his illness enabled him to become the kind of spokesman for kidney research and organ transplants that cyclist Lance Armstrong had become in his fight against cancer. Mourning desired to play for a club in contention for an NBA crown. Riley concurred, "Zo sincerely wants to win a championship."[36]

The Miami Heat signed Mourning on March 1, 2005, as a reserve center for O'Neal. In 37 games that season, Mourning averaged 7.6 points, 5.4 rebounds, and two blocked shots. He started some games because of O'Neal's injuries and played power forward when O'Neal returned as center. His playing time was reduced due to his physical limitations, but he contributed powerfully and helped the Heat make the 2005 NBA playoffs.[37]

Mourning changed his playing style from a scorer to defender upon rejoining the Heat. Before his surgery, he had touched the ball often at the offensive end, averaging 20 points. Defense proved his most valuable asset to the Heat. Mourning adjusted well to Miami's "aging star-laden roster." O'Neal called him "the hardest working big man I've ever seen, a family-dedicated guy, a community-dedicated guy."[38]

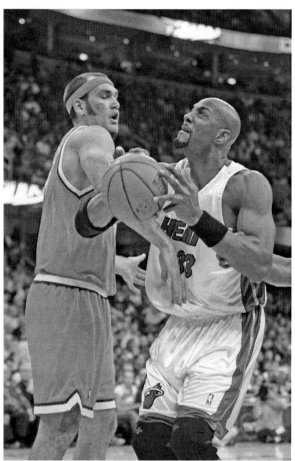

Alonzo Mourning of the Miami Heat is fouled by Scott Pollard of the Cleveland Cavaliers at Quicken Loans Arena in Cleveland on April 5, 2007. Miami defeated Cleveland, 94–90, in overtime to secure a playoff spot (courtesy Icon Sports Media).

Mourning's tenacious defense, steady offense, and general hustle lifted Miami to the second best Eastern Conference record during the 2005–2006 season. The Heat, led by guard Dwayne Wade, finished 52–30 under Riley. Mourning played a valuable role as a reserve for O'Neal and started 18 consecutive games in November and December when O'Neal had a sprained ankle. He helped "fill O'Neal's colossal shoes," averaging 17.7 points and 7.9 rebounds while preserving the Heat's Southeast Division lead.[39]

When the Heat trounced the Portland Trail Blazers, 100–79, on November 23, the warrior-like Mourning did not play like a kidney transplant recipient. He amazingly came out of nowhere to block a two-handed dunk shot by 7-foot 1-inch Portland center Joel Przybilla. Although the Orlando Magic edged the Heat, 80–77, three nights later, Mourning tallied 15 points and 21 rebounds. On November 28 at Miami, he blocked nine shots in 24 minutes in a 107–94 rout of the New York Knicks. During O'Neal's absence, "Zo set the bar very high" defensively. Stan Van Gundy, who coached the Heat until early December, boasted Mourning's performance merited him a starting position in the All-Star Game.

Upon O'Neal's return, Riley limited Mourning to under 20 minutes per game against tall teams. Since Mourning had averaged around 30 minutes per game through mid–December, Riley was worried that the extensive workload would diminish his stamina. "We can't let his huge heart and stubbornness get the best of him,"[40] Riley declared. Although playing just 20 minutes per contest two years after his transplant, Mourning miraculously finished the 2005–2006 regular season leading the NBA with a career-high 59.7 shooting percentage, ranking third in blocked shots at 2.7 per game, and averaging 7.8 points and 5.5 rebounds in 65 games.

Miami blitzed through the Chicago Bulls, New Jersey, and the Detroit Pistons in the 2006 NBA playoffs and won its first-ever NBA Championship, defeating the Dallas Mavericks in the NBA Finals, four games to two. Although a reserve center behind O'Neal during the NBA Finals, Mourning contributed eight points, six rebounds, and five blocks in the decisive Game 6 of the series. The Heat became just the third team to overcome an 0–2 NBA Finals deficit to "transform South Beach into the pinnacle of the NBA universe."[41]

In 2006–2007, Mourning helped Miami return to the playoffs, averaging 8.6 points and 4.4 rebounds and recording an excellent 56 percent field-goal percentage. Chicago, however, swept the Heat in the first playoff round. Mourning played in just 25 games the next season, averaging six points, 3.7 rebounds, and 1.7 blocked shots, and became Miami's all-time scoring leader. He tore his patellar tendon in his right knee on December 19, 2007, during the first quarter against the Atlanta Hawks. The injury ironically occurred on the fourth anniversary of his successful kidney transplant and ended his stellar NBA career.[42]

Mourning, who retired from the NBA as a player at age 38 on January 22, 2009, stated, "I feel like I have physically done all I can for this game." On March 30, 2009, the Heat retired Mourning's number 33 jersey. No other Miami player has a jersey retired by the organization. Mourning remains with the Heat as Vice-President of Player Development and Programs.

During his illustrious 15-year NBA career, Mourning tallied 14,311 points (17.1 average) and made 7,137 rebounds (8.5 average) in 838 regular-season games. He connected on 52.7 percent of his shots and recorded 2,356 blocked shots, averaging the most blocks in NBA history with 2.8 per game. In 95 playoff games, Mourning averaged 13.6 points, seven rebounds, and 2.3 blocked shots.[43] He intimidated opponents, possessed a strong work ethic, and was one of the hardest working and toughest NBA players. His intense style made him one of the NBA's best combined shot blockers, rebounders, and scorers.

In his book, *Resilience: Faith, Focus, Triumph* (2008), Mourning details his personal struggles to overcome FSGS and rejoin the NBA. He also expresses his commitment to increase public awareness of kidney disease and do everything he can to help those who have it. Mourning hoped to inform Americans about high blood pressure, diabetes, family history, and other risk factors, let them know the warning signs of kidney disease, stress the importance of regular doctor visits, and highlight organ donation. He warned that many people with kidney disease did not even know it.[44]

Mourning maintains a broad interest in philanthropy and social betterment. He represented the NBA as their mouthpiece on prevention of child abuse and participated in the NBA's Healthy Families America program. His Alonzo Mourning Charities, established in 1997, has raised nearly $10 million to aid in the development of children and families living in at-risk situations and provide support and services enhancing the lives of promising youth. A National Kidney Foundation spokesman, Mourning in 2001 launched Zo's Fund for Life that has raised over $2 million for kidney research, education, and testing. Funds are allocated toward research for a kidney disease cure, education for doctors and the general public, testing for early detection, and defraying costs for those not able to afford medication.[45] He founded "Zo's Summer Groove," an annual charity event benefiting the Miami-based Children's Home Society and 100 Black Men of South Florida.

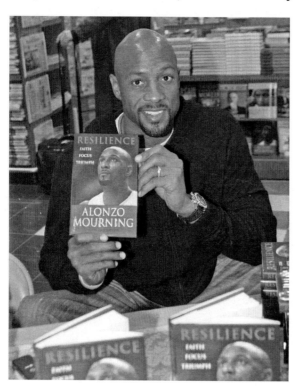

Alonzo Mourning holds a copy of his autobiography, *Resilience: Faith, Focus, Triumph*, at a book signing at Hudson News in Union Station in Washington, D.C., on November 23, 2008. Random House published his book in September 2008 (courtesy Georgetown Sports Information).

In 2001, *USA Today Weekend Magazine* honored Mourning with their Most Caring Athlete Award. Mourning received the J. Walter Kennedy Citizenship Award in 2002 and was named to the Hampton Roads Sports Hall of Fame in May 2009, honoring southeastern Virginia athletes and coaches.

# WILMA RUDOLPH

"I acquired this sense of determination, this sense of spirit that I would never, never give up, no matter what else happened," recalled Wilma Rudolph, who surmounted a formidable medical hurdle to achieve track stardom. Rudolph contracted polio at an early age and found it difficult to walk. Courage and relentless determination helped her transcend that affliction to become one of the world's great sprinters.

Rudolph was brought up in an impoverished African American family in the segregated South. Wilma Glodean Rudolph entered the world two months premature on June 23, 1940, in St. Bethlehem, Tennessee, weighing just four and one-half pounds. Rudolph was the sixth of eight children of Edward Rudolph, a railroad porter, and Blanche Pets Rudolph, a domestic in homes of white families. Her father already had 14 children from a previous marriage. Rudolph's family struggled with poverty, never earning more than $2,500 a year, and moved to a wooden frame house in Clarksville, Tennessee, with no electricity.[1]

Rudolph suffered many childhood maladies due to her premature birth. "I was sick all the time," she remembered. Rudolph contracted polio at age four, suffered double pneumonia twice, and had scarlet fever and whooping cough. Although surviving the illnesses, she lost the use of her crooked right leg for several years. Her right foot was twisted inward.[2] Polio, a highly contagious, infectious, debilitating disease caused by a filterable virus for which there was no immunization or curative treatment, often caused paralysis and struck many children before Dr. Jonas Salk created the polio vaccine in 1955. Polio weakened Rudolph, leaving her partially paralyzed and unable to walk without a brace.

When Rudolph was five years old, doctors fitted her right leg with a cumbersome steel brace to keep it straight. Rudolph was supposed to wear the brace the entire day and wore a brown Oxford shoe with it. The brace, however, made her self-conscious of her infirmity and that "something was wrong with her." "Psychologically," she felt, "wearing that brace was devastating." Rudolph always wanted to be like everyone else. "All I can remember is being ill and bedridden," she recalled. Her mother feared "she would die."[3]

From 1946 to 1950, Rudolph rode the Greyhound Bus 50 miles weekly to receive four hours of treatments on her leg at all-black Meharry Medical College of Fisk University in Nashville. The Clarksville hospital did not treat her because of the Jim Crow segregation laws. In hopes that Rudolph might regain full use of her crippled left leg, doctors pulled, turned, twisted, and stretched the limb and gave it a therapeutic massage in a hot whirlpool. During the rest of the week, her mother and three older siblings massaged it several times daily. The discouraged Rudolph did not notice any significant improvement for a long time.[4]

The desire to walk like everyone else became a driving force in Rudolph's life. When her parents were not home, Rudolph often took off her braces, and her brothers and sisters would let her know when her parents were returning. "I'd hurry and put the braces back on," she said. "Rudolph learned how to fake a normal walk," trying to convince her family that she was improving. Rudolph hoped "People were going to start separating me from that brace." She watched her siblings perform various household chores, portraying herself as their "gimpy-legged cheerleader."[5]

Rudolph missed all of kindergarten and first grade because of her health problems and was tutored at home by her mother, who had not completed elementary school.

The illnesses kept her isolated from other Clarksville children and made her lonely. "Neighborhood children teased her, calling her 'cripple,' and excluded her from their activities."[6] Although her siblings naturally supported her, she felt isolated and rejected.

In 1947 at age seven, Rudolph entered second grade at Cobb Elementary School. The segregated school suffered from substandard facilities, curriculum, and materials. Rudolph was apprehensive about attending school and especially meeting children her own age. Upon attending school for the first time, she disclosed, "I was terrified." Not accustomed to being around other children, the sensitive and insecure Rudolph, who yearned to be like her classmates and be accepted by them, "lived in a mortal fear of being disliked."[7] Rudolph's "competitive spirit" facilitated her recovery. As a child, she longed "to be able to run, jump, play, and all the things the other kids did in my neighborhood."[8] Mrs. Allison, Rudolph's second grade teacher, boosted her self-esteem and confidence. Although never completely conquering her insecure feelings, Rudolph gradually gained acceptance from her peers. She admitted, "That was the most important thing that could have happened to me."[9]

At age nine, Rudolph astonished the members of the Baptist church which her family attended regularly by walking by herself down the center aisle without a brace. Although still receiving medical treatment at Meharry, she considered the church walk "a big moment in her young life. It signaled to everyone, young and old, that she was more than the brace on her leg."[10]

Rudolph began walking even better at age 11, wearing a specially made high-top orthopedic shoe. The shoe allowed her to walk, but she could not run, jump, or skip like other youngsters. With perseverance, Rudolph became more mobile and athletic. By age 12, she walked normally without the aid of crutches, the leg brace, or corrective shoes. Rudolph's mother returned the leg brace to the Nashville hospital. Rudolph shot hoops with her siblings in the backyard and raced in the streets against her peers. "I was challenging every boy in our neighborhood at running, jumping, everything," she recalled. Rudolph finally experienced the joys of real health.

Rudolph's life took an important turn when the new, segregated Burt High School was constructed in Clarksville. Rudolph was introduced to organized sports for the first time, fell in love with basketball, and aspired to make the varsity basketball team.[11] Rudolph's protective mother originally did not want her to play basketball because the sport might be too physically demanding, but relented by seventh grade. Rudolph was very small for her age and had not participated on any athletic teams. She made the varsity basketball team as a junior high student, but did not appear in any games as a seventh grader and only briefly in two lopsided games as an eighth grader. Coach Clinton Gray kept her on the team only because her older sister, Yvonne, also played on it. Rudolph, however, learned much about the game by watching and studying the starting players.

When Rudolph was attending eighth grade, Gray started a girls' track and field team, mostly to maintain the condition of the basketball players during the spring.

Rudolph joined the squad and astonished everyone by winning the 50-, 75-, 100-, and 200-meter dashes and the relays against Springfield, Columbia, and Murfreesboro. Her victories came from natural ability, not hard work or training. Still Rudolph's first love remained basketball. Rudolph practiced hard, and considered herself a better shooter, rebounder, and defender than some of the starters. She constantly pestered Gray about when she would start. Gray began letting her scrimmage against the starters, but kept her on the bench that season except for cameo appearances. He nicknamed her "Skeeter" because she was tall, skinny, possessed long limbs, and resembled a mosquito in perpetual motion.[12]

During her sophomore year, Rudolph finally made starting guard on the varsity basketball team. She helped Burt finish 11–4 and win the Middle East Tennessee Conference title. The 5-foot 11-inch 100-pounder scored 32 points at a round robin tournament held at the crowded Burt gymnasium, converting all her shots. She became a celebrity at school for the first time. Rudolph tallied 803 points in 25 games, establishing a scoring record for girls' basketball in Tennessee.[13] After Rudolph scored 26 points in the victorious opening game of the Tennessee High School Girls' Championships in Nashville, Burt was eliminated in the semifinals.

Rudolph, meanwhile, blossomed as a track and field sprinter, competing in the 50-, 75-, 100-, and 200-meter dashes and the relay in informal meets as a freshman. She competed in around 20 races that spring, triumphing every time. After sweeping the conference competition as a sophomore, Rudolph sensed, "I felt unbeatable."

Rudolph's first sectional track and field meet at Tuskegee Institute in Tuskegee, Alabama, however, revealed her vulnerability. The Tuskegee Relays attracted outstanding athletes from across the South, and she lost every race. Rudolph tasted the agony of defeat in track for the first time and confessed, "It left me a total wreck." The losses, however, taught her how to lose and convinced her that she needed to train extensively daily to enjoy track and field success.[14]

Ed Temple, the women's track and field coach at Tennessee State University, realized that Rudolph possessed the potential to become a great runner and invited her to practice at the Nashville campus in the summer of 1956. Temple trained high school runners who would eventually compete for Tennessee State. The students ran about 20 miles daily for two weeks on the university's roads, using cross-country to help build their endurance and confidence. They ran varying distances thereafter, learned proper running techniques, and perfected relay routines. Rudolph performed well as a sprinter and relay team runner for the Tennessee State Track Club Tigerbelles.[15]

Track and field afforded Rudolph the first opportunity to compete in integrated competitions. Tennessee State won the National Amateur Athletic Union (AAU) Track and Field Championships in Philadelphia that August. Rudolph entered the 75-yard and 100-yard dashes and the 440-yard relay in the girls' junior division. She won all nine races, including qualifying heats, and demonstrated potential as an

Olympic athlete. Brooklyn Dodger star Jackie Robinson, who witnessed Rudolph's impressive performance, told her, "Don't let anything or anybody keep you from running." She realized, "For the first time in her life she had a black person to look up to as a real hero."[16]

Rudolph worked with Temple and on her own, frequently missing classes to practice. As a 16-year-old high school junior in 1956, she qualified for the U.S. Olympic team in the 200 meters and 4×100-meter relay at the Olympic Trials in Seattle. Before the 200-meter race, Mae Faggs, a Tennessee State senior, assured Rudolph of making the team if she kept up with her in the race. Rudolph finished in a dead heat with Faggs to share first place in the 200 meters. Following the race, Faggs told Rudolph, "We've all known you had it in you."[17]

Tennessee State became the first institution to have six members, including the entire American women's relay squad, qualify for the U.S. Olympic team. The relay team consisted of Faggs, Margaret Mathews, Rudolph, and Isabelle Daniels. Rudolph preferred performing the relays to running the 200 meters. Barely 16 years old, she was the youngest woman to make the U.S. Olympic track and field team, coached by Nel Jackson of Tuskegee Institute.

In her initial appearance at the 1956 Summer Olympic Games in Melbourne, Australia, Rudolph finished a disappointing third in the quarter-final round of the 200 meters and was eliminated. "I had let down everybody back home and the whole United States of America,"[18] Rudolph believed. Furthermore, "She was very disappointed in her performance" and "was miserable about her poor showing."[19]

The 400-meter relay gave Rudolph an opportunity for redemption. Rudolph ran the third leg of the 400-meter relay with Faggs, Mathews, and Daniels, helping the Americans place third for a bronze medal. The Americans clocked 44.9 seconds, only .4 seconds behind gold-medalist and record-setting Australia. Rudolph even passed two runners on her leg. Daniels nearly caught the Russians on the anchor leg, just missing second place. The bronze medal performance surprised some experts. According to Rudolph, "Not many people at the games expected us to do as well as we did." The American relay team members wrote their coach Temple, "We are even prouder to bring home to you a world record," noting, "It was the first time in the history of the games that three teams broke the world's record in the same event."[20]

Rudolph left the Olympic Games with mixed feelings. Although "disappointed" about not making the 200-meter finals, she relished the bronze medal and the Olympic experience, especially "the travel, the glamour, the excitement." Burt High School gave Rudolph a special welcome home. Rudolph showed classmates her bronze medal and vowed, "I'm going to go for the gold"[21] at the next Olympic Games.

During her junior year, Rudolph averaged 35 points in basketball for a team that sometimes surpassed the century mark. Burt enjoyed one of the best seasons in Tennessee history, finishing undefeated and capturing the state championship. Burt defeated Merry High School of Jackson in the final seconds, as Rudolph tallied 25 points. Rudolph won all of her track and field races that spring, observing "that a lot of girls were dropping out rather than run against me."[22] Her Olympic experience intimidated them.

The tragic death of Nancy Bowen, her best friend and Burt's leading basketball scorer, in an automobile accident following the junior-senior prom, depressed Rudolph for several weeks. But she trained again at Tennessee State University that summer and set new girls' division AAU records in the 75-yard and 100-yard dashes and 300-yard relay at the National AAU Track and Field Championships in Cleveland, Ohio. "It was great motivation for her."[23]

During her senior year, the 6-foot, 100-pound Rudolph became pregnant by her steady boyfriend, football-basketball star Robert Eldridge. She kept it secret for weeks until informing her older sister, Yvonne, who was residing in St. Louis, Missouri. Yvonne broke the news to Rudolph's mother, who assured Wilma, "She'd stick with me." Rudolph's father forbade her from seeing Robert again, but consoled her by saying, "Everybody makes mistakes."

The pregnancy forced Rudolph to drop out of basketball and skip track and field her senior year, which should have been her best. She graduated from Burt in May 1958 and gave birth to a daughter, Yolanda, two months later in Clarksville. Yvonne cared for the baby in St. Louis from September to December 1958 so Rudolph could attend Tennessee State University. Her mother subsequently cared for Yolanda in Clarksville.

Rudolph entered Tennessee State in September 1958, majoring in elementary education and minoring in psychology. To stay in school, she needed to maintain her grades to keep her scholarship and worked two hours daily, five days a week, at various jobs around campus. Rudolph nearly dropped out of Tennessee State several times as a freshman, but did not quit. The situation improved markedly within a year.[24]

Under Temple, Rudolph starred in track and field. At the time, the Tigerbelles dominated American women's track and field. As a freshman, Rudolph won the 50-yard dash in 6.2 seconds at the 1959 National Indoor AAU Track and Field Championships in Washington, D.C., and triumphed in the 100 meters at the 1959 National Outdoor AAU championships. She also won a silver medal in the 100 meters and ran on the victorious relay team at the Pan-American Games in Chicago, Illinois. "My speed was tremendous after I had the baby," Rudolph discovered. "I was much faster than before."[25]

In 1960, Rudolph became the best American female sprinter. She set two American records with 11.1 seconds in the 100-yard dash and 25.7 seconds in the 220-yard dash at the National Indoor AAU Track and Field Championships in April at Chicago. Rudolph repeated her AAU title in the 100-yard dash at the National Outdoor AAU Track and Field Championships in Corpus Christi, Texas,[26] and was invited to the Olympic Trials at Texas Christian University in Fort Worth in July.

Rudolph excelled at the 1960 Olympic Trials. She set a women's world record of 22.9 seconds in the 200-meter dash, becoming the first American female to hold a world mark in a running event. Rudolph also qualified for the U.S. Olympic team in the 100-meter dash and the 4×100-meter relay and was delighted when Temple was named Olympic coach. "Somebody up there was taking care of me this time around," she recalled. Experts projected Rudolph to capture three gold medals. "I knew if I didn't win three, it would be my fault alone," Rudolph realized. "Everything was in place for me."[27]

The Summer Olympic Games, held at Rome, were televised globally for the first time in 1960, enabling many Americans to watch Rudolph for the first time. Over 80,000 people jammed the Olympic Stadium for the sprints. The day before her first race, however, Rudolph landed in a hole after jumping through the spray from a sprinkler. She suffered a severe ankle sprain and experienced considerable pain. "I thought that I had broken it," she said. Before Rudolph's 100-meter race, though, Temple assured her, "everything was going to be all right."

Despite the sprained ankle, Rudolph became the first American female to win three gold medals in the same Olympic games, prevailing in the 100 meters, 200 meters, and 4×100-meter relay. Her triumphs came in very dramatic fashion. In the semifinals of the 100 meters, Rudolph equaled the world record with an eleven-second clocking. "The crowd never stopped chanting, "Vil-ma ... Vil-ma...""[28] The International Olympic Committee, however, disallowed the record because, according to Rudolph, the wind at her back exceeded 2.2 miles an hour.

In the wind-aided 100-meter finals, Rudolph repeated the eleven-second time for her first Olympic gold medal. Dorothy Hyman of Great Britain edged Giuseppina Leone of Italy for second place. Maria Itkina of the Soviet Union led the first 25 meters, but Rudolph steadily gained momentum by midpoint. "By seventy meters, I knew the race was mine, nobody was going to catch me," Rudolph recollected. She triumphed by around five yards. Although disappointed the International Olympic Committee again disallowed her world record, she was ecstatic about winning her first gold medal. No American woman Olympian had gold medaled in the 100 meters since Helen Stephens in 1936.

Over the next three days, Rudolph rested her ankle for the 200-meter race. "I'd be running curves for the first time since I had sprained it,"[29] she knew. Rudolph set an Olympic record of 23.2 seconds in favorable wind conditions in the opening heat of the 200-meter dash and captured the gold medal with a 24-second clocking in the 200-meter finals. Rain, along with a fierce head wind, slowed the times in the finals. Jutta Heine of Germany finished strong to edge Hyman for second place at 24.4 seconds. Despite the rain, Rudolph triumphed easily without experiencing any problems with either her ankle or the start.[30] The winning time, however, perturbed Rudolph because "it was more than a second slower than her world record time."[31]

Rudolph's Olympic career ended three days later with a third gold medal. Rudolph anchored the victorious U.S. 400-meter relay team, which also included

Tennessee State University runners Martha Hudson, Barbara Jones, and Lucinda Williams, Temple lauded Rudolph before the relay race, observing, "She gets over those starting blocks and — boom — all that harnessed energy explodes into speed."[32]

The 400-meter relay team set a world record of 44.4 seconds in the semifinals and snared the gold medal with a 44.5-second clocking in the finals. Rudolph bobbled the baton exchange from Williams, temporarily dropping the Americans to third, but "accelerated quickly and passed the two front runners in the first fifteen yards." According to Temple, "She was so determined, that I don't believe anyone could have stopped her." The Soviet Union earned the silver medal, while Poland finished third. "We wiped them all out, and we set a world's record in the process,"[33] Rudolph exulted.

Rudolph's moment in Olympic glory gave her the greatest satisfaction of her illustrious athletic career. Upon breaking the tape, Rudolph beamed, "The feeling of accomplishment welled up inside of me." No American woman had earned three Olympic gold medals. Rudolph realized, "That was something nobody could ever take away from me." After Rudolph received her gold medal on the

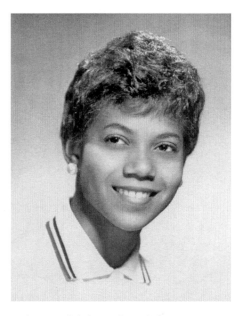

Wilma Rudolph graduated from Tennessee State University in May 1963 with a B.A. degree in elementary education and a minor in psychology (courtesy Tennessee State University Sports Information).

victory stand, the crowd mobbed her. The European press likened Rudolph to a gazelle, highlighting her grace and speed. Temple boasted, "She's done more for her country than what the United States could pay her for."[34]

During the next three weeks, Rudolph competed in several European track and field meets. She prevailed in the 100-meter dash and anchored the come-from-behind victory in the 4×100-meter relay in the British Empire Games at London. When the baton was passed to her with 100 yards to go, Rudolph trailed the leader by around 40 yards. The determined Rudolph "poured it on and ran the fastest anchor leg of her life, catching up (at the very tip of the tape) and winning the race." Track and field meets followed in Stuttgart, Amsterdam, Athens, and other European cities. Rudolph became an instant celebrity in Europe and the United States, being given ticker-tape parades. Clarksville honored her with the first integrated parade in that city's history.[35]

During the winter 1961, Rudolph ran shorter distances at indoor events. She did not enjoy competing indoors and "felt like an Amazon in an arena, performing for the blood-thirsty crowds." At the Los Angeles Invitational in January, "Wilma won [the 60-yard dash] without bothering to remove her wristwatch, and there was some indication she could have carried her purse." The following month, Rudolph set a world record of 6.9 seconds in the 60-yard dash during the Millrose Games at Madison Square Garden in New York. The next night, she established a world record of 7.8 seconds in the 70-yard dash at the Mason-Dixon Games in Louisville, Kentucky. At the New York Athletic Club meet in New York in February, Rudolph bettered her world record in the 60-yard dash with a 6.8-second clocking. Vivian Brown, however, upset her in the 200-yard dash at the National AAU Indoor Track and Field Championships.[36]

Rudolph dominated outdoor competition in 1961. She ran in the first Drake Relays event for women, winning the 100-yard dash in 11.1 seconds in April, and captured the 100-yard dash in 10.8 seconds at the National AAU Outdoor Track and Field Championships in Gary, Indiana, her third consecutive victory in that event. Rudolph equaled her 100-meter world record and anchored the victorious U.S. relay team in a USA-USSR dual meet at Moscow. She broke her 100-meter world record a few days later with an 11.2-second clocking at an invitational meet featuring Olympians at Stuttgart. Rudolph married William Ward, a fellow Tennessee State runner, in 1961, but they divorced the following year.

In 1962, Rudolph's track and field career culminated at its pinnacle. "Give them something to remember you by," Rudolph thought. She won her fourth consecutive national AAU outdoor 100-meter title easily with a 10.8 second time.[37] Rudolph's last race, the USA-USSR dual meet at Stanford University in Palo Alto, California, brought one of her most stunning victories in the 4×100-meter relay. The Soviet Union usually performed better in the relays than the sprints. After winning the 100-meter dash, Rudolph overcame a formidable Russian lead on the anchor leg of the 4×100-meter relay to give the United States a dramatic triumph. "Wilma got the baton as the Russians zoomed past her." The Russians took a sizable lead before Rudolph accelerated. Suddenly, "Wilma kicked in the speed and caught the Russian anchor leg to win the race."[38] The crowd gave her a resounding ovation.

Rudolph had just run her last race, sensing the time had come to retire.[39] Tex Maule of *Sports Illustrated* wrote, "No one in Palo Alto could match the incomparable Wilma Rudolph Ward for effortless grace and poise." After signing autographs for about an hour, Rudolph gave her track and field shoes to a little boy. "I didn't hang up my spikes," she said. "I gave them away."[40] She married Robert Eldridge, Tennessee State basketball star and father of her first child, in July 1963. They had three more children, Djuanna, Robert Jr., and Xurry, before their 1981 divorce.

Rudolph won numerous accolades. In 1960 and 1961, the Associated Press selected her Female Athlete of the Year. Althea Gibson was the only African American woman to win that award previously. Besides being named the 1960 United Press Athlete of the Year, Rudolph won the 1960 Babe Didrikson Zaharias Award as the nation's outstanding female athlete, the 1961 Christopher Columbus Award by the Italian press as the most outstanding international athlete, and the 1960 *Los Angeles Times* Award for Women's Track and Field. In 1961, she received the James E. Sullivan Award as the nation's top amateur athlete. The AAU named Rudolph an All-America in track and field in 1956, 1957, 1959, 1960, 1961, and 1962. Rudolph was elected to the Black Sports Hall of Fame in 1973, the National Track and Field Hall of Fame in 1974, the International Women's Sport Hall of Fame in 1980, the U.S. Olympic Hall of Fame in 1983, and the National Women's Hall of Fame in 1984.

In May 1963, Rudolph graduated from Tennessee State University with a B.A. degree in elementary education and minor in psychology. Despite her track and field success, she shifted jobs quite often. Rudolph returned to Clarksville to teach at Cobb Elementary School and coach track and field at Burt High School. She later directed a community center in Evansville, Indiana, and worked for the Job Corps in Poland Spring, Maine. Rudolph joined Operation Champion, a program making professional training available to star athletes from the ghettos. Her other positions included working for the Watts Community Action Committee in Los Angeles, being assistant director for Mayor Richard Daley's Youth Foundation in Chicago, coaching women's track and field and being special consultant for minority affairs at DePauw University in Greencastle, Indiana, and becoming a vice president of Baptist Hospital in Nashville.[41]

New American Library published Rudolph's autobiography, *Wilma: The Story of Wilma Rudolph,* in 1977. NBC made her story into a television movie starring Cicely Tyson. The book and movie inspired handicapped youths who otherwise might never have worked to overcome their physical problems.

The Wilma Rudolph Foundation, a nonprofit community-based amateur sports program organization based in Indianapolis, offered free coaching, academic assistance, and support for disadvantaged children. Rudolph, who considered the foundation her legacy, loved working with children. "It's the motherly instinct in me," she said. Rudolph served as a motivational speaker for American youth, stressing the importance of being oneself and having self-confidence. She considered her greatest achievement "knowing that I have tried to give something to young people" and observed, "It's a good feeling to know that you have touched the lives of so many young people."[42]

In July 1993, President Bill Clinton honored Rudolph, Arnold Palmer, Kareem Abdul-Jabbar, Muhammad Ali, and Ted Williams as "The Great Ones" at the first National Sports Awards. ESPN ranked Rudolph forty-first on its list of the twentieth century's greatest athletes and her amazing triple win at the 1960 Summer Olympic Games as the century's second most important event in women's sports.[43]

Rudolph died on November 12, 1994, at her Brentwood, Tennessee, home after battling a brain tumor and lung cancer. She grew up with a medical disability in extreme poverty in a racially oppressive environment and inspired many others by overcoming these obstacles to become the fastest woman runner in the world. Rudolph believed in herself and her abilities, denying that the phrase, "I can't," ever applied to her. Always quiet, reserved, dignified, friendly, and humble, Rudolph rose from physical disability to Olympic glory through the efforts of her devoted family and her own firm determination to strengthen her body. She insisted, "The triumph cannot be had without the struggle. And I know what struggle is."[44]

Historian Maureen Smith reflected, "Wilma Rudolph's story is more than the races she won and world records she established." She overcame numerous medical obstacles to become "the epitome of triumph" at "a time period that did not

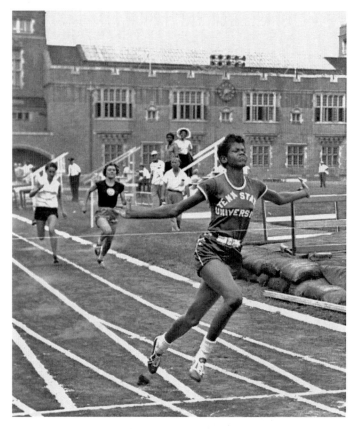

celebrate African American women, in athletics and in American society." Rudolph paved the way for numerous African American track stars, including Edith McGuire, Wyomia Tyus, Evelyn Ashford, Valerie Brisco-Hooks, Florence Griffith-Joyner, Jackie Joyner-Kersee, Gail Devers, Gwen Torrence, and Marion Jones. In 1989, she observed, "For the first time, I'm beginning to see that young black women are making a large contribution in sports." Rudolph concluded, "And that makes me very happy."[45]

**Wilma Rudolph of Tennessee State University is shown here crossing the finish line in a sprint, circa 1959 or 1960, at Franklin Field on the University of Pennsylvania campus in Philadelphia, site of the Penn Relays (courtesy Tennessee State University Sports Information; Charles L. Blockson Afro-American Collection, Temple University).**

# *Childhood Illnesses*

## SCOTT HAMILTON

"I can do this. I can skate,"[1] beamed Scott Hamilton, who was fortunate to be alive. Doctors diagnosed him with Schwachmann-Diamond syndrome, a partial paralysis of his intestinal tract. Hamilton, who exhibited remarkable athleticism, amazingly became a premier figure skater in the 1980s, helping the American men soar to heights not reached in over two decades.

Hamilton grew up in a very caring, relatively affluent family. Scott Scovell Hamilton, who was born on August 28, 1958, in Toledo, Ohio, was adopted six weeks after his birth by Ernest and Dorothy Hamilton, Bowling Green State University professors of biology and family relations, respectively. His father recollected, "Everything went beautifully with Scotty until he was two years old." Hamilton then contracted a mysterious disease and suddenly stopped growing. Tests indicated that he suffered from malnutrition because his body was not digesting and absorbing food properly. One doctor misdiagnosed his problem as celiac disease, an inability to tolerate certain basic foods. For one year, Hamilton was put on a gluten- and milk-free diet. "But all that did, in effect, was to starve the poor little kid," his father recalled. Although largely bedridden for several years, Hamilton "never really felt sick," but "just felt short."[2]

Throughout his childhood, Hamilton visited clinics and children's medical centers frequently as doctors prescribed various unsuccessful treatments and special diets. The hospitalizations and physician visits did not illuminate why he was struggling. in 1966, doctors misdiagnosed his illness as cystic fibrosis because of one recessive gene and gave him just six months to live. "We grew more and more desperate,"[3] his father revealed.

Hamilton's parents took him to see specialists at Children's Hospital in Boston. Physicians correctly attributed his condition to a rare incurable malady, Schwachman-Diamond syndrome, a paralysis of two-thirds of his intestinal tract complicated by severe respiratory problems. This pancreatic disorder interfered with his food digestion, made him unable to absorb nutrients, and stunted his growth to five foot three inches. The hospital prescribed a vitamin-enriched, high-protein diet plan and moderate exercise program.

Hamilton returned home to Bowling Green, where his condition stabilized within a few months. Eight-year-old Hamilton was "terribly frail, his growth forever stunted." He accompanied his older sister, Susan, to watch an ice skating event, still with a feeding tube extending from his nose to his stomach, and astonished his father by remarking, "I'd like to try skating."[4]

Hamilton began figure skating at a relatively late age ten. "He loved it, and he went at it with a vengeance." From the outset, Hamilton skated with confidence and unusual speed and progressed rapidly, demonstrating natural ability. He took skating lessons and entered local and regional sub-juvenile competitions within six months. Although short and underweight, Hamilton felt equal to everyone else for the first time in his life because "I didn't have far to fall." His illness disappeared within a year. Hamilton soon grew and gained weight, although he remained considerably smaller than his peers. Doctors were amazed with his miraculous recovery and attributed it to the beneficial effects of intense physical activity and the coolness of the rink. "The more I gave to skating," Hamilton sensed, "the more it gave back in the form of emotional and physical strength."[5]

From the outset, Hamilton was primarily attracted to two aspects of figure skating, namely, the athleticism necessary for speed and jumps and the art of entertaining an audience. But he also needed to perfect the technique of inscribing figures in the ice, patterns used to demonstrate the skater's control, position, and balance.

Rita Lowery served as Hamilton's first skating coach in 1968 and 1969, giving him four skating lessons a week, split between freestyle and school figures. Hamilton found the compulsory figures, which comprised a majority of the scoring and required enormous patience and discipline, very tedious, boring, and the biggest obstacle to his success. "All I wanted to do was fly across the ice," he explained. After winning the Tri-State Free Skating Competition in Port Huron, Michigan, in the spring of 1969, he beamed, "I was ecstatic." A month later, the *Bowling Green Sentinel-Tribune* ran a nationally syndicated story headlined, "Boy Beats Death Prediction, Skating Uplifts Life of Miracle Child."[6]

At age 13 in the summer of 1972, Hamilton left Bowling Green to train with Pierre Brunet, former Olympic gold medalist and school figures specialist, in Rockton, Illinois. According to Hamilton, skating became "the centerpiece of my life." Although showing promise as a skater, Hamilton lacked motivation and self-discipline. Despite having enormous ambition, he approached his training regimen lackadaisically and performed more perfunctory in competitions. "The off-ice stuff was more important than on-ice things,"[7] he admitted.

Hamilton, meanwhile, attended Bowling Green High School and two other high schools his senior year, receiving sporadic education in between training, competing, and touring. His parents, meanwhile, were struggling financially, as his mother underwent a radical mastectomy for breast cancer and could not work. "More than half of my father's $16,000 salary," Hamilton noted, "was eaten up on my skating bills."[8] His mother wanted him to skate for just one more year. Hamilton ranked seventh among juniors and needed to improve markedly before competing at the senior level. "I actually skated with a sense of urgency," he acknowledged. Hamilton noted, "My intensity and desire doubled."[9] He won the junior title at the 1975 nationals in Colorado Springs, converting a triple Salchow and both double Axels.

Following high school, Hamilton briefly quit skating and arranged to attend Bowling Green State University. The family mortgaged their large house. Frank McLoraine, a wealthy Chicago attorney, and Helen McLoraine, an investor, miraculously volunteered to sponsor Hamilton as a potential Olympic athlete so that he could train under school figure specialist Carlo Fassi at the Colorado Ice Arena in Denver. Hamilton's parents had discussed his skating potential and their financial situation with the McLoraines in Chicago. The McLoraines agreed to defray Hamilton's training expenses, including the coaches' fees. "Mom felt she was living on borrowed time," Hamilton recalled, and wanted him to have the best skating training available. She surmised, "The combination of the McLoraines, who she grew to love, and Carlo, who had a great track record, was unbeatable."[10] The McLoraines became "a second set of parents" for Hamilton and wanted him to develop his skating, character, and responsibility.

Fassi gave Hamilton a true understanding of compulsory school figures. Hamilton traced figures very intricately.[11] Fassi's wife, Christa, was Hamilton's choreographer. After finishing first in the U.S. Men's Junior Figure Skating Championships, Hamilton qualified for senior competition in May 1976. He placed a disappointing ninth in the men's singles, however, at the 1977 U.S. National Figure Skating Championships in Hartford, Connecticut.

His mother's declining health influenced him to pursue skating career full time. Although Dorothy's melanoma was spreading, she gave him unstinting emotional support. Her death on May 18, 1977, dealt him a severe personal setback and profoundly affected his sense of purpose and his attitude toward skating. Hamilton experienced remorse for not having given his best in return for her personal sacrifices. "Everything I do is pretty much for my mom," he wrote. "She gave and gave and gave and sacrificed and sacrificed and really I gave nothing in return."[12]

Hamilton developed an obsession to skate well and become a world-class figure skater. During the next several years, his renewed dedication paid dividends with steadily improving national rankings. In 1978, with newfound inner strength and a technical breakthrough triple Lutz-double toe combination, he placed third in the men's singles competition at the U.S. Figure Skating Championships and a respectable eleventh in his first World Figure Skating Championships. The following year, he finished fourth at the U.S. Figure Skating Championships.

The senior level demanded greater commitment. Hamilton ranked ninth and needed to leap at least six spots to make the world team, which would represent the United States at the 1980 Winter Olympic Games. He promised Fassi to begin attaining his potential.[13] Although Fassi had schooled him well in compulsory figures, Hamilton needed help with his free skating. He had perfected a triple Salchow and triple toe loop, but needed another triple jump and greater consistency. Fassi sent him to Hamilton, Ontario, to train with coach Ronnie Shavers and choreographer Neil Carpenter. Hamilton worked very hard that summer, vowing to make the world team.

In August 1979, Hamilton trained under free skating specialist Don Laws at Lake Placid, New York. Laws worked Hamilton into even better shape and built his confidence. Hamilton attempted to become the first American to perform a triple Lutz in the short program at the Midwestern Figure Skating Championships in Chicago. Charlie Tickner, Scott Cramer, and David Santee, the three world team members from the previous year, competed against him. Hamilton's turning point came there. "I had the short program of my life," Hamilton beamed, landing a revolutionary Triple Lutz combined with a double toe. The short program enabled him to finish third behind Tickner and Santee. "Suddenly, I had the arsenal to compete with the best skaters in the country," he explained.

Hamilton performed well at the international Norton Skate Championships at Lake Placid in September 1979. "All those ghosts and setbacks from my past seemed to vanish," he observed. After finishing fourth in the figures, Hamilton won the short program with this triple Salchow, double loop combination. He converted a triple Lutz, three triple toe loops, and three triple Salchows to defeat Cramer and realized, "The spot on the Olympic team was now mine to lose."[14]

In a close contest at the 1980 U.S. Figure Skating Championships in Atlanta, Hamilton finished third in both the short and long programs to make the world team and U.S. Olympic figure skating team. One international figure skating judge, however, warned that Hamilton had no chance to succeed because his 5-foot 3-inch, 115-pound frame was not big enough to impress the judges on the ice.

In recognition of Hamilton's perseverance and ability to overcome seemingly insurmountable obstacles, the U.S. team captains selected him to carry the U.S. flag and lead the entire team into the arena in the opening day Olympic ceremonies at Lake Placid. According to Hamilton, others noted, "I had overcome terrible obstacles, sickness and all, and that my mother had died at a crucial point in my career, and that I was the smallest male Olympian there." An ecstatic Hamilton felt "ten feet tall." He deemed carrying the American flag "one of the big moments of my life."[15]

At the 1980 Olympic Games, Hamilton finished eighth in the figures, fourth in the short and long programs and fifth overall, drawing a standing ovation from the audience. The thunderous applause even prevented him from hearing his music. His Olympic performance started "his scramble to the top."[16] Gold medal winner Robin Cousins predicted Hamilton would win the next Olympic championship. Hamilton finished fifth in the men's singles at the 1980 World Figure Skating Championships at Dortmund, West Germany.

Between 1981 and 1984, Hamilton did not lose a major national or international competition. In 1981, he easily won the men's singles at the U.S. Figure Skating Championships at San Diego with a program that included challenging jumps and intricate footwork and spins. Hamilton even earned two perfect sixes in an artistic phase of the long program. "It's the best week I've ever had," he beamed.

At the World Figure Skating Championships in Hartford, Connecticut, in March, Hamilton stood third in the men's singles entering the free skating portion. After opening the program with a spectacular triple Lutz, he performed his difficult routine with dazzling flair. Hamilton recollected, "When I hit my last triple Salchow, I felt I had the title." He overtook arch-rival Santee of the United States to win his first world men's senior singles championship. His outstanding freestyle skating made the difference.[17] Hamilton became only the second American to capture the men's crown since 1970.

In 1981, Hamilton also earned an individual gold medal at the first annual Skate America international tournament, sponsored by the U.S. Figure Skating Association. The U.S. Olympic Committee named him Male Athlete of the Year.

Hamilton, over the next three years, practiced hours daily six days a week under Laws at the Colorado Ice Arena in Denver. His grueling training regimen also included regular workouts at a local gym. Hamilton devised original skating programs, too, collaborating with dancer Ricky Harris on a taxing, engagingly whimsical routine set to a medley of big band–era songs. "Skating is the only sport in which your individual personality can come out," Hamilton acknowledged. "It involves how you display yourself and how you impress an audience."[18]

Between 1982 and 1984, Hamilton maintained both the men's senior national and world singles championship titles despite challenges from other superior technicians. In the 1982 U.S. Figure Skating Championships at Indianapolis, Hamilton performed brilliantly in the long program. "With the crowd going nuts," he converted five triples and four double Axels. Legendary skater Dick Button lauded Hamilton's performance as the best of his career. Hamilton impressed judges and dazzled audiences with his very creative, daring free-skating programs. In the 1982 World Figure Skating Championships at Copenhagen, Denmark, Hamilton lacked his usual energy and speed, and yet converted six triples to defend his title. Norbert Schramm of West Germany finished second.

Hamilton won the men's singles at the 1983 U.S. Figure Skating Championships in Cleveland, completing five triples. Hamilton's flair for comedy emerged in his mimicking of a waltz, an innovative, risky routine that captivated both judges and audience. "It was just the kind of decisive victory I needed going into the worlds,"[19] he recollected. Brian Boitano, a wonderful jumper, finished second.

In the 1983 World Figure Skating Championships at Helsinki, Finland, Hamilton skated brilliantly in the long program and easily outpointed Schramm and Brian Orser of Canada with his explosive free-skating. Hamilton gave the competition "special fire" as "the sport's only all-around performer, equally good at athleticism and artistry." The dedicated, athletic Hamilton "brought down the house" in his four-minute performance. He made six triple jumps, including a triple Lutz-triple toe loop combination, "almost spinning himself out of the rink on one," mixed with "some heavy loops and swirls."[20] His virtually flawless execution drew 5.8s and 5.9s, nearly perfect scores from the judges.

Hamilton became the first American men's champion to win three consecutive world titles since David Jenkins from 1957 to 1959 and the first to take three straight world crowns since Ondrej Nepela in 1973. He wore a sleek, form-fitting one-piece suit similar to those worn by speed skaters, discarding the ballet-like skating outfits traditionally worn by male skaters. The innovation was his attempt to change the image of the male skater. Skaters overemphasized ballet, he contended. "Too much artistry by graceful men in jeweled costumes."[21] The three-time world champion stressed the prescribed stunts and technical figures over artistic elements in his free-skating routines.

Hamilton redirected the sport from fashion to athleticism. "Most sports depend on athletic performance, instead of how you look," he observed. "I consider myself an athlete and I want people to look at me and my sport that way." Hamilton crusaded "to bring an aura of masculinity to the sport." His skating demonstrated this "with an almost pugnacious, watch-this-you-guys flair to it."[22]

With Laws, Hamilton developed a new routine exploiting his strengths, speed, and footwork. He termed the program "the Wow-Wow-Wow theory of audience and judge grabbing." The routine showcased the power of his jumps, blinding speed of his spins, and intricacy of his straight-line footwork. He began with technical moves to demonstrate his proficiency, performed dramatic moves to win audience approval, and lastly put the audience in a more ominous mood.

Hamilton selected futuristic music of George Duke's "The Guardian," played on synthesizers, for the attention-grabbing opening section of triple jumps and fleet-footed patterns. In the opening section, he completely integrated action, mood, and music. That portion began "with the crackling sounds of a laser battle." Hamilton chose a suspenseful piece, Hiroshima's "Third Generation," for the slower middle section of combinations and spins. He used modern jazz for the spectacular finale of Russian split jumps, double Axels and Salchows, ending in a blurring scratch spin and inspiring a standing ovation. According to Hamilton, the clean, solid program showed both the audience and judges his skating prowess.[23]

Hamilton's strategy entering 1984 was to finish in the top two in the figures and the top three in the short and long programs. At the U.S. Figure Skating Championships in Salt Lake City in January 1984, Hamilton aspired "to deliver the performance of a lifetime" by making "a clean sweep of all the disciplines." He wanted "to send the strong message" to his competitors that he "was the one to beat." Hamilton presented his new free-skating program for the first time there, explaining his program "exploited my strengths — speed, footwork, a big opening triple Lutz and an athletic resolution." His program "worked to perfection in Salt Lake."[24]

At the Salt Palace Arena, Hamilton "stole the show" with "a rousing long program that brought the crowd to its feet." Hamilton broke a record by being rated first by each of the nine judges in all three school figures, one short program, and one long program, even tallying four perfect sixes for style. No figure had ever received so many perfect marks at the U.S. Figure Skating Championships. "It was a dream nationals, my best ever," Hamilton exulted. "I won every aspect of the competition by every judge." He concluded, "I wanted everyone to know I was ready, in shape and unbeatable." After the U.S. Nationals, *Sports Illustrated* billed Hamilton as "Mr. Gold Medal" and considered him as sure a bet as Secretariat in the Belmont Stakes. Since 1980, Hamilton had won 15 straight championships and was "on an unprecedented roll."[25]

Hamilton's dream of an Olympic gold medal materialized at the 1984 Winter Olympic Games in Sarajevo, Yugoslavia. At the Zetra Ice Arena, Hamilton decisively captured the school figures segment, which accounted for 30 percent of the scoring. All nine judges ranked him first, with the American "painstakingly putting in the bank a big lead that would later pull him through."[26] Orser, his major competitor and Canadian national champion, finished a disappointing seventh in the school figures.

Orser, however, edged Hamilton in the two-minute short program involving seven required elements. The dynamic free skater converted all five triple jumps, recording near perfect scores for technical merit. Six of the nine judges declared Orser the victor in the short program, moving him into fifth place, within "easy striking distance"[27] of Hamilton. An inner ear imbalance and heavy cold hindered Hamilton's performance. Hamilton, who had survived the critical short program, still held a commanding lead entering the long program.

Orser recorded "a knockout" performance in the long four-minute, 30-second program, landing several triples and skating almost flawlessly. He converted five different triple jumps, tallying several 5.9s. For the first time in three years, Hamilton did not win the long program. Sheer athletic stamina helped him complete his long program, which lacked precision because of his illness. Hamilton began his program with a triple Lutz, but did not attempt a triple flip. He planned to make the prescribed five triple jumps, but performed only three. On his final jump, Hamilton executed only a double rather than triple Salchow. He appeared off-balance and the axis on his jumps was tilted. "I couldn't possibly skate any worse than that," he concluded. Hamilton's tentative, uncharacteristically subdued performance brought him the lowest marks for technical merit (5.6 to 5.9) that he had received in several years, but his scores for artistic impression were considerably higher. Hamilton speculated, "There were some lifetime-achievement scores mixed in there."[28] He finished second in the free-skating segment, tallying six 5.9s to Orser's 11.

Although regretting not skating better, Hamilton amassed enough points from the three combined events to fulfill his dream of winning an Olympic gold medal. "Orser had won the evening," but "Hamilton's bank account from the compulsories paid off in gold." Hamilton yelled, "We did it. We won the gold. Life's just wonderful."[29] Orser received the silver medal, while Jozef Sabovtchik of Czechoslovakia took the bronze medal.

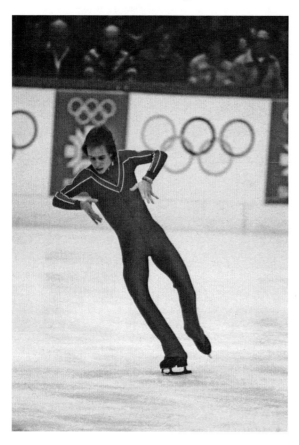

Although not skating his best, Scott Hamilton won the gold medal in men's figure skating on February 16 at the 1984 Winter Olympic Games in Sarajevo, Bosnia, Yugoslavia (courtesy Manny Millan/Icon SMI).

Tears filled Hamilton's eyes during the medal award ceremony. "This is for you, Mom," Hamilton mouthed on the medals' stand. "The medal was definitely hers as much as mine," he insisted. "She kept the faith when I was a sick little boy and doctors were telling her I had only a year to live," he recalled. His parents had sacrificed financially to let him continue skating. The victory proved even sweeter because Hamilton had finished ninth the last time she had seen him skate. Hamilton, carrying a large American flag to thank the American public, took two victory laps around the arena to thunderous applause. His gold medal in men's figure skating was the first for an American since David Jenkins in 1960. "I had passed my biggest and most important test of all,"[30] he beamed.

At a press conference, Hamilton admitted, "They didn't see me at my best today, but they saw the best I had in me." The three-time world champion, nevertheless, had soldiered on "with as much brio as he could muster under difficult circumstances." He disclosed having taken antibiotics for a persistent ear infection that upset his balance. Hamilton made no excuses for his below-average performance. "I felt like I was skating with twenty-pound weights on my shoulders," he reflected. He had still made that night "the most memorable program of my life."[31]

Hamilton brilliantly defended his singles title at the World Figure Skating Championships in Ottawa in March 1984. He led after the figures portion and took revenge against Orser by winning the short program. Orser, however, won the long program again. Hamilton left Canada a four-time world champion, with Orser finishing second. After winning his seventeenth consecutive amateur competition, he acknowledged, "This is the career achievement I'm most proud of."[32] His last amateur performance came at the International Stars on Ice show in Bowling Green, Ohio, where he had started skating 16 years earlier. Shortly afterward, he retired as an amateur skater.

The major ice shows gave Hamilton lucrative financial offers. Hamilton began skating professionally with the Ice Capades in August 1984, performing twice each show. He missed the

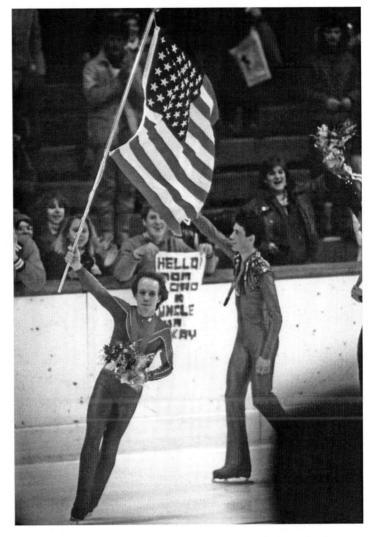

Scott Hamilton carried the American flag around the rink after winning the gold medal for men's figure skating at the 1984 Winter Olympic Games in Sarajevo. Brian Orser, the silver medalist, skates behind him (courtesy Manny Millan/Icon SMI).

amateur competitions and the sense of achievement that comes with a victory, but enjoyed skating before enthusiastic, sell-out crowds. "It's not the same high-high," Hamilton noted. "You like being in front of them, and you like showing off and you like the applause." Two years later, he co-founded, co-produced, and performed in Scott Hamilton's American Tour. This highly successful traveling company was later renamed the Stars on Ice Tour.[33] Hamilton also competed in World Professional Championships and became a figure skating analyst for CBS and NBC television.

Hamilton, meanwhile, received widespread recognition for his achievements.

The Philadelphia Sports Writers Association gave him the 1984 Most Courageous Athlete Award. In 1988, he became the first male figure skater recipient of the Jacques Favert Award. The U.S. Olympic Hall of Fame and the World Skating Hall of Fame enshrined him in 1990. Six years later, the U.S. Sports Academy named him the Mildred "Babe" Didrikson Zaharias Courage Award recipient for demonstrating courage, perseverance, grace, and strength in overcoming adversity to excel in sports.

In March 1997, doctors diagnosed Hamilton with cancer during his Stars on Ice Tour. Several months of abdominal pain had convinced him to seek medical advice. A CT scan revealed a large very large tumor, caused by testicular cancer, had spread to Hamilton's abdomen. Hamilton underwent a rigorous combination treatment of chemotherapy and surgery. Several months of chemotherapy shrank his tumor from the size of two grapefruits to that of a golf ball, whereupon in late June it was removed surgically, with one of Hamilton's testicles. The cancer went into remission. Hamilton vividly recounted his remarkable life story and battle with cancer in *Landing It: My Own Life On and Off the Ice* (1999). In March 2010, the BIO Channel premiered *Scott Hamilton: Return to the Ice*, a two-hour special chronicling his skating comeback after battling cancer.[34]

Hamilton, who began feeling more like himself again, resumed training in August 1997 and returned to rehearsals for the Stars on Ice Tour. He started promoting early cancer detection, performing in a *Back on the Ice* CBS television skating special with several other stars in Los Angeles in late October 1997 to raise money for the new Taussig Cancer Center in Cleveland. The center advocates public education about cancer prevention, chemotherapy, and survival coping skills. His physical endurance increased substantially by the time the Stars on Ice Tour resumed after Christmas. After converting every jump at the Anaheim Pond in January, Hamilton beamed, "My confidence was restored."[35] In February 1998, he served as figure skating analyst for the Nagano, Japan, Winter Olympic Games on CBS. Hamilton skated to fund ongoing cancer research and a program to support patients and their families. In 2001, he retired from the popular Stars on Ice Tour.

Hamilton married Tracie Robinson, a nutritionist, on November 14, 2002. They have two sons, Aidan and Maxx, and reside in Franklin, Tennessee.

Hamilton in 2008 co-authored with Ken Baker another book, *The Great Eight*, in which he relates how skating taught him happiness, and shared eight secrets that he practiced daily "with repetition, focus, and discipline" to help him overcome numerous challenges and disappointments. His recipes for success include not giving up when things get hard, trusting in God, moving forward when you are discouraged, having "open, honest communication" about those things that bother you, thinking positive when negative situations arise, putting others before yourself, and trying new things and making changes in your life.[36]

Hamilton has experienced additional bouts with cancer. In November 2004, he was diagnosed with benign brain cancer and was treated at the Cleveland Clinic.

Surgeons in June 2010 took out a benign brain tumor, which would have caused him blindness if left untreated. Hamilton was hospitalized that November to stop the bleeding in an artery that had been nicked during the removal of his brain tumor. Doctors stemmed the bleeding, but operated on an aneurysm that developed a few days later.

Throughout his skating career, the charismatic, energetic Hamilton overcame formidable challenges. He compensated for his small stature by developing impressive jumping techniques, extended lines, intricate footwork, and the ability to entertain audiences. Hamilton attributed some success to his small size. "My size is perfect for skating. I have a lower center of balance. I don't have

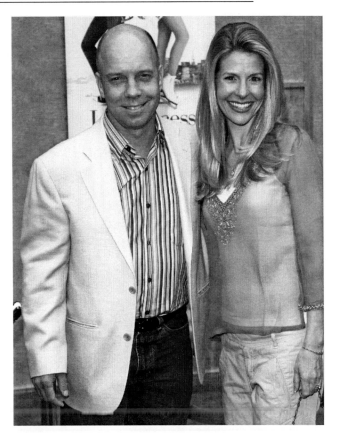

Scott Hamilton and his wife, Tracie Robinson, attended the Hollywood premier of Walt Disney Pictures' *Ice Princess* at the El Capitan Theater in Los Angeles on March 13, 2005 (courtesy Featureflash/Shutterstock.com).

as much body to adjust when I make a mistake, and not as much body to get tired."[37] Hamilton's self-deprecating sense of humor and friendly, easygoing manner made him the most popular figure skating champion in decades.

Hamilton's eight consecutive national and world titles assured his place as the preeminent international figure skater of the early 1980s. Hamilton changed the nature of figure skating. Throughout the 1970s, balletic performers John Curry and Robin Cousins dominated men's figure skating. Hamilton viewed figure skating as a sport rather than an art form. The fragile-looking skater created surprisingly athletic free-skating routines in an energetic style that won over judges and audiences alike. He also extended the dimensions of ice entertainment as cofounder, performer, and producer of the Stars on Ice Tour. His enthusiasm for figure skating, his generosity to younger skaters, and his personal hardships made him a beloved figure. Through grappling with a devastating disease and aiding others similarly affected, he seized a seemingly insurmountable obstacle as an opportunity for positive gain.

# Bobby Jones

"When a person is that ill, it tends to breed in them a kind of inner toughness and scrappiness" summarizes the inspirational story of Bobby Jones. Jones contracted a gastrointestinal digestive ailment that doctors believed would kill him before he was fully grown. The frail, awkward Jones developed into the greatest amateur golfer ever and the only golfer to capture all four major tournaments in the same year.

Jones, unlike most athletes in this book, came from an elite background. Robert Tyre Jones Jr. was born on March 17, 1902, in Atlanta, and grew up in privileged circumstances. His father, Robert Sr., starred in baseball at the University of Georgia before becoming a prominent Atlanta attorney, while his mother, Clara, was a homemaker. The Joneses' first child, William, had died in 1901 after three agonizing months of illness, devastating them.

Jones's early life involved a battle for survival. Doctors wondered whether Jones would live beyond infancy. Jones was very frail with a severe digestive ailment until age five. Jones recalled having "a spindling body," weighing slightly over five pounds at birth and suffered lengthy "operatic fits of colic." The digestive problem greatly distressed his parents and doctors. The perplexed doctors prescribed "a strict diet of boiled egg whites," pablum, and black-eyed peas. "I didn't eat any real food," Jones recollected, "until I was five years old."[1]

Jones, whose medical condition was exacerbated by his mother's worry, weighed under 40 pounds at age five. Mark Frost, his biographer, wrote, "Clara's heightened anxiety about her lost first child played a major part in shaping and disrupting the nervous system of her second; his elusive and fragile 'condition' might have been a self-fulfilling projection of his mother's hyperactive concerns for him." Jones's frailty convinced his parents to have no more children. Since "childhood diseases were a deadly threat, Clara kept the boy cloistered in their home, a virtual prisoner to her fears."[2] Until age five, Jones seemed the least likely candidate for competitive athletics. Sportswriter O.B. Keeler observed, however, "Some hardy inherent fighting quality in the frail little chap asserted itself," because he soon "was eating everything he could bite."[3] The battle for survival made Jones a perfectionist.

In the summer of 1907, his parents rented rooms in the home of Mrs. Frank Meador in exclusive East Lake, near East Lake Golf Course. They hoped the fresh air and exercise would strengthen him physically, and they began taking golf lessons with club professional Stewart Maiden. Jones began golfing with a discarded, badly nicked old cleek on a course he and playmate Frank Meador built on a dirt lane beside the Meador house. Since they were not old enough to go on the East Lake Course, they peered through the course gate to watch the golfers perform.[4] By the next summer, Jones trailed his parents around the golf course carrying one club.

Jones quickly demonstrated an extraordinary golf talent. He learned the game by watching and imitating Maiden's classic swing and style and seeking his advice. Jones idolized the Scotsman and "tagged him all over the links." Maiden, "a good role model," utilized a simple swing.[5] After following Maiden for several holes, Jones ran to the thirteenth green near the clubhouse and practiced with mashie and putter. In 1908 at age 6, Jones captured a six-hole tournament, defeating Perry Adair and Alexa Stirling. The following year, he bested Adair in a 36-hole contest. In 1912, Jones captured his first formal tournament, the AAC's Junior Championship. He shot an 80 for 18 holes at age 11 at East Lake. He rushed to the fourteenth green to show the card to his very proud father, who "with wet eyes, hugged his son like no other." Golf became more serious than just a game to Jones, who initially confronted "that invisible opponent, 'Old Man Par.'"[6]

Several tournament victories soon followed. In 1915, Jones won the Druid Club Championship with a course record 73 and his initial gold medal. Keeler observed, "He wants to be perfect — stone dead." Linkster Jim Barnes predicted, "This kid will be one of the world's greatest golfers." That August, Jones astounded the golf world winning the Georgia State Amateur title at the Capital Country Club in Atlanta. He changed his attitude completely, growing more confident in himself and his game. Jones said, "I began to play hard aggressive golf,"[7] striking the ball forcefully. In June 1917, the 5-foot 4-inch, 165-pounder became the youngest Southern Amateur tournament winner at the Roebuck Springs Country Club in Birmingham. He already had developed a strong chunky body, powerful wrists, chest, and shoulders.

At age 14 in 1916, Jones became the youngest golfer ever to enter a major tournament. The "'new kid from Dixie' became an overnight sensation" in the medal-qualifying rounds in his first U.S. Amateur Championship at the Merion Cricket Club in Haverford, Pennsylvania. Jones burst on the national golfing scene, leading the entire field in the morning qualifying round with a 74, and was suddenly "cast in the limelight." The Georgian defeated 1906 champion Eben Byers in the first round and rallied to best reigning Pennsylvania state champion Frank Dyer in the second round. He led defending national champion Robert Gardner in the third round before succumbing to pressure, five and three. Gardner made miraculous recoveries on the sixth, seventh, and eighth holes, deflating Jones's spirit. "I wanted to go off and pout," Jones admitted. "I didn't half try on any shot thereafter."[8] Jones, nevertheless, quickly attracted international fame as the nation's child golf prodigy.

Jones experienced "seven lean years," being winless in 11 U.S. Amateur and U.S. Open Championships from 1916 through 1922. The Georgian considered those years a valuable learning experience, claiming they "didn't seem so lean and prepared him for the subsequent 'fat years.'" He told Keeler, "I must play every shot for all that is in it." Although cool and calculating, he seethed inside. Jones pressured himself too much with his perfectionist attitude and struggled controlling his temper. Bernard Darwin wrote, Jones "set himself an impossibly high standard," regarding it "an act of incredible folly" to "make a stroke that is not exactly as it ought to be made."[9] It took Jones another seven years to "detach himself from playing against an opponent, think only of the job in hand, play the best he could, and leave the rest to Fate." Jones needed to understand that "matching shots with the most debonair of human adversaries is at the best a feeble and uncertain pattern, compared with the iron certitudes of 'Old Man Par.'"[10] Major tournaments proved so stressful that Jones could not eat properly, would lose several pounds, and chain smoked.

Jones ended runner-up in major tournaments more often than other contemporary golfers. He finished second to S. Davidson Herron in the 1919 U.S. Amateur at Oakmont, Pennsylvania. Jones also placed second in the 1919 Canadian Open and won the 1920 Southern Amateur. "Defeat will make him great," Barnes predicted. "He has to be perfect."[11] Jones, who often golfed 18 holes in under three hours, steadily gained experience, physical strength, and emotional maturity.

The nadir of his career came in the 1921 British Open in St. Andrews, Scotland. He led after two rounds, but shot an uncharacteristic 46 for the first nine holes of the third round. After recording a six on the tenth hole, he drove his tee shot on the eleventh hole into the bunker. Following several futile attempts to blast the ball out, he put the ball in his pocket, tore his scorecard to shreds, and left the course. The tournament withdrawal signified "the most inglorious failure" of his golfing career. Jones resolved "never again to breach the highest ethics of sportsmanship."[12]

After capturing the 1922 Southern Amateur, Jones finished a single stroke behind Gene Sarazen at the 1922 U.S. Open Championship in Chicago and lost badly to Jess Sweetser in the 1922 U.S. Amateur at Brookline, Massachusetts. The Georgian did not believe that he could become a champion. According to Jones, "Tournament golf only began to gall when anything but an outright win looked like failure to me, and to everyone else."[13]

During this phase, education supplanted golf. Despite his golf achievements, Jones considered the sport a game played only three months a year and concentrated on furthering his education. An outstanding student, he graduated from Tech High School at age 16 in 1918. After earning bachelor's degrees in engineering from Georgia Institute of Technology in 1922 and in English literature from Harvard University in 1924, he attended Emory University Law School in Atlanta for one year, passed the state bar in 1928, and joined his father's law firm. He married childhood sweetheart Mary Malone on June 17, 1924, and had three children, Clara, Robert III, and Mary Ellen.

Jones gradually conquered his temper by learning to accept imperfect shots, allowing his great talent to blossom. He never won major tournaments until controlling his temper. Friends, admirers, and sportswriters still pressured him enormously, terming him "as good a golfer as anybody else" and "perhaps the best shotmaker among the amateurs."[14]

Before 1923, Jones performed better in stroke competition than at match play. He began winning match-play competition when he vowed to forget about his opponent and play for pars. Keeler advised Jones in match play to compete against "Old Man Par" and concentrate on scores, signifying "complete detachment from surrounding circumstances to produce a fine round of golf."[15]

Jones usually competed only in major championships. He improved his game dramatically between 1923 and 1930, capturing 13 of 21 majors and finishing second four times, including two playoff losses. His first major title came at age 21 in the 1923 U.S. Open Championship at the Innwood Course in Long Island. Jones led by three strokes after three rounds, but struggled with two bogeys and a double bogey on the last few holes. "I had the championship in my pocket and chucked it away,"[16] he moaned. Bobby Cruickshank trailed by one stroke entering the eighteenth hole, but finished with a magnificent birdie to tie.

Jones told Keeler, "I'm no champion. Anybody who finished like I did can't hope to be a champion. I'm a dirty yellow dog." Keeler replied, "You are a dirty dog only if you think you are." Jones learned "the secret of winning championships," realizing he needed to beat himself, not Cruickshank. With new resolve, Jones captured an exciting 18-hole playoff with Cruickshank by two strokes. He led Cruickshank by one stroke entering the final playoff hole. Jones gambled with a courageous shot over the lagoon guarding the front of the green. The ball landed just seven feet from the hole,[17] ensuring his victory.

Jones compiled a phenomenal record in the subsequent "eight fat years," capturing at least one major championship annually from 1923 through 1930. He became the first and only golfer to win the U.S. Amateur tournament five times. Jones competed in eight U.S. Amateur Championships, prevailing in 1924, 1925, 1927, 1928, and 1930 and being edged in 1926. He defeated George von Elm resoundingly, 9 and 8, to take the 1924 U.S. Amateur at Ardmore, Pennsylvania, and captured the 1925 U.S. Amateur at Oakmont, Pennsylvania. Johnny Goodman upset him in the first round of the 1929 U.S. Amateur at Pebble Beach, California, stunning the golf world.[18] Atlantan James J. Haverty attributed Jones's victories "to a high order of mental capacity, concentration and self-control, supported by youthful enthusiasm, great determination, superb ambition, and modesty of demeanor." He called Jones "the greatest golfer in the world, because of his antecedents, his blood, and his youthful, praiseworthy ambition."

Jones enjoyed tremendous success against professionals, dominating the U.S. Open tournament for nearly a decade. He competed in 11 U.S. Opens from 1920 through 1930, winning in 1923, 1926, 1929, and 1930, finishing second four times, and missing the top ten only in 1927. Jones lost two U.S. Open playoffs, including the 1925 to Willie MacFarlane in Worcester, Massachusetts. At the eleventh hole in the first round, his ball accidentally moved when he addressed it. He assessed himself a penalty stroke over the objection of United States Golf Association (USGA) officials, insisting, "There is only one way to play this game."[19]

Jones won the British Amateur in 1930 and the British Opens in 1926, 1927, and

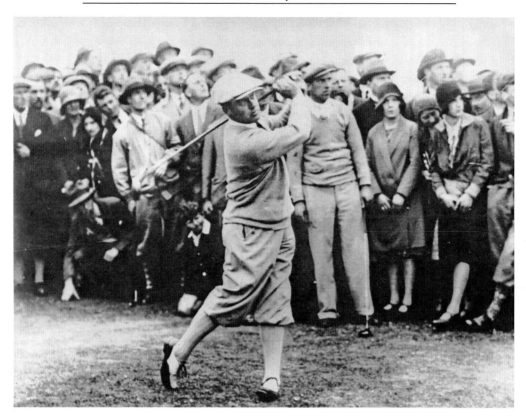

Bobby Jones, shown here teeing off at a major golf tournament circa 1930, set a record by winning 13 major tournaments, including five U.S. Amateurs, four U.S. Opens, three British Opens, and one British Amateur, between 1923 and 1930 (courtesy Kenan Research Center at the Atlanta History Center).

1930. In his last 11 British and U.S. Opens during this span, he triumphed seven times and finished second four times.

Jones's 1926 U.S. and British Open victories made him the first golfer to attain both feats in the same year and unquestionably the world's top golfer. The Georgian shot a record 66 in the qualifying round of the 1926 British Open near London and edged Al Watrous by one stroke, becoming the first amateur to take the title since Harold Hilton in 1892. He made the best iron shot of his career on the seventeenth hole in the final round. Watrous already had landed his second shot on the green. Jones's 175-foot shot landed inside Watrous's ball. Watrous, who three-putted the hole, "essentially handed the trophy to Bob on that definitive hole."[20] Jones won the 1926 U.S. Open near Columbus, Ohio, birdieing the final hole with a drive measured at 310 yards.

The following year, Jones repeated as the British Open and U.S. Amateur champion. He shot a spectacular 68 in the first round of the British Open, his first round below 70 in a major championship. Jones led throughout the tournament, recording an aggregate score of 285 to prevail by six strokes. "Never before had such a low score been recorded in the national events of either Britain or America." Jones told the crowd afterward that "winning the championship on the Old Course had been the 'ambition of his life.'" He routed Chick Evans, eight and seven, to take the 1927 U.S. Amateur title at Minneapolis. He also played on the triumphant 1926, 1928, and 1930 U.S. Walker Cup teams, captaining the last two squads.

The most dramatic moment for Jones came at the 1929 U.S. Open in Mamaroneck, New York. Jones led entering the final round, but shot a calamitous seven on the eighth hole and struggled thereafter. "The balance of the round was an agony of anxiety," he lamented. After pulling his third shot on the last hole, Jones sank "a villainous, curling, sidehill 12-foot putt"[21] for a par to tie Al Espinosa. Sportswriters lauded Jones's memorable shot, which brought a thunderous roar from the crowd. Keeler claimed if Jones "hadn't sunk that putt, there wouldn't have been any Grand Slam in 1930." Grantland Rice called it "Golf's Greatest Putt." The next day, Jones won the 36-hole playoff with Espinosa by 23 strokes for the title. He performed "the best golf of the tournament,"[22] recording a 72 and 69 for a 141 tally. Espinosa never recovered from shooting a disastrous eight on the eleventh hole the day before.

In March 1930, Jones captured the Southeastern Open at Augusta, Georgia, by a decisive 13 strokes. "I played the best golf I ever played in any tournament," he admitted. At age 28, Jones defied 50-to-1 odds by becoming the only golfer to capture the Grand Slam, winning all four majors in 1930. In one of the supreme twentieth century athletic achievements, he won the British Amateur, British Open, U.S. Open and U.S. Amateur the same year. This feat has never been replicated.

The British Amateur had eluded his grasp. Jones termed the 1930 British Amateur "the most important tournament of his life." The format at the challenging, windy St. Andrews course required eight 18-hole rounds of match play, followed by a 36-hole final. Jones played seven matches, edging defending champion Cyril Tolley, Jimmy Johnston, and George Voigt. The dramatic Tolley match was deadlocked after 18 holes and ended with the Britisher stymied on the first playoff hole. Both players' balls landed on the same side of the nineteenth hole, but Jones's putt completely blocked Tolley's ball. "I felt the same exultation and desperate urgency I should expect to feel in a battle with broadswords or cudgels," the exhausted Jones noted. "The great battle had ended," relieving his "almost unbearable" tension. Darwin recollected, "It was the devil of a match."[23]

The Johnston and Voigt contests were decided by two strokes. Jones lurked "on the verge of defeat three times," but responded each time with "sizzling, sub-par golf." In the Johnston match, he converted "a curling, eight-foot putt" on the final hole. Voigt led Jones by two holes with five remaining, but the Georgian seized the advantage on the final hole. Jones realized, Keeler observed, "At every crisis he stood up to the shot with something I can define only as inevitability and performed what was needed with all the certainty of a natural phenomenon."[24]

Jones defeated Syd Roper, Cowan Shankland, George Watt, and Eric Fiddian in the uneventful 18-hole morning matches. Jones eagled the fourth hole against Roper, converting a dramatic, 140-yard shot. Scotsman Sir James Lieshman noted, "He cannot be beaten here."[25]

Jones's self-confidence built as he held a four-hole advantage over 1923 Amateur champion Roger Wethered in the morning round of the 36-hole final. The match concluded at the twelfth hole in the afternoon round, with Jones prevailing, seven and six. Almost 15,000 witnessed the afternoon match. "I don't think I was ever so happy about any golf event in my life," Jones beamed. He confessed, "I have never worked harder or suffered more in trying to get it." After the British Amateur, Keeler told Jones, "You managed to extract every possible ounce of drama from the performance." Jones countered his concern was "to extricate myself from the many perilous situations I encountered on the way." He sighed, "This championship had taken a big load off my chest."[26]

Jones began brilliantly in the 1930 British Open at Hoylake, shooting rounds of 70 and 72, exhibiting "stolid patience." He shared the lead with Henry Cotton and Macdonald Smith after the first round, tapping in numerous short putts for pars. At the halfway mark, Jones led Fred Robson by one stroke and Smith by three strokes. Archie Compston, who trailed Jones by five strokes, caught the Georgian early in the third round. Jones's five-stroke lead evaporated completely in four holes. Compston shot a 68 to seize a one-stroke advantage in the third round, while Jones struggled with a 74. One British writer observed Compston played "like a frenzied giant."[27] Compston, however, fell out of contention with an 82 on the final round.

Jones, meanwhile, performed better on the first few holes of the final round, but shot a disastrous seven on the eighth hole. "I was in a daze," the badly shaken Georgian recollected. On the sixteenth hole, he hit a spectacular second shot from a bunker that landed just two inches beyond the hole and made a birdie three. Jones recorded a 72 for a 291 overall score, withstanding challenges from Leo Diegel and Smith to capture the British Open by two strokes. His "sheer doggedness" brought victory. According to Jones, "These last two British championships were the hardest ones."[28] New York City welcomed Jones back to the United States with a ticker-tape parade.

Jones's sternest test came in the 1930 U.S. Open at Interlachen in Minneapolis. Walter Hagen, Horton Smith, Harry Cooper, Johnny Farrell, and Tommy Armour contended in what Hagen termed "the greatest field ever assembled on any golf course." The temperatures exceeded 100 degrees during the first round, the warmest Jones could ever remember.[29] He recorded a 71 in that round, trailing Macdonald Smith and Armour by one stroke.

Jones made a legendary "Lily Pond Shot" on the ninth hole of the second round. The green was situated about 30 yards beyond a lake. Jones pushed his tee shot on the right bank of the lake, requiring a hard shot to reach the green. He flinched upon seeing two young girls break as though to run across the fairway and half-topped the ball. The ball skidded across the pond, bounced off a lily pad floating in the lake, and amazingly hopped up short of the green. Jones birdied that hole and shot a 73 for the round, two strokes behind Smith. He denied, however, that "the stroke of luck actually decided the championship," asserting, "My game was coming in at just the right time."[30]

Jones played sensationally through the first 16 holes of the third round and appeared destined for the lowest score ever in a U.S. Open round. "This was the one time that I played at my very best in a championship," he recalled. Although bogeying the final two holes, he still surged ahead with a sizzling 68 for a five-stroke advantage over Cooper. Smith, though, played brilliantly on the first nine holes of the final round to catch Jones. During the last round, Jones double-bogeyed three par-three holes, giving up "six precious strokes." He partially redeemed those lapses, following with birdies on the first and last holes and two birdies on the middle one. The "intensely competitive" Jones seemingly recovered his composure, showing the crowded gallery that he had refused "to accept defeat or disaster." Rice described the Jones-Smith battle as "one of the great epics of golf."[31]

The lead over Smith diminished to one stroke, as Jones bogeyed the seventeenth hole. Jones, who left his tee shot 40 feet below the eighteenth hole, confessed, "I was quivering in every muscle" when preparing to putt. The crowd roared after he miraculously birdied the hole, sinking the 40-foot putt, providing overwhelming melodrama. "The heart that would not break had tipped the clubs with fire."[32] Jones waited in the clubhouse for Smith to finish his round. Smith needed an eagle on the final hole to tie Jones, but parred instead. Jones won that tournament by two strokes over Smith, recording a 287 and becoming the first golfer to capture three majors the same year.

After the U.S. Open, Jones experienced two close calls with death. A lightning bolt struck a big double chimney above his head near the locker room entrance of the East Lake Golf Course. Jones miraculously escaped with a minor shoulder scratch. The second scare occurred while Jones was walking to the Atlanta Athletic Club to deliver a speech. An unoccupied car, parked at the top of a hill near the club, started rolling downhill, jumped a curb, and was headed directly toward Jones. A pedestrian yelled, "Look out, mister." Jones recalled, "I made a broad jump that would have done credit to Jesse Owens." The automobile crossed over the spot where Jones had been and hit the clubhouse wall. "I would have been crushed between the automobile and the building had not the lone pedestrian warned me,"[33] Jones claimed.

The final Grand Slam tournament, the anticlimactic 1930 U.S. Amateur, was held in mid–September at the Merion Cricket Club in Haverford, Pennsylvania, one of Jones's favorite courses. Francis Powers of the *Chicago News* penned, "There goes another race by the Four Horsemen of the Apocalypse over the fairways of Merion, and this time their names are Jones, Jones, Jones, and Jones." Jones stood at "the top of his form now, and nobody could approach him." His toughest match came in the

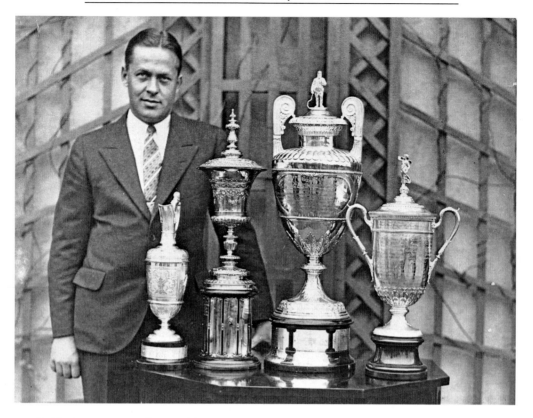

Bobby Jones, pictured here with his 1930 trophies, became the only golfer to ever win the Grand Slam, taking the British Open, the British Amateur, the U.S. Open, and the U.S. Amateur in the same year (courtesy Kenan Research Center at the Atlanta History Center).

first round, when he eliminated Canadian champion C. Ross Somerville, five and four. Jones termed the crucial seventh hole, which he barely won, "the break of the tournament." He reflected, "I managed to play my best golf in the very first match" when "I needed it most."[34]

Jones ousted Canadian Fred Hoblitzell by the same score that afternoon, routed Sweetser, nine and eight, in the semifinal round, and vanquished Eugene Homans, eight and seven, in the final round to capture the U.S. Amateur. "No golfer faced a more torturing task than that of playing against Bobby Jones that day." Jones called the U.S. Amateur "the easiest to win of the Big Four," never experiencing "any sort of trouble."[35]

At least 18,000 spectators, a then-record golf gallery, stormed the eleventh green. "The fans swarmed in worship around their hero." When Homans congratulated him, Jones finally sensed "the wonderful feeling of release from tension and relaxation that I had wanted so badly for so long a time," and observed, "Nothing remained to be done." *New York Times* sportswriter William Richardson described Jones's walk to the clubhouse as "the most triumphant journey that any man ever travelled in sport."[36]

Sportswriters lauded Jones's fourth major title in the same season within four months. Keeler dubbed it the "Grand Slam," borrowing a bridge term. George Trevor of the *New York Sun* wrote that Jones had stormed "the impregnable quadrilateral of golf, that granite fortress that he alone could take by escalade, and that others may attack in vain, forever." Wells Twombly pictured the Grand Slam as "a sports masterpiece that even an America plunging into financial ruin could not help but celebrate." George Greenfield penned, "Jones is as truly the supreme artist of golf as Paderewski is the supreme artist of the piano."[37]

Most people erroneously assumed Jones would turn professional, but the Georgian never intended to make the game a career. On November 13, 1930, he retired from serious golf competition, "having no more worlds to conquer."[38] Jones viewed golf as "a means of obtaining recreation and enjoyment," and explained that his law profession now required greater attention and energy. "I might have become a better golfer had I kept on," he realized. "But I am certain I could have added nothing of significance to the record."[39]

Golf historians rank Jones, who never accepted monetary prizes in open events, the greatest amateur golfer ever. Jones played in few amateur events annually, competed nationally and internationally for only 11 years, and retired from competitive golf at age 28 to practice law in his father's Atlanta firm. "His strength was driving, putting, and an ability to get out of trouble," the *New York Times* eulogized. "He was an imaginative player, and he never hesitated to take a chance."[40] Jones's sportsmanship even supplanted his extraordinary playing record, setting an exceptional standard. His outstanding skill, amateurism, and personality appealed to Americans.

Jones fulfilled a lifelong dream of planning his own golf course. Although the nation was gripped in an economic depression, he joined New York City financier Clifford Roberts and renowned architect Alister MacKenzie in designing, building, and organizing the Augusta National Golf Course and modeled it after St. Andrews in Scotland. They helped transform an Augusta botanical garden "into the most celebrated golf course in the nation."[41] Upon completion of the magnificent course in December 1932, they began building the Augusta National Golf Club membership.

In 1934, Jones and Roberts established the first Augusta National Invitation Tournament, later renamed the Masters. The Masters became the first leg of the modern professional Grand Slam. "It was Bobby's epitaph." According to Jones, the prestigious tournament enabled Americans "to see the world's best players in action on a first-class golf course." It became a fitting tribute to golf's greatest amateur, whose exploits made it a major sport. As Walter Hagen reflected, Jones brought "huge galleries out to watch tournaments" and "created the golf craze in America."[42]

After Jones underwent several operations, doctors in 1948 diagnosed him with a very painful, crippling spinal cord disease that eventually confined him to a wheelchair. The USGA in 1953 lauded Jones's "unselfishness, superb judgment, nobility of character, and unwavering loyalty to principle." A perfectionist who put family and profession ahead of golf, he combined incredible strength of character with tremendous personal magnetism, exhibiting modesty and a generous fighting spirit.

Jones received numerous accolades. The Amateur Athletic Union (AAU) in 1930 gave Jones its first James E. Sullivan Memorial Award for having done the most during the year to advance the cause of sportsmanship through his performance, example, and influence as an amateur athlete. In a 1950 Associated Press poll, sportswriters and sportscasters named Jones the greatest golfer of the first half of the twentieth century. A 1952 Professional Golfers Association (PGA) poll designated him the half-century's top amateur golfer. Six years later, Jones became the second American to receive the Freedom of the City Award at St. Andrews, Scotland. He was inducted into the World Golf Hall of Fame in 1974.

Jones, who died of an aneurysm on December 18, 1971, in Atlanta at age 69, battled for survival to become the greatest golfer of his era. "All the odds on the health side" were "against me from the beginning," he knew. But the sport gave him four decades of "exciting experiences."[43] His 13 major championship victories rank third all-time behind Jack Nicklaus and Tiger Woods. No golfer amassed as many major titles so quickly. The Augusta National Golf Course and the Masters Tournament perhaps remain his greatest legacies.

# DORIS HART

"The only antidote for the poison of self pity is faith, courage and patience," affirmed Doris Hart, who fought back from adversity to become a tennis star. "As a child Doris Hart was certainly not a candidate for sports immortality."[1] Hart was diagnosed with a serious infection in her right knee as a toddler and faced the prospect of being crippled for life. She strengthened her knee by playing tennis and became the best player in the world, winning the women's singles at all Grand Slam tournaments.

Doris Hart, who experienced a modest middle-class upbringing, was born on June 20, 1925, in St. Louis, Missouri, and encountered leg problems through early childhood. When Hart was only 15 months old, her parents, Robert and Ann, noticed that she limped and favored her right leg. Hart had fallen and bumped her knee. "It became badly infected," Hart wrote, "and took a long time to heal."[2]

Dr. David Todd, the family physician, had gone on a hunting trip. A baby specialist misdiagnosed Hart's knee infection as rheumatism, advising heat treatments with a special apparatus. The infection spread rapidly up her right leg, triggering severe cramps. "It must have hurt dreadfully," she said. The baby specialist feared that gangrene would occur and gravely endanger her life. Two other baby specialists were consulted. To save her life, doctors recommended amputating her right leg.

Her father, Robert, did not give consent to the amputation and consulted Dr. Todd, who rushed back to St. Louis. Dr. Todd diagnosed Hart with having osteomyelitis, an inflammation of the bone and bone marrow in her right leg, caused by bacterial infection. Hart remembered, "My poor leg appeared lifeless," and feared that "the poison could easily reach the heart."[3] Dr. Todd needed to operate on her quickly to save her life and did not have time to move her to a hospital. He performed her emergency surgery on the Harts' kitchen table, draining the poison while Robert and a nurse held her arms and legs stationary.

Dr. Todd visited Hart daily for weeks thereafter, but her recovery proved slow. The doctor's incision did not drain very well. Too weak to move, Hart was carried from room to room. Ann massaged Hart's right leg muscles daily, hoping to strengthen them. Hart suffered various maladies, including a severe case of scarlet fever, requiring a mastoid operation. Although able to stand on her left leg with the aid of tables or chairs, she still could not put pressure on her right leg.

The leg massages, encouragement from Hart's family, and her personal determination helped her nearly regain normal use of her right leg. Hart initially put weight on her right toes and then eventually on her entire right foot. Suddenly one morning, after crawling on the floor, she stood up in Ann's presence. Hart recollected, "There I was, standing in the middle of the room, all by myself, with a big smile on my face. Even I knew that I had accomplished something important." Although Hart began to walk, Dr. Todd believed that she would never run or participate in active sports. "My leg had little strength and the knee was quite sensitive."[4]

In 1929, the Harts moved to Coral Gables, Florida, and operated the Miami Beach Kennel Club. Hart was glad that her family relocated to a warmer, year-round climate. "I'd never have been much of a tennis player otherwise," she explained. Swimming in the warm Atlantic Ocean, combined with the abundant sunshine, helped strengthen her right leg. Her father took her to the beach daily so she could swim in the salt water. Her leg improved rapidly. Faith, courage, and patience, Hart reflected, "saved me from being a cripple and helped me over the many hurdles that hedged my tennis career."[5]

Hart underwent an operation for a bilateral hernia at age 10 and spent several weeks recuperating at Victorian Hospital and at home. From her bed, she saw tennis being played at Henderson Park and "fell in love with the game." Henderson Park was located across the street from her residence. "Its location might have been arranged by the Hand of Providence, spouting out my future to me, had I but known it," she wrote. Hart fantasized about playing tennis and even admitted, "At times I had visions of becoming a champion at the sport!" Dr. Jones ordered her not to participate in sports for three months. Robert bought her a second-hand tennis racket for $5 and promised to teach her to play tennis when her health improved. "I was so excited that I had to be restrained from jumping out of bed," Hart recalled. "I could hardly wait to hit the ball with my new racket."[6]

Hart became a tomboy, aided by her older brothers, Bob and Bud. Despite having bowed, wobbly legs, she began playing tennis with Bud at Henderson Park at age 10 as therapy. Bud initially taught her how to play the racquet sport and practiced long hours on grass surfaces with her. Her enthusiasm for tennis rapidly intensified. She watched others play and took lessons from Arnaud Pyform.[7] Since Bud brushed and swept the court, officials waived their 25-cent hourly fee.

Bud's constant encouragement and challenges to improve helped Hart develop an all-court game with various properly executed strokes. Due to her limp, Bud instructed Hart "to concentrate on her serve and the drop shot — lessons that served her well her entire career."[8] Hart never would have attained her tennis stardom without him. "I loved the game from the very beginning and could not stay away from the courts," Hart recollected. "All the best players congregated at Henderson, so we got great matches."[9] She subscribed to several tennis magazines, avidly followed the tennis results, and participated in a mixed doubles night league at Henderson Park, winning a trophy at age 11. E.J. Harbett, Miami Beach professional Ike Macy, and Mercer Beasley instructed her.

Hart's right knee problems still limited her court mobility. The surgery left her knee scarred and right leg thinner than her left. Sportswriters erroneously claimed that Hart had made a gallant recovery from infantile paralysis. "I guess it makes a better story that way,"[10] Hart observed. The smiling, slim, rangy, 5-foot 9½-inch Hart compensated for her knee problems with an excellent serve and developed a fluid style and full-court game. "Slim and wiry, she packs a deceptive wallop in her drives, and she can really power the ball on her first serve," ABC Sports Director Harry Wismer wrote. "Doris likes an attacking game, eschewing defensive tennis. She employed "a smashing service" and liked "to charge the net." *Boston Globe* columnist Bud Collins noted, "She moved very well, despite the early handicap of her legs, and had an excellent disposition. She was effective at the net, or in the backcourt."[11]

In 1938, 13-year-old Hart won the Memphis women's and girls' singles titles easily and took the Arkansas State Open crown. After finishing runner-up in the Southern Junior Championships, she lost in the first round of the National Junior Championships. At that tournament the following year, Hart dominated her first- and second-round opponents. She upset Dorothy Wightman in the third round and Sissy Madden in the fourth round, providing her "first real taste of victory against a better opponent."[12] Pat Canning Todd of California eliminated her in the semifinals. In 1942, Hart became the first southern female to take the U.S. Lawn Tennis Association's girls' 18 singles championships and successfully defended her crown the following year. She graduated from Gesu High School in Miami in 1945 and entered the University of Miami, where she excelled in tennis.

Hart joined the elite tennis players, ranking sixth nationally in 1942. After rising to third in 1943, she slipped to sixth in 1944 and 1945. Hart ranked fourth in 1946, trailing only Pauline Betz, Margaret Osborne, and Louise Brough. At the 1946 U.S. Women's Singles Championships, she eliminated Osborne in the quarter-finals and Mary Arnold in the semifinals. Hart, however, lost to Betz, 11–9, 6–3, in the finals, but reaching the finals at the U.S. Nationals was "the greatest thing that had happened in her tennis career." Hart valiantly forced Betz to 20 games before losing the first set. "But the Betz jinx prevailed."[13]

In 1947, Todd defeated Hart, 6–3, 3–6, 6–4, in the 1947 French Women's Singles finals. After losing to Osborne, 6–2, 6–4, in the 1947 Wimbledon Women's Singles finals, Hart combined with Todd to upset Osborne and Brough for the Women's Doubles title. When Betz turned professional that year, some insiders expected Hart to begin winning Grand Slam singles crowns. "It's a pleasure not to have to worry about Betz," Hart sighed. She made it to the 1948 Wimbledon Women's Singles finals, losing to Brough, 6–3, 8–6.[14]

Hart's first Grand Slam crown came in the 1949 Australian Women's Singles Championship at Adelaide, where she defeated Nancy Bolton, 6–3, 6–4, in the finals amid temperatures ranging from 90 to 104 degrees. The weather suited the Floridian's game. Hart underwent two eye operations to remove irritating cysts in 1949, causing her to miss the Wimbledon Tournament that year. But she realized, "My sight was much more important than the tennis tournament."[15] Osborne defeated her, 6–4, 6–1, in the 1949 U.S. Women's Singles finals.

By 1950, Hart's comeback had provided an inspirational sports story. Atlantis described Hart as "an amazing" player, whose "sheer courage and determination" catapulted her among the world's premier players. It termed her game "splendid" and argued, "Her ground strokes are about as good as any in the game today." Hart's "choice of shot and her ability to pick the openings, coupled with the tremendous will to win, concentration, and steadiness,"[16] augmented her prowess. Fatigue occasionally limited her effectiveness on the court.

After playing tennis extensively in Africa in early 1950 and losing to Brough, 6–4, 3–6, 6–4, in the 1950 Australian Women's Singles Championship, Hart took the 1950 French Women's Singles title, besting Todd, 6–4, 4–6, 6–2, in the finals. Later that year, Hart captured the U.S. Clay Court Women's singles title, routing Shirley Fry, 6–1, 6–2, but Osborne defeated her, 6–4, 6–3, in the finals at the 1950 U.S. Women's Singles Championships.

Hart reached the finals of the French Women's Singles tournament from 1951 through 1953, out-dueling Fry, 6–4, 6–4, to win in 1952 and losing to Fry, 6–3, 3–6, 6–3, in 1951 and to Maureen Connolly, 6–2, 6–4, in 1953. The crowd booed Hart and Fry for arriving late for the 1952 French Women's Singles finals, not realizing the chauffeur had failed to pick them up on time. The delay disrupted the concentration of both players. "Imagine having over ten thousand people giving you the Bronx cheer!"[17] Hart recollected.

In 1951, Hart snared her only Wimbledon Women's Singles Championship. After being seeded number three, she deliberately skipped the Queen's Club tournament. "I was going all out and made up my mind that this had to be my year to win," Hart vowed. She did not lose a set before the semifinals. Beverly Baker Fleitz surprised Osborne in the quarter-finals and Fry upset Brough in the semifinals, smoothing the path for Hart. In her third Wimbledon Women's Singles finals, Hart played superb tennis, routing Fry, 6–1, 6–0, in just 34 minutes. Collins labeled the thrashing "one of the worst beatings in the tournament's history."[18] Hart recounted, "I started off with a bang," disrupting Fry's base-line game with tailspin drives, attacking service, and decisive volleys. "I was playing tennis as if I were in another world," she beamed. "I could do no wrong." Hart added, "For once in my life I had played my best tennis when it counted most." Fry agreed that Hart deserved this turn of fortune. The Duchess of Kent gave the beaming Hart the prestigious winning trophy. "It was the most thrilling moment of my life," Hart wrote. "I had finally accomplished my main tennis objective after many years of struggle and devotion to the sport."[19]

Hart scored a trifecta at Wimbledon in 1951, snagging the Women's Doubles and Mixed Doubles titles. She lost only one set in the three events, the loss occurring in the Mixed Doubles with Frank Sedgman. *Sports Illustrated* noted how Hart's three triumphs came on the same day, courtesy of rain delays.[20] Brough prevented her from repeating as champion in the 1952 Wimbledon Women's Singles, ousting her in the semifinals. Connolly bested her, 8–6, 7–5, at the 1953 Wimbledon Women's Singles finals.

Hart aspired to win the U.S. Women's Singles championships. Connolly, the junior champion from California, defeated her in the 1951 U.S. Women's Singles semifinals. Hart led 4–1 in the first set when rains began. To her dismay, the umpire refused to halt the match. Hart lost six consecutive games before the match was suspended. "The rains made the court quite slippery, and this favored Maureen greatly," Hart claimed. Hart could not reach Connolly's deep baseline drives or utilize her drop shot effectively. The match resumed the next day. "'Little Mo' raked the sidelines with her ground strokes, never permitting Miss Hart to gain the initiative," Associated Press sportswriter Will Grimsley observed. "When Doris rushed to the net, she often was passed or sent scurrying to the baseline by a well-placed lob."[21] After upsetting Hart, 6–4, 6–4, Connolly triumphed over Fry in the finals.

In the finals at the 1952 and 1953 U.S. Women's Singles Championships, Connolly prevailed over Hart in straight sets. The margins were 6–3, 7–5, in 1952 and 6–2, 6–4, in 1953, making her a bridesmaid for the fourth time in that tournament. Hart feared becoming "the Champion of Runner-ups, and quite possibly the world's most unlucky player." Her quest to capture that title intensified after losing in the Women's Singles finals four times in five years. "To be Queen of Forest Hills is the ultimate goal of all the women players' careers," Hart insisted. She yearned for that honor and "was determined not to give up," believing that eventually her dream would be fulfilled.[22]

Hart's dream finally came true at age 29 in her fifteenth attempt for the U.S. Women's Singles crown in 1954, when she met 31-year-old Brough in the thrilling finals. "This might be my last chance to win," Hart realized. "It was now or never!" The playing conditions were ideal, and the stadium was filled. Hart lost the first set, 8–6, but neither finalist performed well. She missed most of her ground shots and struggled with serves. The momentum shifted in the second set, which Hart took easily, 6–1. "I was determined to find myself," she remembered, "and fought, concentrated, as I never had before in all my life."[23]

Hart and Brough played much better in the third set, each holding service. Hart regained much of her confidence and stroked more freely. She sharpened her serve and played more aggressively. Hart came "perilously close to a sixth defeat," but overcame Brough to win her first National Championship. She trailed, 6–5, and survived three match points when Brough hit her second serve into the net. Hart won that game to knot the score, 6–6, and sensed, "The tide was turning in my favor." Both players were physically and mentally exhausted. The nervous Brough played more cautiously and defensively. "I was fighting on courage alone," the struggling Hart admitted. She broke Brough's serve in the thirteenth game, seizing a 7–6 lead.[24]

Hart captured the next game to take the set, 8–6. She won the first point, Brough the next. Hart scored aces on the next two serves to seize a 40–15 advantage. Brough hit the second rally of the next point into the net, finally ending the match. "I was stunned by my victory," recollected Hart, who received a tremendous ovation. Her "long frustrated dreams of being national champion had come true."[25] Hart, so emotionally drained that she could hardly speak, thanked her family, especially Bud, who had flown to see her play.

The 1954 U.S. Singles Championships marked new experiences for the 29-year-old Hart and 31-year-old Vic Seixas, who had easily captured the U.S. Men's Singles title, defeating Rex Hartwig of Australia in four sets. *Sports Illustrated* termed the pair "Forest Hills' most experienced runners-up." Hart had played in five U.S. Women's finals and Seixas had performed in two U.S. Men's finals without achieving any victories. In 1955, Hart successfully defended her U.S. Women's Singles crown, vanquishing Pat Ward, 6–4, 6–2.

After failing to get to the quarter-finals in her first two major tournaments, Hart reached that round in her last 32 Grand Slam singles tournaments. The initial two tournaments came when she was just 15 and 16 years old. She competed in 18 Grand Slam singles finals, triumphing six times, and captured the 1955 U.S. Singles Championships in her final majors appearance.[26]

Hart and Fry, meanwhile, amassed Wimbledon Women's Doubles titles from 1951 through 1953. During that span, they established a tournament record by winning both the semifinal and final round matches without losing one game. In 1951, they upset Brough and Osborne in straight sets. "Amazingly enough," Hart wrote, "I still produced the same brand of 'dream tennis' that I had displayed in the singles, and

Shirley was now completely relaxed and playing wonderful tennis. We worked well together."[27]

Hart paired with Fry to set a record by taking four consecutive French Women's Doubles titles from 1950 through 1953. They lost only one set in those finals during that span, deposing long-time rivals Brough and Osborne, 1–6, 7–5, 6–2, in 1950. Gigi Fernandez and Natasha Zvereva tied that record four decades later as French Women's Doubles champions from 1992 through 1995.

Hart and Fry also captured the U.S. Women's Doubles crowns from 1951 through 1954. In the 1951 U.S. Women's Doubles finals, they ended the record streak of Brough and Osborne at nine championships and 41 matches. Hart and Fry survived a furious 6–2, 7–9, 9–7 struggle, avoiding two match points while trailing 5–2 in the third set. In the 1955 U.S. Women's Doubles finals, Brough and Osborne ended the Hart-Fry streak of four championships spanning 20 matches.[28]

Hart captured the Women's Doubles titles with Todd at Wimbledon in 1947 and France in 1948 and with Brough in Australia in 1950. She also took the U.S. Women's Clay Court Doubles crowns in 1944 and 1945 with Betz, 1950 with Fry, and 1954 with Connolly, and the U.S. Women's Indoors Doubles in 1947 and 1948 with Barbara Schofield.

Hart teamed with Sedgman of Australia to capture the 1951 and 1952 Wimbledon Mixed Doubles Championships and U.S. Mixed Doubles Championships. At both 1951 tournament finals, they swept Nancye Bolton and Mervyn Rose of Australia in straight sets. Although physically exhausted after performing in the singles matches, she claimed that mental fortitude gave her physical strength. Hart, ecstatic, said, "It was no longer Heart-break Court for me!"[29]

Hart combined with Seixas to win the Wimbledon and U.S. Mixed Doubles titles from 1953 through 1955 and the Wimbledon Mixed Doubles crown in 1956. They especially wanted to win the 1954 U.S. Mixed Doubles Championship because both had captured the U.S. Singles titles that year. Hart stressed, "We both hoped to make it a grand-slam year." After dropping the first set, 4–6, to Osborne and Ken Rosewall, they won the next two sets, 6–1, 6–1, to take the match. Only once before had an American man and woman snared the Singles, Doubles, and Mixed Doubles crowns in the same year. Alice Marble and Don Budge had accomplished the rare combination in 1938. "It was quite a feat,"[30] Hart beamed. Her 1955 Mixed Doubles titles marked the first time a player had won five consecutive Mixed Doubles crowns. Hart also took the U.S. Indoor Mixed Doubles with Bill Talbert in 1947 and 1948 and the U.S. Hard Court Mixed Doubles with Eric Sturges in 1948.

Hart's triumphs at both the 1951 Wimbledon and 1954 U.S. Women's Singles, Women's Doubles, and Mixed Doubles tied records held by Hazel Hotchkiss Wightman, Mary Kay Browne, Suzanne Lenglen, Marble, Brough, and Osborne. "I had certainly hit the jackpot that time,"[31] Hart enthused.

Hart, the fifth winningest female player of all time, recorded 35 Grand Slam women's singles, women's doubles, and mixed doubles championships. Her Grand Slam career victories equaled Brough and trailed only Margaret Court (62), Martina Navratilova (56), Billie Jean King (39), and Osborne (37).[32] Hart, Court, and Navratilova remain the only tennis players to win all 12 major tennis titles. They captured every possible singles, same-sex doubles, and mixed doubles crown from the four Grand Slam tournaments. Hart's Grand Slam titles included six women's singles, 14 women's doubles, and 15 mixed doubles. Hart, one of only 12 to win all four singles titles, ranked first nationally in 1954 and 1955 and among the U.S. Top Ten from 1942 to 1955.[33]

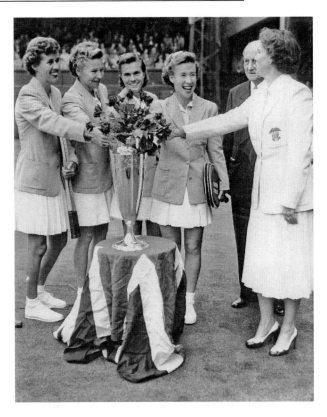

Doris Hart (far left) is shown here after winning the mixed doubles championship with Vic Seixas on June 12, 1954, at Wimbledon in London. Other ladies pictured include Louise Brough (second from left), Shirley Fry (third from left), Maureen Connolly (second from right), and Mrs. Margaret DuPont (far right). Lord Templewood (in back right) presented their winning trophies (courtesy Zuni Press/Icon SMI).

Between 1946 and 1955, Hart excelled for the United States against Great Britain in the Wightman Cup matches. She won all 14 singles matches and eight of nine doubles matches against the British and captained the triumphant 1970 U.S. Wightman Cup team.

Hart retired as an amateur after capturing the 1955 U.S. Women's Singles title, having taken 22 American singles and doubles championships on various surfaces. In singles competition, her record included 8–1 in the Australian Championships, 28–5 in the French Championships, 43–8 in the Wimbledon tournament, and 57–13 in the U.S. Championships. Although not keeping most of her Grand Slam trophies, she explained, "I know what I did and I made great friends, and that's all that really matters."[34]

In 1955, Hart wrote her autobiography, *Tennis with Hart*, received the U.S. Lawn Tennis Association Service Bowl, and turned professional. She joined the Spalding Tennis Advisory staff, conducting tennis clinics for the sporting goods company.

Hart taught tennis for 28 years in Pompano Beach, Florida, and played the sport until 1990, "when her right leg became too painful." The International Tennis Hall of Fame inducted her in 1969, lauding her 35 Grand Slam titles as "a lofty achievement" in a "sterling career."[35] Hart also was elected to the University of Miami Sports Hall of Fame in 1967 and the Florida Sports Hall of Fame in 1978.

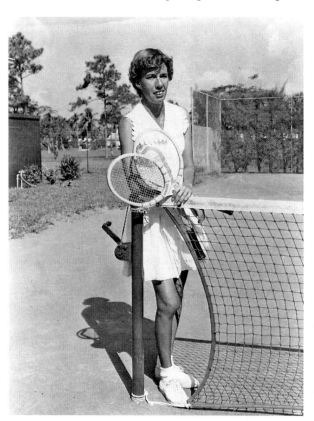

In December 1999, *Sports Illustrated* named Hart the eighth greatest sports figure in Florida history, noting her 35 Grand Slam tennis crowns and her being "one of two players, male or female, to pull off hat trick — titles in singles, doubles, mixed doubles — at all four majors." Floridians Deion Sanders, Emmitt Smith, Steve Carlton, Chris Evert, Bob Hayes, Rowdy Gaines, and Deacon Jones finished ahead of her.

Doris Hart, pictured here in the 1960s, joined the Spalding Tennis Advisory staff after turning professional in 1955 and conducted tennis clinics for the sporting goods company (courtesy International Tennis Hall of Fame and Museum).

Hart's family provided invaluable support in helping her overcome adversity to fulfill her tennis dreams. In her autobiography, Hart acknowledged, "Without my family I could not have had a tennis career, certainly I could never have reached championship heights."[36] Robert had financed his daughter's training from court fees to professional instruction, while her brother, Bud, had played tennis with her, counseled her, and taught her. Ann had set aside her own work to travel with her, sacrificing in pursuit of her daughter's goals.

# *Physical Disabilities*

## JIM ABBOTT

"Always believe. Anything is possible"[1] exemplified the amazing life of Jim Abbott, who defied the odds to become a major league baseball player. Abbott was born a congenital amputee with just one hand and spent his childhood and early adulthood proving doubters wrong. The multi-sport star not only fulfilled his dream of pitching in the major leagues, but even hurled a no-run, no-hit game.

Abbott, who grew up in a working-class family, struggled from the outset. James Anthony Abbott was born September 19, 1967, in Flint, Michigan, with a right arm ending about halfway between the elbow and the wrist and without a right hand. He had a rounded stub at the end of his right arm where the wrist would normally be, and with one small, finger-like protrusion where his right hand should be. Abbott later commented, "The only thing really missing is fingers." Doctors fitted him at age five with a fiberglass and steel hook-type prosthesis, an artificial hand, with clamping metal hooks. Youngsters called him cruel names, including "Captain Hook" and "Crab." Abbott, who was told that his hand looked like a foot,[2] hated the prosthesis and stopped wearing it within a year.

His parents, Mike, a sales manager for a beer company, and Kathy, a lawyer specializing in educational issues, gave him valuable support. They let him discard the prosthesis at age five. Abbott claimed that his parents never tried to make too much of his missing hand. When neighborhood youngsters taunted him, "his parents sent him right back out to play." "They never shielded me,"[3] he remembered. According to his father, Abbott never rued, "I wish I had two hands." As a child, Abbott claimed, "I never felt limited." He admired how his young parents, who had married as 18-year-olds just out of high school, handled his situation. "They were alone. There were no support groups."[4]

When Abbott developed an interest in sports, his parents realized their son's natural athleticism. They tried to guide him toward soccer, a sport that does not require the use of hands except for the goalie and would make his handicap less important. Since Abbott loved baseball much better, however, his parents bought him a glove. Others warned Abbott that he could not be a pitcher, but he adamantly disagreed.

"I had to learn to do it with one hand because that's all I had,"[5] he recalled. His father soon taught him how to develop a fluid and natural pitching motion and delivery and throw a baseball left-handed, with the palm of his glove resting on the stub.

Abbott's instantaneous glove-switching technique was described as legerdemain, letting him pitch with his left hand while balancing the inside of his glove on his nub. After delivering each pitch, Abbott quickly slipped his hand inside the glove and switched the glove to his left hand so that he could catch or field balls. When fielding the ball, he cradled the glove with his right arm and threw.

Abbott worked on his pitching motion daily while tossing a ball against the brick wall of his family's house. He repeated that maneuver thousands of times by himself, switching the glove to his left hand to catch it at closer and closer ranges until the transfer became natural.[6] When a grounder was hit to him, Abbott jammed his left hand into the glove, fielded the ball, shed the glove, and threw to first base. He perfected the motion as a youngster. "It was just all I knew," he said. Abbott's split-second glove-switching technique was crucial to his success in baseball, where his fielding ability often was questioned. Although his pitching skill was not doubted, he always needed to prove that he could throw runners out. His mother Kathy recalled, "What he did we took for granted."[7]

Abbott, who idolized University of Michigan star Rick Leach, debuted as a pitcher for Lydia Simon Real Estate at age 11 in a Little League game. After hurling a five-inning no-hitter in his initial start, he became a local media celebrity. If family members and friends had not encouraged him, he admitted, "I might have been crushed and never gone on." Abbott believed, "He could do anything he wanted."[8]

When Abbott was a freshman at Flint Central High School, opponents quickly challenged his fielding ability. One coach ordered eight consecutive batters to bunt after Abbott had struck out 10 batters. The first batter reached base safely, but Abbott threw out the next seven hitters. He pitched four no-hitters and played the outfield and first base when not pitching.

As a senior, Abbott batted .427 with a team-high seven home runs, resting the bat handle on his right wrist and then grasping the wrist and the bat with his left hand. The gifted, one-armed hurler averaged two strikeouts per inning and fewer than two hits allowed per game. Abbott explained, "I've been blessed with a pretty good left arm and a not-so-great right arm."[9] His feats included throwing out a speedy runner at home plate on a 270-foot fly to left field, belting a 330-foot game-winning home run to center field, and clouting a three-run game-winning homer in extra innings in the nightcap of a doubleheader.

Despite his handicap, Abbott became a multi-sport scholastic superstar. He paced the Flint Central intramural basketball league in scoring. Bob Holec, his baseball coach, persuaded him to play football his junior year. Abbott needed several weeks to learn to control the snap, but quarterbacked Flint to the state semifinals as a senior. He hurled four touchdown passes in one playoff game and averaged 37.5 yards a punt. Holec said, "He's a tremendous competitor" and "doesn't think he has a hand-icap."[10]

The Toronto Blue Jays in 1985 drafted Abbott as a high school senior in the thirty-sixth round, but he rejected the team's $50,000 offer. Scouts indicated that Abbott would have been selected in the third or fourth round if he had been born with two hands.

The University of Michigan recruited the 6-foot 3-inch, 210-pound Abbott, whose tall, powerful physique was tailor-made for pitching, on a baseball scholarship. Scouts timed Abbott's fast ball in the low to mid-eighties. Abbott made his initial appearance in the seventh inning against the University of North Carolina. A runner tried to steal home against him after his third pitch, but he threw the runner out by 20 feet. The Wolverines took the lead in the eighth inning and won, 6–3, giving Abbott his first collegiate victory.[11] Abbott fared 7–2 as a freshman, clinching the regular-season 1986 Big Ten Conference title game for the Wolverines and winning the Most Courageous Athlete Award from the Philadelphia Sportswriters Association. The same year, the American Sport Art Museum and Archives gave Abbott the Mildred "Babe" Didrikson Zaharias Courage Award for demonstrating courage, perseverance, grace, and strength in overcoming adversity to excel in sport.

Abbott finished 11–3 his sophomore year, leading Michigan to the 1987 Big Ten Conference crown and making All-American. He did not yield an earned run in 35 consecutive innings. Abbott "dazzled a troop of major league scouts," allowing only one hit in six innings in a 2–1 victory over Indiana University and defeated Purdue University in the Big Ten Tournament. *Sports Illustrated* wrote, "He's being appreciated more and more for his ability than his disability." Abbott won the 1987 Golden Spikes Award, baseball's equivalent of the Heisman Trophy, as the nation's outstanding amateur baseball player by the U.S. Baseball Federation. He became the first baseball player to win the James E. Sullivan Award as the nation's best amateur athlete by the Amateur Athletic Union (AAU), outpolling Olympic gold medalists and world record holders Jackie Joyner-Kersee and Greg Louganis.[12]

Following his sophomore season, Abbott was selected to the American baseball team at the 1987 Pan-American Games in Indianapolis. Before the games, the United States played Cuba in an exhibition series. Abbott pitched the third game in Havana, helping Team USA defeat the heavily favored Cubans in baseball for the first time in 21 years. Team USA also traveled to Japan, where Abbott learned more about life with a disability. "They said in their country a little boy with one hand wouldn't be allowed to play, wouldn't be allowed to even get this far. And that just made me hope my playing has opened some eyes,"[13] he said. The U.S. contingent chose Abbott to carry the American flag in the opening ceremonies of the Pan-American Games, providing his biggest thrill. Abbott posted a 2–0 record with a sparkling 0.00 earned run average (ERA). Abbott averaged more than a strikeout per inning against formidable international competition for the second-place Americans.

Abbott returned to Michigan for his junior year, winning eight of 11 decisions. During three seasons with the Wolverines, he compiled a 26–8 win-loss record and a 3.03 ERA. Abbott hurled 13 complete games and six shutouts, recording 186 strikeouts in 234 innings pitched.

Major league clubs still questioned Abbott's skills. National League (NL) squads did not draft him because of concerns about his hitting and bunting abilities. Some teams wondered if a one-handed player could field. Others doubted how he would handle major league pressure and the constant media scrutiny. Abbott welcomed the skepticism as a challenge, never viewing himself as a liability.

The California Angels in June 1988 surprised some baseball pundits by making Abbott their first-round draft choice, the eighth player chosen overall. The Angels, who sought a left-handed pitcher, believed that Abbott possessed the best combination of intelligence, arm, athletic ability, and poise of any American left-hander. "If there's something I've learned about Jim Abbott," Angels scouting director Bob Fontaine explained, "it's never say he can't do anything."[14] Abbott's fast ball was clocked at 90 to 94 miles per hour. Angels minor league director Bill Bavasi acknowledged, "He's the only guy we ever drafted that we knew going in what he had inside." Abbott welcomed his selection, reflecting, "All I ever wanted was a shot."[15]

Before signing a $200,000 a year contract with California in August 1988, Abbott starred for the 1988 U.S. Olympic team. Baseball was a demonstration game at the 1988 Summer Olympic Games in Seoul, South Korea. "He's the hardest thrower on my staff," Olympic coach Mark Marquess beamed. In pre–Olympics exhibition games, Abbott won seven of eight decisions with a 2.59 ERA. At the Olympic Games, the U.S. defeated South Korea, Australia, and Puerto Rico and triumphed over Japan, 5–3, in the championship game at Chamsi Baseball Stadium in Seoul in September. In the finale, Abbott celebrated his twenty-first birthday, allowing only seven hits and retiring 11 of the final 12 batters. He led the Americans to a gold medal and made a spectacular defensive play in his championship-clinching performance.

Skeptics questioned whether Abbott could make the major leagues, but the lefthander made the Angels' 40-player roster. The Angels planned to send Abbott to Midland, Texas, in Class AA to supplement his slider and his 94-mph fastball with a more effective curveball. Abbott drew international attention, as newspapers, magazines, television, and radio media featured his story. Many people were moved upon learning about a 'disabled' person playing major-league baseball at spring training. *Sports Illustrated* noted, "Rarely has there been so much clamor over the debut of a rookie who wasn't on his organization's major league roster." Abbott, who already had spurned three book offers and a movie deal before throwing his first professional pitch, took the media attention in stride. "All I'm trying to do is pitch the best I can,"[16] he said.

In his first exhibition appearance at Yuma, Arizona, Abbott blanked the San Diego Padres on two hits over three innings, striking out four and walking none.

Upon entering the fourth inning, he struck out outfielder Thomas Howard and 1984 Olympian Gary Green. Infielder Tim Flannery grounded out to end that frame. California catcher Lance Parrish boasted that Abbott possessed "as strong an arm as any left-hander I've caught. His motion is so fluid, the ball just kind of explodes."[17] Abbott pitched so well in spring training that he skipped the minor leagues entirely and joined the Angels' starting rotation for opening day, just the tenth time since 1965 that a pitcher moved directly to the major leagues without any minor-league experience.

Abbott's major league debut in Anaheim, California, against the Seattle Mariners on April 8, 1989, proved disappointing. Seattle hit Abbott hard, as he lasted just four and two-thirds innings in a 7–0 loss. In Abbott's next home appearance five days later, the Oakland A's bested him, 5–0. His first major league victory came on April 24, when he edged the Baltimore Orioles, 3–2, at Anaheim. "That night I had the most incredible euphoria," Abbott recalled. "I just wanted to hold onto it." He added, "There's nothing better than pitching a game and doing well. Nothing."[18]

In 1989, Abbott compiled 12 wins and 12 losses with a 3.92 ERA and 115 strikeouts in 181 innings pitched. The Angels scored only 23 runs in his 12 setbacks. Abbott struggled in 1990 with a 10–14 mark and a 4.51 ERA, leading the American League (AL) in hits surrendered with 246. The Angels tallied just 96 runs in his 33 starts and merely 15 runs in his 14 losses, the sixth-worst run support in the junior circuit.

The 1991 season marked a major turning point for Abbott. Abbott started out poorly, losing his first four decisions with a 6.00 ERA. "It was the toughest thing I've gone through baseball-wise," he admitted. Reporters, however, did not blame those losses on his lack of a right hand. Abbott knew that finally he had arrived. "It was all about pitching—this guy stinks," he admitted.

Abbott worked on his pitching mechanics, hoping to improve his performance. Angels manager Doug Rader and pitching coach Marcel Lachemann advised him to depend more on his power pitches, rely less on off-speed deliveries, and utilize more often the inside of the plate. Team psychologist Ken Ravizza taught Abbott to relax by conversing with himself on the mound. Teammates, his parents, and his fiancée, Dana Douty, also encouraged him. Abbott regained his self-assurance and throwing rhythm in May and became one of the major league's premier pitchers, winning 14 of 18 decisions with a 2.95 ERA from May through September. "There's so much more confidence," he explained. "I like to go home and read the statistics now that I'm not ashamed of my own."[19] Abbott notched a career-best 18 wins with 11 losses, a 2.89 ERA, and 158 strikeouts in 222 innings pitched. He was named to the AL All-Star team and placed third in the AL Cy Young Award balloting.

Although having a mediocre 7–15 record in 1992, Abbott ranked fifth in the AL with a 2.77 ERA. He logged at least seven innings in 22 of his 29 starts, allowed a career-low 12 home runs, and committed no errors in 46 chances. Abbott used his superb slider and fastball to strike out 130 batters, second best on the Angels' staff.

In a *Baseball America* poll, AL managers ranked his slider second best to that of Roger Clemens. Abbott's winning percentage declined largely because the Angels gave him only 2.55 runs per game, the lowest mark in the AL in 22 years. "He pitches his heart out every time," Angels batting coach Rod Carew observed. "But he pitched with incredibly bad luck."[20]

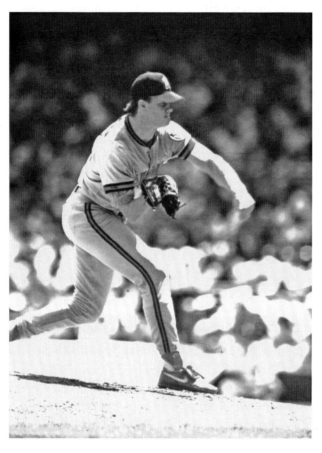

Jim Abbott, the one-handed first-round draft pick of the California Angels in 1988, pitched for the Angels from 1989 to 1993, compiling an 18–11 win-loss record and a 2.89 earned run average in 1991 (courtesy National Baseball Hall of Fame Library, Cooperstown, N.Y.).

Following the 1992 season, Abbott became involved in a contract dispute with the Angels. In December, California traded Abbott to the New York Yankees for first baseman J.T. Snow and two pitching prospects. The trade surprised Abbott, who had expected to spend the remainder of his career with the Angels. Abbott "felt a real sense of rejection," but liked joining a better team. "I'm excited to play for a club that wants to win."[21]

The 1993 season brought Abbott a few glorious moments. On April 12, Abbott won his Yankee debut, 4–1, over the Kansas City Royals in the home opener at Yankee Stadium in what an Associated Press reporter described as one to "cheer and cherish." The complete game victory saw him throw only 85 pitches, surrender eight hits, strike out four batters, and walk none. "I couldn't ask for more," Abbott exulted. "It's a tremendous rush, one I will remember for a long time." Royals pitcher David Cone concurred, "He was great."[22] On May 29, at Yankee Stadium, Bo Jackson of the Chicago White Sox broke up Abbott's no-hit bid late in that game. Otherwise, Abbott struggled during the summer, as he inexplicably lost some velocity on his fastball.

Abbott, who never let his disability affect his desire, joined baseball lore by hurling a 4–0 no-hitter against the Cleveland Indians on September 4 at Yankee Stadium.

He had lost five of his previous six starts. Abbott became only the ninth player in the 90-year Yankee history and the first franchise pitcher in a decade to achieve that gem. Tom Verducci of *Sports Illustrated* wrote that Abbott now headed the list alphabetically among pitchers with no-hitters. "Should you then delineate the no-hitters to their inspirational value, the same one would lead the list."

Abbott throttled a formidable Cleveland Indian lineup that featured six players hitting .298 or better, masterfully working the outside corner more and throwing more breaking pitches. Yankee infielders rescued Abbott several times. Third baseman Wade Boggs dove to his left to stop Albert Belle's hard grounder and made a perfect throw to first baseman Don Mattingly in the seventh inning. In the ninth frame, the 27,225 spectators stood and cheered as Abbott retired Kenny Lofton on a ground ball, Felix Fermin on a 390-foot drive to Bernie Williams in left center field, and Carlos Baerga on an easy roller to shortstop Randy Velarde. After Velarde fired the ball to Mattingly, Abbott exulted, "How about that, baby!" Abbott, who hurled five other career shutouts, walked five, struck out three, and induced 17 ground balls in that historic gem. Verducci marveled at Abbott's masterpiece, reminding readers "that he was born without a right hand."[23] "I'm thrilled to death," Abbott beamed. "I never thought about pitching a no-hitter." His teammates signed the pitching slab and gave it to him, while his hat and ball were sent to the National Baseball Hall of Fame in Cooperstown, New York.

Yankee manager Buck Showalter, normally stoic, almost hit his head on the dugout roof. "The last couple of innings," Mattingly recalled, "I had these huge goose bumps on my forearms." Yankee reliever Paul Gibson aptly described Abbott's feat: "He's done something only a select group of people have ever done the history of the game, and he did it by overcoming the kind of physical challenge that would make most kids quit Little League."[24] Chris Bosio of the Seattle Mariners hurled the only other AL no-hitter that season. The remainder of Abbott's season proved anticlimactic. Abbott finished 1993 with 11 wins, 14 losses and a 4.37 ERA and a career-low 95 strikeouts.

Following the 1993 season, Abbott was embroiled in a contract dispute with the Yankees. Arbitrators awarded him the $2.35 million New York offered rather than the $3.5 million he sought. In the strike-shortened 1994 campaign, he fared 9–8 with a 4.55 ERA. Abbott compiled a lackluster 20–22 record over two seasons with the Yankees.

Abbott signed a one-year contract with the Chicago White Sox as a free agent in April 1995. He excelled on a mediocre pitching staff, posting a 6–4 record and a 3.36 ERA. The first-place California Angels reacquired Abbott and reliever Tim Fortugno for four minor league prospects on July 27. Abbott, caught off guard by the transaction, relished rejoining the Angels. "How many times do you get a chance to be in a pennant race, to have a chance to fulfill a dream?"[25] he asked. Abbott won five and lost three in his second stint with the Angels and finished the strike-shortened season 11–8 with a 3.70 ERA. The Angels' fortunes, however, collapsed in September. California blew the biggest lead in the shortest time in major league history, squandering a 10½ game lead in 35 days and losing the AL Western Division title to the Seattle Mariners in a playoff game.

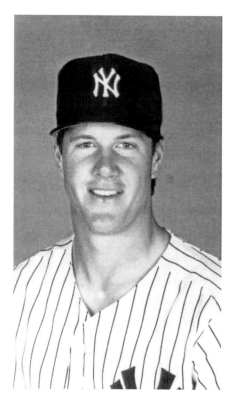

Jim Abbott pitched for the New York Yankees in 1993 and 1994, hurling a no-hitter against the Cleveland Indians on September 4, 1993, at Yankee Stadium. He became only the ninth pitcher in the storied 90-year Yankees history to accomplish that feat (courtesy National Baseball Hall of Fame Library, Cooperstown, N.Y.).

Abbott struggled the remainder of his major league career. In 1996, he continued losing much of his velocity and experienced one of the worst seasons in major league history with a 2–18 mark and 7.18 ERA. "Most observers," *Sports Illustrated* wrote, "thought his considerable reservoir of talent and courage was exhausted." After a hiatus from baseball in 1997, Abbott signed a minor league contract with the Chicago White Sox in May 1998. He ascended rapidly through their farm system. "He spent three months riding buses around North Carolina (with the Class A Hickory Crawdads and the Winston-Salem Warthogs), pitching in the Alabama humidity (with the Double A Birmingham Barons) and toiling in an old stadium in rodeo-rabid Alberta (with the Triple A Calgary Cannons)."

Chicago recalled Abbott from Calgary of the Pacific Coast League on September 2. Abbott joined White Sox third baseman Robin Ventura, who had played on the gold-medal-winning 1988 U.S. Olympic squad. He won his five starts, including victories over the Cleveland Indians and the New York Yankees, in a hitter's era. "Neither he nor the White Sox can explain his success."[26] Abbott, however, left the White Sox when Ventura became a free agent after the 1998 season.

The Milwaukee Brewers (NL) signed Abbott as a free agent in January 1999. Abbott won only two of 10 games with a 6.91 ERA and was released on July 23, ending his major league career. During his major league career, he compiled 87 wins, 108 losses, and a 4.25 ERA and struck out 888 batters in 1,674 innings with 31 complete games and six shutouts.[27]

Abbott, whom sportswriters followed closely, rejected offers for the film and book rights to his story. The media often compared him to one-armed outfielder Pete Gray of the St. Louis Browns in 1945. Abbott discouraged those comparisons, countering, "I didn't grow up wanting to be another Pete Gray. I grew up wanting to be another Nolan Ryan."

Although serving as a role model for many handicapped youngsters, Abbott still refused to acknowledge that he suffered a handicap. "I just don't think all of this about me playing with one hand is as big an issue as everyone wants to make it," he insisted. "I just accept it." Abbott denied that courage was "playing baseball with one hand" and contended, "Courage is fighting a war, being a parent of a child who is very sick, facing death."[28]

Abbott's athletic achievements nonetheless amazed sports fans and inspired countless numbers of Americans with disabilities, who flocked to ballparks to see him pitch. Abbott, who lives in Corona del Mar, California, served as a motivational speaker, hired by Prudential, Exxon, and Wells Fargo to tell his story. He was deluged with letters, many from young people with hand disabilities and from parents of children who had lost limbs. Abbott receives several e-mails or letters a month, "all of them heart-wrenching, many of them about children who are missing a hand, or part of a hand, or feeling in a hand. He responds to each one personally." Abbott, who still meets and speaks with disabled people, said, "It's a difficult spot, because I know what they're going through and I know how far a little help can go."[29] He inspires youngsters by recounting how he handled his situation. Youngsters relate to his story. Abbott counsels them to never consider themselves handicapped, imploring them to believe, "Anything is possible." He philosophizes, "You can do anything you want if you put your mind to it." Abbott gives each child acquaintance hope, affirming, "Hope for a life free of sympathy and self-pity."[30]

In 2012, Abbott's inspirational autobiography, *Imperfect: An Improbable Life*, was published. The book centered on Abbott's no-hitter, but spun stories about his family and related how numerous disabled people wrote him for encouragement and guidance. Abbott wrote, "I knew how far a little boy or girl could run with 50 words of reassurance." He recalled visiting one boy who had suffered a stroke and was confined to Anaheim Hospital. Abbott, the boy, and his mother suddenly began to cry. "I sat in the bed," Abbott recalled, "and we talked about courage, about getting better, and about believing in himself." Similar visits ensued. "I was inspired," Abbott recollected. "They pushed me back onto the field and into my own battles. I was going to be just like them." He remembered, "What drove me were the low expectations people had for me. I insisted on showing them what I could do."[31]

When Abbott pitched, his lack of a hand gradually slipped into the background. Spectators became less conscious of the physical difference between Abbott and the other players. Abbott, who symbolized courage and determination, assured disabled youngsters, "I'm just like you."[32] His success enriched the sports world in a thrilling, irreplaceable way.

# DUMMY HOY

"The small deaf boy with big dreams, going off to play professional baseball against all odds"[1] defines "Dummy" Hoy, who persevered with a handicap to excel in major league baseball. Hoy contracted meningitis as a very young child, leaving him deaf and mute. He did not let that obstacle impede his quest to become an excellent major league baseball player, developing a system of signals to communicate with teammates.

Hoy was brought up in a middle-class agricultural setting. William Ellsworth Hoy was born in rural Houckstown, Ohio, on May 23, 1862, and grew up on a farm there with his parents, Jacob and Rebecca, three brothers, and one sister. He contracted meningitis at age three, leaving him deaf, mute, and unable to attend public schools. Deaf-mutes often were nicknamed "Dummy" in the 1800s because they could not speak. Hoy grew up when few deaf people had learned to vocalize and before signing was considered true language. When Hoy was 10 years old, his parents sent him to the Ohio State School for the Deaf in Columbus. The highly intelligent, hard-working Hoy completed both grade school and high school in seven years and graduated as class valedictorian at age 18.[2] The Ohio School for the Deaf had instituted baseball by 1872, affording Hoy an opportunity to begin developing his playing skills.

Economics delayed Hoy's start in professional baseball. When Hoy graduated, his father persuaded him to return to Houckstown and become a cobbler. After assisting a Houckstown shoemaker, Hoy earned sufficient cash to purchase the business. The number of customers declined during the summer months, when rural area residents often went without shoes. Hoy frequently played baseball with the local youngsters outside his shop when business waned.[3]

A Findlay, Ohio, resident noticed Hoy playing baseball outside his shop. "Disappointed at finding I was a deaf mute he continued on his way," Hoy recalled. The passerby, however, returned the next day to scout Hoy and asked him to play for his nearby Kenton, Ohio, team against arch-rival Urbana. Hoy accepted the scout's invitation and performed well against Billy Hart, a former professional pitcher. "Dummy had no trouble solving him for some base hits."[4]

Several professional teams declined to sign the 24-year-old Hoy because of his handicap. Hoy began his professional baseball career with Oshkosh, Wisconsin, in the Northwestern League in 1886, agreeing to a contract for $75 a month. He faced an uphill battle. "His deafness prevented him from hearing the crack of the bat, or any verbal communication by umpires or teammates. But he was determined to prove he could succeed."[5] Oshkosh manager Frank Selee was reluctant to sign "a deaf-mute who communicated only with a pad and pencil." The deaf-mute found his first few months in Oshkosh especially difficult. "Often he was the butt of ridicule by his fellow players. But Hoy persisted and let his play speak for itself."[6]

Hoy's contract permitted him to leave the Oshkosh team on August 1 if "work was piling up at his cobbler's shop." Hoy, however, closed his cobbler's shop when Oshkosh paid him $300 for the remainder of the 1886 season. Selee retained Hoy because of his innate playing ability and aggressive on-field attitude. Although batting only .219, Hoy impressed spectators with his speed and defensive skills. "His outstanding outfield play convinced Selee to renew Hoy's contract." Hoy made one sensational catch while "balancing on the shaft of a buggy parked inside the stadium" or "leaping astride the horse."[7] His intelligence, quickness, and alertness helped him cope with his handicap.

During the off season, Hoy notified Selee about his hitting problems. Since Hoy could not hear the umpire call strikes or balls, he had to turn around to lip-read what the umpire had called. Moundsmen often threw the next pitch before Hoy was ready. Hoy arranged for Selee to hand signal

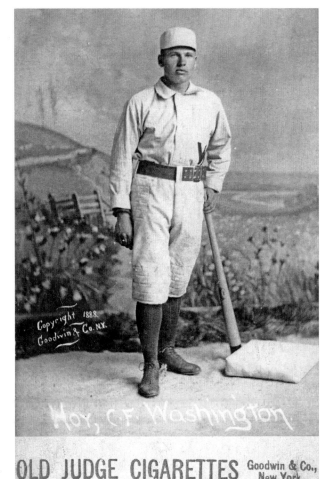

Dummy Hoy of the Washington Statesmen, the first deaf major league player, is pictured here standing at the plate, circa 1888, on a Goodwin & Company Old Judge Cigarette card. Hoy played an instrumental role in the development of hand signals for batters, base runners, outfielders, managers, and coaches (courtesy National Baseball Hall of Fame Library, Cooperstown, N.Y.).

from the third base coaching box whether pitches were strikes or balls, thus pioneering the creation of hand signals. Selee quickly raised his right hand for each strike and left hand for each ball, enabling Hoy to be ready for the next pitch. "Opposing pitchers, who previously had savored Hoy's uneasiness in the batter's box, suddenly found themselves facing a solid, concentrating hitter."[8] Hoy also utilized the out and safe signals from American Sign language. He enjoyed a stellar season in 1887, raising his batting average to .367, stealing 67 bases, and leading Oshkosh to the Northwestern League pennant.

Hoy began his major league career with the struggling Washington Statesmen of the National League (NL) in 1888, becoming the third deaf major league player following pitchers Ed Dundon and Tom Lynch, and the first deaf major league position player. The diminutive, 5-foot 4-inch, 145-pound Ohioan, who batted left-handed and threw right-handed, ranked among the era's smallest major league players. During the late 1880s, most players lacked formal education. Baseball historian Thomas Lonergan, who saw Hoy perform in St. Louis in 1891, called him "one of the brainiest ballplayers I ever saw."[9]

Hoy, who played with six major league teams, was among 29 players to compete in four of the five acknowledged major leagues, the NL, Players League (PL), American Association (AA), and American League (AL). Upon joining Washington in 1888, Hoy posted instructions on the clubhouse wall for teammates to avert possible collisions with his fellow outfielders, second baseman, and shortstop on fly balls. His instructions were: "Whenever I take a fly ball I always yell (actually squeak) I'll take it — the same as I have been doing for many seasons, and of course the other fielders let me take it. Whenever you don't hear me yell, it is understood I am not after the ball, and they govern themselves accordingly."[10]

The Washington club traveling secretary unfortunately forgot to notify Hoy about an exhibition game in Paterson, New Jersey. When the Statesmen assembled in the lobby for the trip, Hoy did not appear. Teammates went to Hoy's room and tried unsuccessfully to rouse him by knocking loudly, raising their voices, squeezing a little guy inside the transom, squeezing a bellboy over the transom, and throwing several plugs of tobacco and playing cards at him. "Finally, a set of keys was sent through the transom tied to a bed sheet and dragged across Hoy until it caught in his night shirt, whereupon he sleepily awoke to find a bunch of playing cards lying all over him. Thinking his mates were playing a trick on him, he quickly grabbed a pitcher of water and flung it at the heads peeping at him from the transom."[11] The team always informed Hoy thereafter of any changes in traveling plans.

Hoy and several teammates bolted to the Buffalo Bisons (PL) in 1890. The PL was formed to improve player pay and working conditions, challenging the reserve clause. Hoy disliked the reserve clause, which forced a player to sign with his own club or not play at all. "Hoy was one of the few early players willing to contest his tendered salary in public, and to withhold signing in hopes for negotiation of a higher wage." The Bisons, as well as the PL, disbanded after one season because of revenue problems.[12]

Hoy's first experience with a winning team came with player-manager Charlie Comiskey's St. Louis Browns (AA) in 1891. When the AA folded after the 1891 season, Hoy returned to the weak Washington Statesmen in 1892 and 1893. Washington traded Hoy to the Cincinnati Reds (NL), where he played from 1894 to 1897 and enjoyed his longest stint with any one club.[13]

Hoy competed for the Louisville Colonels (NL) in 1898 and 1899, teaming with player-manager Fred Clarke, shortstop Honus Wagner, and pitcher Rube Waddell. When Louisville was dropped from the NL, he performed with the Chicago White Stockings in 1900 and 1901, the latter year in the fledgling AL. Hoy rejoined the Cincinnati Reds for his final major league campaign in 1902 and completed his professional baseball career with the Los Angeles Looloos of the Pacific Coast League (PCL) in 1903. Although still a major league-caliber player, Hoy aspired "to see another part of the country."[14]

Hoy, who demonstrated "acknowledged intelligence and savvy understanding of the game's subtleties," exhibited numerous all-around skills. He usually batted at or near the top of the lineup, reached base often, was an excellent baserunner, and scored frequently. Hoy compensated for his lack of size and power with speed, hitting .300 twice and scoring 100 runs nine times. He batted .274 in 1888, setting rookie records for games, plate appearances, hits, singles, and walks. Hoy hit .298 with Buffalo in 1890, .299 and .298 with Cincinnati in 1894 and 1896, and .304 and a career-best .306 with Louisville in 1898 and 1899. He possessed a keen eye and a very small strike zone, ranking second in the NL with 69 walks in 1888, leading the AA in walks with 119 in 1891, and pacing the AL in walks with 86 in 1901.[15]

Hoy also performed well in several other offensive categories. Besides finishing second in the AA in runs scored with 136 in 1891, he recorded over 20 doubles each season from 1894 through 1897, ranked second in the NL in triples with six in 1898, and shared the club lead with four home runs in 1896. Hoy clouted the second grand-slam home run in AL history on May 1, 1901, and helped lead Chicago that season to the first AL pennant. In 1901, he also finished fourth in the junior circuit in runs scored with 112 and on-base percentage with .407. His on-base percentage topped .400 five times.

Speed and superior base-running abilities were among Hoy's greatest assets. "I never saw him picked off," Lonergan observed. "There"ll never be another like him." Hoy followed his natural base-running instincts rather than watching the coaches. "I had to go solo," he explained. "I was always mentally figuring in advance all possible plays on the bases and in the field." As a rookie in 1888, Hoy led the NL with 82 stolen bases.[16]

Hoy exhibited an uncanny ability to take extra bases, often moving from first base to third base or scoring from second base on singles. He capitalized on his speed, recording 30 or more stolen bases in 11 of his first 12 major league seasons and registering 594 career stolen bases. Hoy stole 487 bases from 1886 through 1897, when runners were credited with a steal whenever they took an extra base on a hit or an out. He pilfered just 107 bases after the statistic was redefined to its present meaning in 1898.[17]

Despite being deaf and among the shortest outfielders in major league history, Hoy exhibited extraordinary defensive leadership and excelled as a center fielder. Historian Stephen Gould called center fielders "generals of the outfield," letting the left and right fielders know who should handle each fly ball. Lonergan likewise lauded Hoy's exceptional outfield skills. "Hoy was as swift as a panther in the field." Lonergan affirmed, "I have seen balls hit for singles that would have been doubles or triples with other players fielding them." Lonergan added, "With men on the bases, Hoy never threw to the wrong spot. No player ever returned a ball faster from the outfield."[18]

Hoy, who read lips superbly, taught his outfield teammates sign language to facilitate communication. Left fielder Tommy Leach, Hoy's Louisville roommate in 1899, recalled Hoy and his wife "could read lips so well they never had any trouble understanding anything I said." Leach waited for Hoy's reaction when fly balls were hit. "You listened for him and if he made this little squeaky sound, that meant he was going to take it." Leach remembered, "We hardly ever had to use our fingers to talk, though most of the fellows did learn the sign language." Right fielder Sam Crawford, who played alongside Hoy at Cincinnati in 1902, recalled, "I'd have to listen real careful to know whether or not he'd take a fly ball." Crawford recollected, "He'd make a kind of throaty voice, kind of a little squawk, and when a fly ball came out and I heard this little noise I knew he was going to take it. We never had any trouble about who was to take the ball."[19]

Hoy, considered the first center fielder to play his position very shallow, capitalized on his anticipation skills and quickness to run

HOY, C. F., Washington
Copyrighted by GOODWIN & CO. 188?
OLD JUDGE
CIGARETTES.
GOODWIN & CO., New York.

Dummy Hoy, shown here fielding a ball for the Washington Statesmen on a Goodwin & Company Old Judges Cabinet Cigarette card, circa 1888, excelled defensively as a center fielder and set a major league record by throwing out three Indianapolis Hoosier runners trying to score from second base on singles on June 19, 1889 (Library of Congress).

down balls hit behind him. "He used his speed and cunning in the outfield to great advantage, becoming one of the great 'fly hawks' of the early game." During the 1893–1894 winter season, Hoy made a sensational, ninth-inning catch in a thick gray San Francisco fog. When he made a spectacular catch, "fans would stand *en masse* and wave their arms and hats wildly, knowing Hoy couldn't hear their cheering."[20]

Hoy owned a rifle arm and exhibited uncanny throwing accuracy. He developed strong hands and forearms by milking cows on the family farm during the off-season and uncorked a baseball from different distances at a certain brick in the barn wall. Hoy "could throw strike after strike to home plate from center field." He nailed three Indianapolis Hoosiers runners trying to score from second base on June 19, 1889, uncorking perfect strikes to catcher Connie Mack at home plate. This "seldom-equaled feat" was considered "Hoy's own proudest achievement."[21] Jim Jones of the New York Giants and John McCarthy of the Chicago Cubs were the only other major league outfielders to duplicate Hoy's accomplishment.

Hoy consistently ranked among league leaders defensively, finishing in double figures in outfield assists every season except 1902 and compiling 328 career assists. He paced NL outfielders in assists with 27 in 1896 and in putouts with 359 and total chances in 1897. In 1900, Hoy topped Western Association outfielders with 337 putouts, 45 assists, and a .977 fielding percentage. His 45 outfield assists established a record for any league. No other outfielder has ever paced the major leagues in all three categories.[22]

Hoy was well-liked, popular, and honest. "The fans loved him." Umpires never ejected the gentlemanly, polite outfielder, whose "integrity almost cost him his job." A heated argument arose between Hoy's manager and the umpire in one game around dusk when a ball was hit toward the center fielder. The umpire had ruled that Hoy caught the ball on one bounce and called the batter safe at first base. When the manager insisted that Hoy had caught the ball, the umpire turned to the center fielder to see if he had caught the ball. Hoy indicated that he had trapped the ball on the bounce. "Hoy's teammates were furious."[23]

Hoy and Luther "Dummy" Taylor of the New York Giants were the only deaf-mutes to gain major league acclaim. Taylor won 117 major league games, including 27 in 1904, in nine major league seasons. The Reds played the Giants on May 26, 1902, before 5,000 fans at Cincinnati in the only major-league game in which two deaf players ever competed against each other. In the first inning, 40-year-old Hoy led off for Cincinnati and greeted 26-year-old Taylor in sign language, "I'm glad to see you."[24] He singled to center field in the first frame and was the only Reds player to collect two hits, scoring one run and walking once. Taylor surrendered three unearned runs in the eighth inning before being relieved. New York, however, rallied for five runs in the ninth inning to win, 5–3.

Hoy's professional baseball career ended with Los Angeles (PCL) in 1903. Hoy appeared in all of the Looloos' 211 games with 210 base hits, 156 runs scored, 46 stolen bases, and 413 outfield putouts to help Los Angeles win the PCL pennant.

Despite his belated start, Hoy amassed near Hall of Fame credentials in 14 major league seasons. In 1,796 major league games, nearly all as a center fielder, he batted .287 with 2,044 hits, 1,426 runs scored, 248 doubles, 121 triples, 40 home runs, and 726 runs batted in (RBI). Most of his home runs were hit inside the park. Hoy compiled an excellent .386 career on-base percentage and, upon his retirement, ranked second to Billy Hamilton with 1,004 walks. Defensively, Hoy in 1899 broke Mike Griffin's major league career record of 1,459 games as a center fielder, in 1901 surpassed Tom Brown's mark of 3,623 outfield putouts, and in 1902 broke Brown's record of 4,461 outfield chances. Hoy held the major league record for most games played in center field (1,726), most putouts (3,958), and most total chances (4,625). Jesse Burkett broke his record for career putouts in 1905, Clarke for career total chances in 1909, and Tris Speaker for most games as a center fielder in 1920. Hoy ranked second to Jimmy Ryan in outfield games played (1,795), third in outfield double plays (72), and seventh in outfield assists (173).[25]

Some baseball historians believe that umpires began using hand signals on balls and strikes and that managers started signaling to batters for the benefit of Hoy and other deaf players. Newspaper clippings dating back to 1888 link Hoy with using hand signals. According to Steve Sandy and Richard Miller, Hoy "invented the basic hand signals of baseball: those used by outfielders to avoid collisions on fly balls; those from the manager or coach to batters to indicate bunt, hit, or other options; and the umpires' signals for strikes and balls." Paul Helms, Hoy's nephew, claimed that umpires, managers, and players found baseball hand signals so useful that they became standard practice.[26] Historian Lee Allen wrote that Cincinnati players signaled strikes to Hoy by raising their right arms. Other baseball historians, however, deny that Hoy influenced the creation of signals. Hoy could read the lips of an umpire only a few feet away and might not have needed a manual signal. Cy Rigler may have created signals for balls and strikes while umpiring in the Central League on April 30, 1905. Bill Klem, a colorful umpire who began officiating two years after Hoy retired, is credited with introducing hand signals to the NL in 1905, as noted on his National Baseball Hall of Fame plaque.[27]

Hoy, on October 26, 1898, married Anna Maria Lowery, who likewise was deaf and taught the deaf in Ohio. They had three children, Carson, a distinguished Ohio jurist, and Carmen and Clover, who taught in schools for the deaf. After his retirement from baseball, Hoy purchased a 60-acre dairy farm in Mount Healthy, Ohio, near Cincinnati. During World War I, he supervised hundreds of deaf workers. After selling his farm in 1924, Hoy worked as a personnel director for deaf employees at the Goodyear Rubber Company in Akron, Ohio, and was employed by the Methodist Book Concern in Cincinnati.[28]

Hoy, who remained active in deaf, youth, and adult baseball organizations, received belated recognition. In 1951, he became the first deaf athlete elected into the American Athletic Association of the Deaf's Hall of Fame. Hoy was selected to the Louisville Colonels Hall of Fame in 1941 and Cincinnati Reds Hall of Fame in 2003. A baseball field at Gallaudet University in Washington, D.C., was named for him. Several former teammates, including Mack, Wagner, Crawford, and pitcher Clark Griffith, lobbied unsuccessfully for his inclusion in the National Baseball Hall of Fame. His name appeared on the Veterans Committee ballots several times, but he has never been chosen.[29]

Gould contended that Hoy belongs in the Hall of Fame because of "his excellent, sustained play over a long career" and claimed that 12 players from Hoy's era have been chosen with records not exceeding his exemplary statistics. He especially lauded Hoy's "great fielding," "savvy base running," and "more than adequate hitting." "Hoy's deafness," Gould argued, deprived him "of a necessary tool for the later renown that gets men into the Hall by sustained reputation." The press seldom interviewed him, denying him greater recognition. "Few reporters ever bothered to interview Hoy at all, even though he was probably the smartest player in baseball at the time. They were discomfited, didn't know how, or just didn't want to bother with the extra time needed to read and write answers."[30]

On October 7, 1961, the fragile, white-haired, 99-year-old Hoy threw out the ceremonial first ball in Game 3 of the World Series between the Cincinnati Reds and the New York Yankees at Crosley Field. He died of a stroke 69 days later in Cincinnati, five months and eight days short of his 100th birthday, having lived longer than any other major leaguer until Conrado Marrero.[31]

Hoy's baseball accomplishments loom especially large because he could not hear or speak and was the first deaf player to have an extensive major league career. "Hoy started out as the small deaf boy with big dreams, going off to play professional baseball against all odds." The deaf center fielder "proved it could be done," becoming "one of baseball's original 'spark-plugs' and finest 'fly-hawks.'" Hoy's "determination, honesty, character and energy left a lasting impression on all he met. He became a hero to the deaf community and to all handicapped people to aspire to reach for their dreams." Above all, "he was such an exemplary performer and human being."[32]

# HARRY GREB

"The Human Windmill" with "speed, ferocity, endurance, and will to win" summarizes Harry Greb, who did not let a major sports injury impede his boxing career. Greb became blind in his right eye during a 1921 bout with Kid Norfolk, but concealed the injury. He returned to the ring within one week and later became American light-heavyweight and world middleweight champion.

Greb experienced a working-class socioeconomic upbringing. Edward Henry Greb, the only son of Pius Greb, a stonemason, and Anna Wilbert Greb, was born on June 6, 1894, in Pittsburgh and grew up in a strict household. He attended Pittsburgh schools and became an electrician's apprentice at Westinghouse Electric and Manufacturing Corporation in 1910. In 1913, Greb defeated three Pittsburgh amateur boxers to win a tournament at Waldemeir Hall in March. Greb's father had no respect for boxing and wanted him to pursue baseball instead. After just two more amateur bouts, however, Greb was signed to a professional boxing contract by James "Red" Mason and fought professionally until August 1926. In 1913, he battled Frank Kirkwood to a six-round no-decision on May 29 and recorded his first victory over Battling Murphy by technical knockout on July 19.

The 5-foot 8-inch, 158-pound Greb competed mostly as a middleweight, exhibiting an unusual boxing style. The fearless, aggressive fighter was nicknamed "The Human Windmill" because he threw punches in rapid flurries. Although not a hard puncher, he masterfully tantalized opponents. Greb's "unorthodox style frustrated nearly all of his opponents."[1] The New York Sun observed that the Pittsburgh boxer "has two active hands that fly around in all sorts of weird motions," but pointed out, "The top of his head is his most dangerous weapon." Greb wore down opponents with tenacious in-fighting tactics during frequent clinches, rarely absorbing much punishment because opponents were preoccupied defending themselves from his powerful punches. "He punched with accuracy and rapidity, tossing punches from all angles."[2]

Greb stayed in excellent physical condition, averaging 22 bouts annually. His most notable early opponents included light heavyweight champions Battling Levinsky, Mike McTigue, and Jack Dillon, and world middleweight champion Frank Klaus. Before the 1920s, Greb fought twice unofficially for the world middleweight title. He needed knockout victories to capture the crown because these were newspaper-decision bouts, but did not achieve that objective in either fight. Greb dominated Al McCoy at Exposition Hall in Pittsburgh on April 30, 1917, taking all 10 rounds. McCoy, who retained the title, termed it "the worst ring beating he had ever received as a fighter."[3] In his second title bout, Greb lost a very close, 10-round decision to Mike O'Dowd on February 25, 1918, at the Auditorium in St. Paul, Minnesota.

Greb wed long-time acquaintance Mildred Reilly in Pittsburgh on January 30, 1919. They were married four years and had one daughter, Dorothy. Mildred succumbed on March 23, 1923, from a lengthy battle with tuberculosis in Pittsburgh. Although tenacious in the boxing arena, "Greb found his young wife's imminent death unbearable."[4] Greb, who boxed frequently, took a three-month respite. He later was engaged to Pennsylvania native Naomi Braden and planned to marry her in late 1926.

Greb, a southpaw, developed blindness in his right eye while defeating Kid Norfolk on August 29, 1921, at Forbes Field in Pittsburgh. He won a 10-round decision, taking rounds two and six through 10, and wore down Norfolk with very physical

tactics in repeated clinches. "The final rounds were tough, but Greb was able to cap-
italize on Norfolk's tiring and 'lacking steam' in his punches." The *Pittsburgh Post*
noted, "Greb's only mark was a puffed left eye."[5]

Newspapers, however, did not report the damage Greb suffered to his right eye.
Five years later, Dr. Carl McGivern, his personal physician based in Atlantic City,
New Jersey, disclosed that Norfolk had blinded Greb in the right eye with a blow in
their 1921 bout.[6] Gloves featured free-moving thumbs with little padding and considerable flexibility. Norfolk thumbed Greb in the right eye in retaliation for the
latter's tussling and tugging when they were in clinches. Bill Paxton, Greb's biographer,
speculates that a Norfolk punch caused the trauma to Greb's right eye. "A retinal tear
occurred five days later with visual impairment starting up around two weeks after
that. Once he started experiencing the visual problems, it was possibly partial blindness in different quadrants of the eye."

When Greb fought Chuck Wiggins to a no-decision in Cliffside, Kentucky, on
September 5, his vision probably was not yet impaired. His retinal tear, however,
had started by September 20 when he defeated Joe Cox at Coney Island. Greb did
not compete again until outpointing Jimmy Darcy on October 24 in Buffalo, New
York. Greb visited Dr. McGivern in Atlantic City after the Cox bout for treatment.

Greb's last 89 bouts likely were fought with vision in only his left eye. Greb
deliberately kept the blindness in his right eye secret except for notifying family, a
few intimate friends, and his doctor. Otherwise, boxers would have exploited that
knowledge to their advantage and thrown more punches from that side. The boxing
commission might have banned him from further bouts, too.[7]

Greb's unconventional method enabled him to continue boxing with just one
eye. His windmill style involved perpetual motion, letting his left eye view his opponent from different angles. After suffering the eye trauma, "Greb started thumbing
people in his fights and being extra rough." Despite blindness, he still fought "by any
means necessary, even if it meant using some rough tactics he had learned along the
way to help compensate for his handicap."

On March 13, 1922, Greb trounced highly favored Tom Gibbons in 15 rounds
at Madison Square Garden in New York, becoming the top American light heavyweight contender. The 5-foot 9½-inch, 197-pound Gibbons enjoyed a height, weight,
and sight advantage and possessed a powerful knockout punch. Greb, fearless and
undaunted, seized the initiative from the outset and took all but rounds two and
seven. "Greb had set an incredible pace for the entire fight and just never let up."[8]
Greb deliberately tricked Gibbons, lowering his hands to his side and goading his
opponent into throwing a right-hand punch. He constantly landed uppercuts with
his right hand before Gibbons responded. Greb capitalized on his "aggressiveness,
footwork, cleverness and courage." According to the *Chicago Daily Tribune*, "For
nearly the entire fight Gibbons was at the receiving end of the greatest shower of
blows he had ever seen in his life."[9]

Greb challenged American light heavyweight champion Gene Tunney in a 15-round bout at Madison Square Garden on May 23, 1922. The 6-foot, 171-pound Tunney, who had won 29 consecutive contests, was 13 pounds heavier, possessed a height advantage and longer reach, and was three years younger. The Greb-Tunney bout resembled "a cross between a boxing contest and a back-alley mugging."[10] Greb defeated Tunney, taking 12 of 15 rounds. In the first round, his powerful left hook broke Tunney's nose. Greb targeted Tunney's face "with rights and lefts while circling his wounded prey." He attacked Tunney from all angles, moving constantly so he would not receive punches that he could not see and could fight rougher on the inside to compensate for his partial blindness. Tunney, whose nose bled profusely, barely withstood the onslaught. "Greb's speed seemed to increase and his bombardment became more furious." Greb combined his patented "windmill" attack with "grabbing Tunney behind the head with one hand while punching with the other."[11]

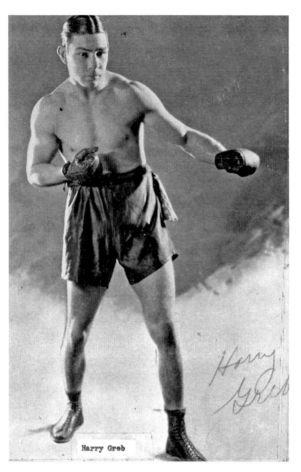

Harry Greb fought more than 300 times from 1913 to 1926, held the middleweight and light heavyweight titles, and defeated every member of the International Boxing Hall of Fame he ever fought (collection of Bill Paxton, www.harrygreb.com).

Greb, benefitting from his conditioning and training, completely dominated Tunney. He unleashed a series lefts and rights, forcing Tunney toward the ropes, and would have scored a knockout if he had "possessed a big punch." Greb dealt Tunney such a thorough thrashing that the latter remained bedridden for a week. After boxing nearly a decade, Greb finally had won a title. "His speed and endurance mixed with almost a decade of experience and a will to win had finally paid off."[12]

Tunney immediately demanded a rematch. Lightweight champion Benny Leonard taught Tunney how to adapt his technique to Greb's scientific style. Tunney had concentrated on Greb's head rather than his body. Leonard instructed Tunney to come underneath Greb's elbows and strike him in his midsection. The tactic proved invaluable in Tunney's rematch with Greb.

Greb defeated Bob Roper on November 10, 1922, in Buffalo, although likely losing the sight in his right eye completely. Roper "may have thumbed Greb's eye at close range, worsening Greb's retinal tear." Doctors examined Greb's eyes at West Penn Hospital in Pittsburgh in early December, but he "was probably fully blind in the right eye."

On January 30, 1923, Greb retained his light heavyweight title against Tommy Loughran in a 15-rounder at Madison Square Garden. He already had defeated Loughran twice. Loughran seized the initiative the first three rounds, but Greb

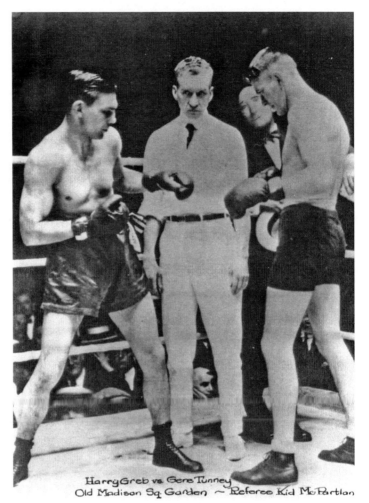

Harry Greb vs Gene Tunney
Old Madison Sq Garden ~ Referee Kid McPartlan

Despite being blind in his right eye, Harry Greb (left) defeated Gene Tunney (right) in 15 rounds on May 23, 1922, at Madison Square Garden in New York City to win the light heavyweight championship. Referee Kid McPartland is shown in the center (collection of Bill Paxton, www.harrygreb.com).

dominated thereafter and "kept Loughran on the defensive" the next nine rounds. Loughran often clung to Greb "to weather the storm, but Greb would just punch away using both hands."[13] Loughran attempted a futile comeback in the last three rounds.

Around 13,000 spectators packed Madison Square Garden for the Greb-Tunney rematch on February 23, 1923. Billy Gibbons, Tunney's manager, warned officials about Greb's fighting style. Greb worried the referee might disqualify him for fighting his normal style. "Greb swarmed all over Tunney" from the outset, punching him in the head. To Greb's dismay, Tunney effectively employed Leonard's strategy of hitting

Greb below his elbows at the midsection. He unleashed persistent, penetrating right-hand blows to Greb's left side through the first five rounds. Greb started dancing more, winning rounds six through 12. Referee Arthur Haley warned Greb after the twelfth round for attempting to butt Tunney in the clinches.

The momentum shifted abruptly in round 14. Tunney landed a right to Greb's face and again crouched to the breadbasket, bringing Greb's hands down. "It was do or die for Tunney now." Tunney landed "a right hand smash that caught Greb's jaw almost flush."[14] The crowd arose "in an uproar." Tunney continued "unleashing a fusillade of punches as the round wound down"[15] to Greb's midsection, forcing the latter on the defensive for the first time.

Tunney recaptured the American light heavyweight title in a controversial split decision. Judge Charles Miles scored Greb the winner, but Haley and the second judge declared Tunney the victor. The difference maker proved Tunney's devastating right to the jaw in the fourteenth round. According to Haley, "Greb's foul tactics, including holding and butting, influenced the verdict which he and the judges gave to Tunney, despite the Pittsburgher's apparent margin on points." Although the crowd backed Tunney, most sportswriters believed either that Greb prevailed or fought to a draw. New York State Athletic Commission chairman William Muldoon insisted that Greb should have been declared the winner.[16]

In a December 10, 1923, rematch with Greb at Madison Square Garden, Tunney retained his American light heavyweight title. He seized the offensive this time, concentrating again on Greb's midsection, and won by unanimous decision, taking nine of the 15 rounds. Greb performed best in the final round, but took only three other rounds. "The Greb-Tunney fights were sensational ring encounters."[17] Greb drew with Tunney in September 1924 and lost in March 1925.

Greb, meanwhile, had challenged Johnny Wilson for the world middleweight championship on August 31, 1923, at the Polo Grounds in New York. Although holding the American light heavyweight championship, he was a natural middleweight and coveted most the elusive world middleweight crown. After considerable reluctance, Wilson eventually agreed to fight Greb, whom he thought was out of shape. Surgeons had operated on Greb for an infection in his right arm. Greb quickly seized the initiative and dominated Wilson. Wilson focused on a body attack, but Greb proved too quick and a "shifty and elusive target."[18] Greb hurt Wilson's left eye with a hard punch in the eighth round, and his nose with a hard punch in round 10. Six rounds later, Wilson's left eye was nearly closed and his mouth was bleeding. By round 15, "Greb was fresh and alert, while Wilson still seemed bewildered." Greb had drubbed the unpopular Wilson, capturing nearly every round. Announcer Joe Humphries declared Greb the new world middleweight champion, fulfilling the latter's dream. According to the *Chicago Tribune*, Greb fought "rings around Johnny Wilson." "My speed would be too much for Wilson," Greb said. "I am Wilson's master,"[19] he boasted.

Greb ruled the world middleweight division from 1923 to 1926, defending his title six times. His first title defense came against Bryan Downey on December 3, 1923, at Motor Square Garden in Pittsburgh. Downey won the first round, but Greb took rounds three through 10, "whaling away at the Columbus tough guy." Greb won the bout easily, having "outfought, outpunched, outgeneraled, and outroughed Bryan Downey."[20]

Greb defended his middleweight title on January 18, 1924, against Wilson in 15 rounds at Madison Square Garden. He controlled the fight, especially rounds nine and 11, losing only the fourth round, and intensifying the pace in the final two rounds. "He finished the fight strong and quick, completely dominating Wilson." The *Pittsburgh Post* reported Greb "dealt a thorough licking to Johnny Wilson."[21]

Greb retained the middleweight title with a one-sided, 12-round technical knockout (TKO) of Fay Keiser on March 24, 1924, at the 104th Regiment Armory in Baltimore. In round 12, Greb put "everything into a right swing, flopped the groggy Keiser to the floor." Keiser was "battered and bleeding, floored with a hefty right to the chin and then arising in a pitiful condition, [until] the referee [Charley Short] humanely stepped in."[22]

Greb's next middleweight title defense came against Ted Moore on June 26, 1924, at Yankee Stadium in New York. Greb won by decision, taking all 15 rounds except the sixth and seventh. The referee disqualified Greb in round six for using dirty tactics after the bell sounded. "Moore had to defend himself against a ceaseless two-fisted attack to the face."[23] He landed one good punch in the ninth round that only enlivened Greb. Greb nearly won by knockout twice in the latter rounds.

Greb fought 22 more times in 1924 and 1925 before defending his middleweight crown against world welterweight champion Mickey Walker on July 2, 1925, at the Polo Grounds. During that span, Greb fought Tunney twice, and Jimmy Slattery and Wilson once each. The fight ranked among the great donnybrooks. Over 60,000 fans witnessed Greb win a 15-round decision. Greb nearly knocked down Walker with a left to the jaw in the second round and captured 12 of the 15 rounds, taking rounds four, 11, 13, and 14 decisively. Walker took only the first and twelfth. The *Pittsburgh Press* called Greb "a master boxer," who "bewildered Walker at nearly every stage, took the hardest raps the heavier puncher landed and still had stamina left to finish with a blaze of speed and glory." The *Pittsburgh Post* concluded, "Walker never had a real chance to win and it was only his indomitable spirit which carried him across to the final bell."[24]

On July 16, 1925, Greb defeated light heavyweight Maxie Rosenbloom in a 10-round decision in Cleveland, Ohio. Rosenbloom fought well the first three rounds, but Greb seized the momentum by the sixth round, flooring him in the seventh.

On August 19, 1925, the one-eyed Greb was involved in an automobile accident with two other cars near Erie, Pennsylvania. When Greb slammed on the brakes to avoid the crash, his car wheels locked and his vehicle slid and overturned.[25] Greb was rushed to West Penn Hospital with two fractured ribs and cuts and bruises on his back and chest. The fractured ribs were near his lung, making breathing difficult. Greb's boxing skills diminished after the accident.

Theodore "Tiger" Flowers, another southpaw, wrested the middleweight title from Greb on February 26, 1926, in a split 15-round decision at Madison Square Garden. By 1926, Greb's vision in his right eye had been completely gone for four years. Greb easily had defeated Flowers, then a welterweight, in a 10-round decision on August 21, 1924, in Fremont, Ohio. No African American had challenged for any boxing title since Jack Johnson won the heavyweight crown in 1908.

The Greb-Flowers match was fiercely contested. Judges Tom Flynn and Charles Mathison ruled for Flowers, while referee Gunboat Smith backed Greb. Flowers did not knock down Greb or punish him seriously. The judges detected "Harry's inability to put usual speed and accuracy behind his windmill attack." Flowers prevailed "not because of how well he fought," but due to Greb's sub-par performance. He became the first African American to capture the middleweight crown. "The final verdict shocked the passionate Greb, who "had finally lost the title that he seemed to 'love more than life.'" Greb rationalized, "I have never been right since that accident last summer." He also believed that he had overtrained for the fight. The *Pittsburgh Post* noted the defending champion "was so far off his accustomed form that it seemed as though his name was not Greb."[26]

Greb's final bout resulted in another closely contested 15-round split decision loss to Flowers on August 19, 1926, at Madison Square Garden. Referee Jim Crowley determined Greb the winner, but judges Mathison and Harold Burnes declared Flowers the victor. Flowers took seven rounds, Greb won six, and the third and seventh were even. Flowers fared best in the middle rounds, while Greb triumphed in rounds one, four, six, 11, 14, and 15. Round eight proved decisive. Greb knocked down the champion onto the canvas and dominated the round, but both judges scored the round for Flowers because of the former's foul tactics. Greb, who continued fighting after the bell sounded, fared best in the last two rounds, but it was too late. The Pittsburgher had not fought as well as anticipated. His unfair tactics, which included "unwarranted pushing and mauling which once sent Flowers through the ropes," also swung the momentum to Flowers.[27] "The crowd," the *New York Times* wrote, "thought that Greb should have received the decision." Paxton concluded, however, "Greb's best years were behind him."[28]

Greb had accomplished much after a ring injury gradually caused blindness in one eye. This injury should have ended his boxing career, but he kept his condition secret. Although boxing professionally for only 14 years, Greb officially fought 294 times with 112 wins, only eight losses, three draws, one no-contest, and 170 no-decisions. Nearly 60 percent of his bouts ended without victory or defeat. Greb was knocked out only once, by Joe Chip on November 29, 1913, at Old City Hall in Pittsburgh. He defeated opponents who outweighed him by over 30 pounds, held the middleweight and light heavyweight titles, and prevailed against all 11 International Boxing Hall of Fame champions he faced. Among world champions, only welterweight Jack Britton and featherweight Johnny Dundee fought more often. Greb engaged in more bouts than heavyweight champions Jim Corbett, Jim Jeffries, Tunney, Joe Louis, Rocky Marciano, and Muhammad Ali combined.

Greb was elected to *The Ring*'s Boxing Hall of Fame in 1955 and the International Boxing Hall of Fame in 1990. In 2001, *The Ring* magazine voted Greb the greatest middleweight of all time. Greb may have been his era's greatest boxer. "Greb battled the past, present, and future champions in the top three weight divisions, beating every single one of them." He defeated middleweight champions Chip, McCoy, Wilson, Flowers, and Walker, light heavyweight champions Loughran, McTigue, Dillon, Levinsky, Slattery, and Rosenbloom, and heavyweight champion Tunney. Tunney observed, "Greb is the gamest man I ever met and the most remarkable product I have ever seen in the ring."[29]

In July 1926, Greb entered the Atlantic City hospital to have his right eye completely removed and replaced with a stone glass eye. Dr. McGivern had feared that the condition would spread to his left eye and make him totally blind. Dr. Gustav Guist, an Austrian eye specialist, performed the surgery.

During early October, the visually impaired Greb was involved in another automobile accident in Pittsburgh. He tried to avoid two farmers whose wagons were obstructing the road. His car plunged over an embankment, opening the wound from the operation and fracturing several bones in his nose. Greb complained of headaches and dizziness.

Tragically, the indomitable Greb died at age 32 from complications during minor surgery. On October 22, 1926, doctors operated on Greb to remove a fractured bone in his nose. Greb was having difficulty breathing. Dr. Weinberg, one of the surgeons, stated, "Evidently a piece of bone extending from the bridge of the nose to the floor of the skull had been fractured in such a manner that a blood clot was formed in the brain."[30] A day after the operation, Greb fell into a coma and died of heart failure in Atlantic City.

On October 27, the *New York Times* notified readers that Greb had a glass eye and had fought with a blind right eye his final five years. Ida Edwards, his sister, disclosed, "Harry didn't want to let anybody know about it" except for family, a few intimate friends, and the surgeons who had operated on him.[31] He had overcome the blindness to win titles in two boxing divisions.

# Part II. Accidents and Injuries

## *Accidents*

### GLENN CUNNINGHAM

"Never quit! Run on!" was the motto of Glenn Cunningham, who conquered adversity to become a legendary track miler. Cunningham's legs were so badly burned in a schoolhouse fire as an elementary school student that doctors predicted that he would never walk again. After being bedridden for nearly two years, he not only learned to walk again, but to run and to shatter the world record for the indoor mile.

Cunningham came from a lower-class socioeconomic background. Glenn Vernice Cunningham was born in Atlanta, Kansas, on August 4, 1909, and had six siblings. His father, Clint, worked as a water-well driller and also performed odd jobs, while his mother, Rosa, was a homemaker. As a seven-year-old, Cunningham attended one-room Sunflower School in Rolla, Kansas, located about two miles from the two-story farmhouse his family rented. On the cold morning of February 9, 1916, he, his 11-year old sister Letha, his 13 year old brother Floyd, and his nine year old brother Raymond headed for school. Margie, his 14-year-old sister, stayed at home that morning to care for two younger siblings, Johnny and Melva.

Glenn, Letha, Floyd, and Raymond arrived at Sunflower School before their teacher, Mr. Schroeder, and their 19 classmates. Letha played on the frozen, sandy, snow-blown schoolyard. Floyd, Raymond, and Glenn entered the school via the side door, which clicked shut behind them. Raymond and Glenn played tick-tack-toe at the blackboard, while Floyd went to put wood inside the big pot-bellied stove to start the fire to heat the room.

After playing games and drawing on the blackboard with Raymond, Glenn started walking toward the rear of the room. Floyd reached over for a five-gallon can he thought contained kerosene and started to pour it on the pot-bellied stove. Glenn smelled something suspicious as Floyd uncapped the can. Unbeknownst to Floyd, the fuel can contained gasoline. The Ladies' Literary Society had met at the schoolhouse the previous night and had rebuilt the fire. They had filled their lanterns with gasoline before returning home and carelessly left gasoline in the can that normally held kerosene to prime the stove.

An explosion occurred, engulfing the building in flames and badly burning the legs of both Floyd and Glenn. Glenn recalled, "A blinding flash seared my eyes and made my head swim. An awful force, as if from hell itself, hurled me painfully back against the wall." Floyd screamed, "I'm on fire." Glenn also was afire and writhed in pain on the floor. He tried to get up, but his legs buckled. "They felt awful — like they had been burned off,"[1] he remembered. Glenn crawled painfully after Raymond, but could not escape the mounting flames. Raymond ran through the smoke to the side door and yelled to Letha to open it up. Letha saw the flames and smoke inside the windows and raced to the side door, jerking it open. Raymond and Glenn rolled over, trying to smother the flames. Floyd staggered to his feet and yelled, "We gotta get home!"[2] They thought their parents would know what to do.

Glenn and Floyd incredibly tried to run the two miles home. Only the top of Floyd's jacket remained. Both of Glenn's pant legs had burned away and deep burns were on his legs. Glenn fell down after staggering only 100 feet. Raymond prodded him to get up and continue the two-mile trek home. Glenn stumbled to his feet and began hobbling again. Raymond kept encouraging Glenn, while Letha prodded Floyd.

Only Margie, Johnny, and Melva were home at the time because Clint had left to pick up Rosa, who had spent the night with an ill neighbor. Raymond ran to get his parents. After opening the front door of the farmhouse, Margie gasped in horror when she saw Letha drag Floyd the last few steps. Floyd collapsed inside the door with a loud groan, falling into Margie's arms. Margie gingerly removed Glenn's clothing, while he howled in pain. Floyd stared glassy-eyed at the ceiling, not making a sound. Margie removed Floyd's burning shoes and temporarily put them in a small sled outside the door. Glenn recalled, "The fire remaining consumed both the sled and the shoes." Margie moved Floyd and Glenn to their parent's downstairs bed. "I remember screaming and not being able to stop,"[3] Glenn recollected.

Mr. Heinrich, a German neighbor who lived alone, clumsily wrapped Glenn's throbbing wounds. Rosa held him down until Dr. Fergusen arrived. Dr. Fergusen examined Glenn, and then talked to Clint and Rosa outside. He warned Clint and Rosa that both of Glenn's badly burned legs might have to be amputated. "If the infection gets too bad," Dr. Fergusen added, "we won't have any choice but to amputate. Regardless, Glenn will never be able to walk again on those legs." Clint and Rosa had trouble accepting the doctor's pessimistic prognostication. Glenn's right leg was nearly three inches shorter than his left leg. His toes were nearly burned off his left foot and both of his arches were damaged. Glenn lost all of the flesh on his knees and shins. Dr. Fergusen tried treating Floyd, but realized, "There's not much we can do" because he was "too badly burned."[4]

Floyd's condition steadily worsened the next several days. Ashen-faced, Floyd did not even notice when family members were in the room. He did not speak, ate little, and seldom moved. If needing assistance, he stared vacantly until someone came. Around midnight each night, Floyd hummed the hymn, "God Be with You Till We Meet Again." He never recovered, succumbing nine days after the explosion.

Glenn's legs steadily worsened and pained him, especially at night. Glenn experienced terrible dreams about the fire and feared that he would never walk again. He wondered whether infection had set in because he could no longer bend either leg at the knee and recalled his legs "were so bad now that I could hardly stand the pain that came from just resting them on the bed." Glenn fantasized about standing, walking, and perhaps even running again. His siblings took turns lifting his legs off the bed to relieve the pain. A huge boil formed on his left hip. Glenn also suffered from a large burn on his right leg, forcing him to remain on his back. An Elkhart visitor told Rosa, "Glenn's going to be an invalid the rest of his life." Glenn, who overheard the conversation, countered, "I'm NOT going to be an invalid." Rosa assured him, "I know she's wrong."[5]

Glenn's legs did not heal the next several months as the infection spread through his legs. Dr. Fergusen changed Glenn's dressings and found the burns "so severe" that he did not rule out amputation. He patted Glenn's shoulder and promised to let him sit on the porch when the weather warmed. Dr. Fergusen tried consoling him, "It takes time, Glenn." Glenn retorted, "You're thinking I'm never gonna get well; my legs are always gonna be like this!" Glenn dreamt about running again, declaring, "I want to walk and run. And I will."[6] But the awful ache in his legs, throbbing boil, and stabbing bedsores threatened to dash his dreams.

Scar tissue covered the wounds after four painful months, "but the legs remained useless, the tendons unresponsive, muscles tight, twisted, powerless." Glenn still believed "those legs would again jump and skip and hop as a boy might command them." Rosa changed his dressings and massaged his legs daily, even though there was little muscle and sinew left to rub. "For hours she kneaded the damaged muscles and flxed the legs. When fatigue forced her to quit, Glenn took over."[7]

In August 1917, Dr. Fergusen tried again to bend Glenn's stiff legs and challenged him to walk. Glenn attempted to bend his legs and take a step, but could not. "My legs wouldn't move,"[8] he recollected. Glenn sobbed as Dr. Fergusen and Rosa lifted him back into bed. Dr. Fergusen decided not to amputate Glenn's legs, but doubted he would ever use them very much.

His parents moved Glenn to an upstairs bedroom to give him a change of scenery. Glenn asked Clint to bring him a sturdy, homemade chair from downstairs to put beside his bed and used that chair as his exercise machine for several weeks in 1917. He pulled himself slowly from his bed to the chair seat and then into an erect position. The bed sores gradually healed, but his legs hurt constantly. The day before Christmas, 22 grueling months after the explosion, Glenn told Rosa he had a present for her and asked her to close her eyes. Glenn slipped from the bed and took his first few faltering steps toward her. "Mother's small gray eyes widened," Glenn said, "Then she made a choking sound as she rushed forward to catch me in her arms. We sank to the floor, hugging one another."[9] They both cried with tears of joy. Glenn repeated his teetering walk for his siblings that afternoon.

On Christmas morning, Clint carried Glenn downstairs. Glenn, who had not seen the downstairs in several months, excitedly shouted, "I'm walking again. I told you I would walk again." Rosa replied, "It has to be a miracle." Glenn later explained, "As long as you believe you can do things, they're not impossible. You place limits on yourself mentally, not physically."[10] The Biblical verse Isaiah 40:31 inspired him: "But those who wait on the Lord shall renew their strength; they shall mount up with wings like eagles; they shall run, and not be weary; they shall walk and not faint."

Dr. Fergusen grew cautiously optimistic upon learning about Glenn's halting steps. The sight of his walking transfixed Dr. Fergusen. "It was a strange limping gait, but Glenn was walking, unaided." Glenn laughed, "I told you I'd walk. Next time, I'll run."[11] Glenn's right leg was still weak and would not straighten out, but his knees were loosening. Intense stiffness replaced the throbbing pain in his legs.

Dr. Fergusen wanted Glenn to exercise. Clint took his family on a wagon to catch rabbits in 1918 and challenged Glenn to walk. Glenn initially balked because exercise made his legs stiffer and more painful. He hobbled slowly forward and nearly fell, muttering, "Can't he understand that I'm still not well?" Glenn limped about a quarter of a mile and then took a dozen steps back toward the wagon when Clint picked him up and carried him the rest of the way. Clint eventually challenged him to run late one afternoon. Glenn wanted to run, but needed someone to assist him. He grabbed the tail of a cow and let it pull him, taking weight off his legs. By the fall of 1918, his legs had strengthened considerably. Clint's words inspired him, "Never quit. Always get out there and try to overcome, no matter what."[12] By 1919, Cunningham even began running again "for the sheer joy of it" and saw his speed gradually return. "We lived on the farm and when we went from the house to the corral, we would run," he recalled. "We ran everywhere, even my brother and I when we went to the country school."[13]

The Cunninghams moved in 1919 from the rental farmhouse to a tent about a mile from Elkhart, Kansas, a town of 2,000 people, 20 miles further west. After residing there for just one year, they spent a year in Colorado. They returned to Elkhart and rented a small frame house near the city. Glenn did not attend school either during his year of rehabilitation or in Colorado and was only in fourth grade as a 12-year-old. He finally had recovered his health after a lengthy battle.

Cunningham scuffled with a larger boy one day at school, knocking him down and punching him several times. The confrontation inspired him to compete against larger boys in athletic competition. Cunningham vowed, "I'll learn to run again! I'm even gonna win races again."[14] Although experiencing a long, harrowing recovery, he had fought back and developed a stronger body.

The following week, 13-year-old Cunningham entered the mile run in the school track and field meet. "I want to win that little medal they got on display in the drugstore window," he told a classmate, "the one for the mile run. It looks like it might be pure gold." "Win? You?" the classmate scoffed. "Don't be a fool, Scarlegs!" Cunningham's parents disapproved of his participation in athletic events. "But he wanted that medal so badly that he sneaked away and entered the race."[15] Cunningham's legs felt stronger despite having several ugly places where the flesh had not grown completely back.

The race took place at a cow pasture at the edge of Elkhart. Cunningham, who wore tennis shoes, faced eight competitors, mostly high school students with spiked shoes. He started out slowly, pacing himself. Cunningham overtook all except two tall front runners after the first lap, but did not know he was supposed to pass them on the outer side of the track. He ran between them rather than around them, moving under their pumping elbows. Cunningham then pulled away from the other runners and crossed the finish line well ahead of the other runners, ducking the string stretched across the track. One spectator yelled to him, "You gotta break the string to win." He whirled back and touched the string seconds before two other runners reached it. The crowd roared. Cunningham, who captured the medal, soon realized hundreds of people saw him "win a race no one had thought I'd ever finish."[16]

The thrill of victory quickly turned to emptiness, however, because he never received the medal. Since Cunningham did not claim the medal after the race, Mr. Simmons, his principal, sent it back. Cunningham recalled, "I was so scared after the race that I ran home so my father wouldn't know I had entered." Although disappointed about what happened to the medal, he noted that the race marked "the beginning of my career as a mile runner."[17]

Cunningham's fourth grade teacher inspired him to pursue more education and fulfill his dreams. Cunningham yearned to acquire all the education he could as quickly as possible. He saw a film newsreel featuring Paavo Nurmi, the great Finnish runner, setting a new world record for the mile in four minutes, 10.4 seconds. "Some day, I'm gonna break a record," he told his sister, Melva.[18] Melva snickered.

By age 15, as a junior high student, Cunningham defeated all the local high school runners. He attended Elkhart High School, participating in football, basketball, and track and field, singing in the glee club, and studying the violin. Since his legs were deeply scarred, Cunningham always needed an extensive massage and warmed up for an hour to restore his circulation. Cunningham's endurance and strength compensated for his lack of a smooth or efficient style.[19] Cunningham maintained that pre-race routine throughout his high school career. In his first race as a sophomore, he easily defeated the Elkhart scholastic mile record holder and shattered the local high school record by 18.9 seconds. He, however, disobeyed his coach Bill Mulligan, who had ordered him not to sprint until the stretch. Mulligan refused to let him run the mile again that season.

Mulligan taught Cunningham to stretch out his legs, lengthen his stride, and use a rocking motion with his heel and toe. Cunningham obeyed his coach this time as a junior and won every event, unofficially breaking the world scholastic mile record. Mulligan took him in the fall of 1928 to Chicago to compete against the nation's best runners. Cunningham, however, developed a blister in his heel from walking too much around Chicago and came down with a 104.5-degree fever. A doctor urged him not to run. Nevertheless, Cunningham stubbornly ran the next day and stumbled across the finish line in fourth place. His tortured heel pained him.

As a senior, 20-year-old Cunningham dominated the one mile and other Kansas scholastic races. At the Kansas state meet in Manhattan, he established a new state record for the mile at four minutes, 28.3 seconds. Mulligan again took him to Chicago to compete in the mile at the national scholastic meet at Stagg Field. After trailing in fourth place, Cunningham widened his stride, quickened his pace, and glided past the other runners into first place. The crowd roared as he neared the tape. "I was setting a new world record for the interscholastic mile!" Cunningham beamed. An ecstatic Mulligan shouted to him, "You did it. You broke the record." Cunningham had established the prep record with four minutes, 24.07 seconds for the mile. The citizens of Elkhart were overjoyed.[20]

During the depression, Cunningham attended the University of Kansas and worked his way through to defray his college expenses. NCAA rules banned freshmen from competing in intercollegiate sports, but he still worked out with the team in 1931. His scarred legs unfortunately started hurting again. Track and field coach John "Buck" Barnes ordered him to see the school doctor, who detected nothing seriously wrong. Cunningham discovered many years later that poison from an abscessed tooth that resulted from a baseball injury triggered much of his leg pain and stiffness. He was catching without a mask at baseball practice in 1928, when a tipped ball hit him in the mouth and knocked eight teeth loose. During Cunningham's sophomore year in 1932, an Iowa State University senior miler challenged him to a special race. Barnes urged Cunningham to take the lead by the second lap and to hasten the pace each subsequent lap and sprint toward the finish line on the final lap. Cunningham heard the roar of the crowd in the background, as he easily defeated his challenger.

At Kansas, Cunningham competed in the half-mile, mile, and two-mile races. He won six Big Six Conference titles, two NCAA Championships, and 10 Amateur Athletic Union (AAU) crowns in the one-mile event, with five being outdoor. He recorded his first major victories in 1932, capturing the 1500 meters at the Big Six Conference Championships and NCAA Outdoor Track and Field Championships. Barnes wanted Cunningham to try out for the 1932 U.S. Olympic track and field team. That had been Cunningham's dream since fourth grade. Cunningham made the 1932 U.S. Olympic team by winning the 1500-meter race on June 11 at the Olympic Trials in Chicago in a collegiate record time of four minutes, 11.1 seconds. He traveled 1,600 miles by train to compete in the Summer Olympic Games in Los Angeles, but suffered infected tonsils, a sore throat, and chest pains and finished a disappointing fourth in the 1500-meter race. Luigi Beccali of Italy won the gold medal in a clocking that Cunningham had bested several times. The setback taught him the importance of discipline and perseverance. He knew, "Whatever you attempt, never quit!"[21]

Cunningham, under new track and field head coach Bill Hargiss, enjoyed a banner year in 1933, earning the James E. Sullivan Award as the nation's top amateur athlete. He captured his second NCAA title in the mile in four minutes, 9.3 seconds. Cunningham recorded a rare double by taking AAU outdoor titles in both the 800 meters in one minute, 51.8 seconds, and the 1500 meters in three minutes, 52.3 seconds. He ran over 20 races in Europe and the Orient, winning 11. Cunningham also maintained busy 1934 indoor and outdoor seasons. In 1934, he earned his B.A. degree in physical education from Kansas with the highest academic record in his class.

In 1934, the mile run became the centerpiece of track and field meets, attracting public interest. The span, "the most exciting short period in the history of the 1500 and the mile," resulted in world records. Cunningham engaged in several exciting mile races with Bill Bonthron of Princeton University. Madison Square Garden in New York City turned away thousands wanting to watch Cunningham and Bonthron. "Their exploits made headlines throughout the country."[22] The pair ran some very close indoor races, tying each other in setting a new indoor record of three minutes, 52.2 seconds in the 1500 meters.

The duo met at the Princeton University Invitational Games on June 16, when 25,000 spectators witnessed Cunningham run perhaps the best race of his career. Cunningham, Bonthron, and Gene Venzke competed in the mile, with the Princeton runner heavily favored. Venzke led for the first lap, with Cunningham close behind. Halfway through the second lap, Cunningham seized the lead. Bonthron closed in on Cunningham, "seemingly ready to speed past him at the end of the race." During the third lap, however, Cunningham showed a tremendous burst of speed. "His scarred legs churned wildly" as he entered the last lap. "Around the turn, he opened up an alarming gap of 10 yards over Bonthron." Upon reaching the backstretch, Cunningham led Bonthron by 20 yards and Venzke trailed badly. The crowd began yelling for Cunningham. By the homestretch, Cunningham widened his lead over Bonthron to 40 yards. "He tore through the tape with a time of 4:06.7, a new world record."[23] Cunningham's mark lasted for three years. His lap times were 61.8 seconds, 64.0 seconds, 61.8 seconds, and 59.1 seconds, as his strategy of covering the second half faster than the first half paid dividends. He had run seven of the world's 13 fastest miles and accomplished his boyhood dream of lowering Nurmi's mark.

That summer, however, Bonthron bested Cunningham in other races, including the NCAA and AAU Outdoor Track and Field Championships. When Cunningham speeded up after two laps in the NCAA Championships at Los Angeles, "Bonthron exploded with an unbeatable kick which shot him five yards past Cunningham in the space of about 30 yards." Although both broke the existing world record, Bonthron also defeated him on June 30 at Milwaukee. Cunningham ran the 1500 meters in three minutes, 48.9 seconds, which would have set a new world record. Bonthron, however, covered the distance even faster in three minutes, 48.8 seconds. "It's a strange feeling to break a world's record and still lose,"[24] Cunningham said.

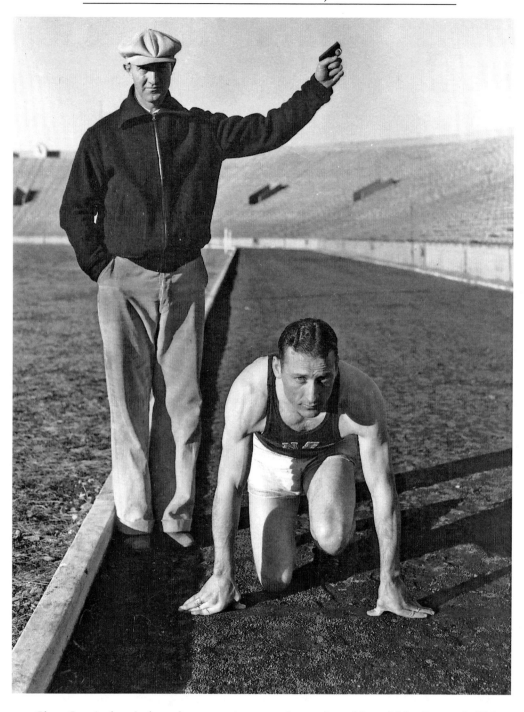

Glenn Cunningham is shown here preparing to run in practice at Memorial Stadium at the University of Kansas in Lawrence, circa 1933, with his track and field coach Bill Hargiss holding the starting gun. He competed in the mile for Kansas from 1931 to 1934, setting numerous records (courtesy Kansas Athletics).

In 1935, Cunningham prevailed in the 1500 meters in three minutes, 52.1 seconds at the AAU Outdoor Track and Field Championships and also won the Wanamaker Mile in four minutes, 11 seconds, with Venzke second and Bonthron third. Cunningham captured the 1500 meters at the 1936 AAU Outdoor Track and Field Championships again and the 1936 Olympic Trials, making the U.S. Olympic team for his second time. Cunningham's strategy of conserving his speed until the latter stages paid dividends. "He hung back, running slowly and not pushing the pace."[25]

Before the 1936 Summer Olympic Games, Cunningham vowed, "I wanted to show the world that I could do much better than I'd done four years before." The 1936 Olympic Games, held at Berlin, were highly politicized by Nazi dictator Adolf Hitler. Cunningham passed several

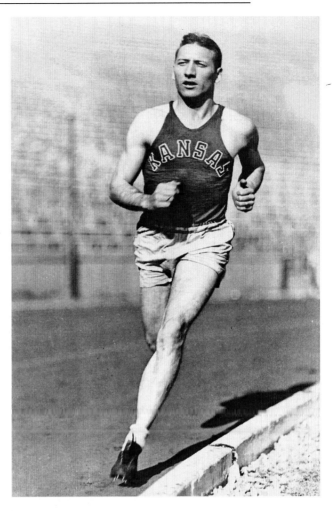

Glenn Cunningham, pictured here finishing a mile race for the University of Kansas, circa 1933, captured rare AAU outdoor titles in both the 800 meters and 1500 meters that year (courtesy Kansas Athletics).

runners, including Eric Ny of Sweden, Friedrich Schaumburg of Germany, Jack Lovelock of New Zealand, and Beccali of Italy, on the second lap of the 1500 meters. The pace became grueling. Cunningham lengthened his stride, pumped his arms harder, and appeared headed for victory. On the third lap, however, he experienced a sharp pain in his legs and was overtaken by Ny. The dampness and Berlin's cold weather had stiffened his legs. Cunningham explained, "I was pouring on the power when suddenly my legs began to hurt." Lovelock whipped past Cunningham and Ny and outsprinted them to the finish, setting a world record of three minutes, 47.8 seconds. Cunningham settled for a silver medal, being clocked in three minutes, 48.4 seconds, and Beccali placed third.[26]

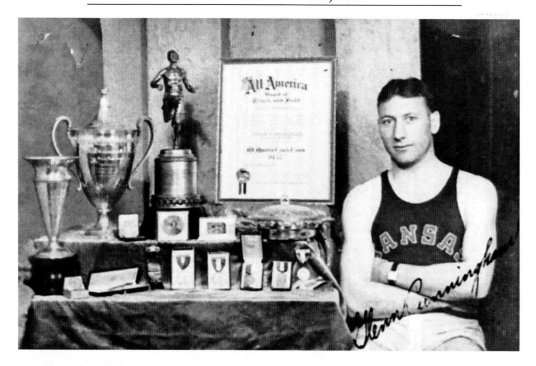

**Glenn Cunningham won numerous awards and trophies while competing in the mile for the University of Kansas. He received the James E. Sullivan Award as the best amateur athlete of 1933 (courtesy University of Kansas Athletics).**

Cunningham had recorded his fastest-ever time in the 1500 meters, breaking the American record. But Lovelock had established a new world record. "I broke the Olympic record for the mile," Cunningham reflected, and "only one person in the world ran faster." The Kansan concluded Lovelock "must be the greatest runner ever." Although disappointed at not winning a gold medal, he had broken the previous Olympic record. Cunningham considered his silver Olympic medal "a major turning point in my life. It was both victory and defeat. It made me realize that sports competition is valuable in many ways, but never an end in itself."[27] Two weeks later, he established a world mark of one minute, 49.7 seconds in the 800 meters at Stockholm, Sweden. In 1936, he also earned a master's degree in physical education from the University of Iowa.

Cunningham added the 1937 and 1938 AAU outdoor titles in the 1500 meters to his résumé, clocking three minutes, 51.8 seconds and three minutes, 52.5 seconds, respectively, to give him five crowns altogether and four consecutive. The Kansan thrived on endurance and pacing, which gave him a significant advantage over other runners. Since no runner could sprint for a mile, he learned how to spread his effort over the distance so that he could "complete it in as short a time as possible without burning out before the finish."[28]

Cunningham, who completed his Ph.D. in physical education at New York University in 1940, boasted 12 of the 31 fastest miles ever recorded by 1938. At the time, Nurmi held the world record of six minutes, 42.8 seconds for one and one-half miles. Cunningham greatly admired Nurmi, but casually remarked to some runners at Madison Square Garden that the Finn's record could be broken by running six 66-second quarters. The bemused runners implored him "to try to beat that record." Cunningham replied, "I wouldn't mind trying." When sportswriters printed those remarks, Cunningham was invited to try to break Nurmi's record at Randall's Island. After racing an exhibition mile at Paterson, New Jersey, he was whisked to Randall's Island. Cunningham broke Nurmi's record, covering the distance in six minutes, 34 seconds. He ran six quarters under 66 seconds and shattered Nurmi's mark by eight and eight-tenths seconds.[29]

Dartmouth College invited Cunningham to run a handicap mile on its new high-banked indoor track on March 5, 1938. The press portrayed him as "less the lissom runner, with his heavy stride and wide-thick shoulders, than a powerful blocking back or a nimble hodcarrier." At age 28, Cunningham, flanked by six Dartmouth runners, showed his endurance on the long, narrow track with difficult turns. One runner retained a good pace for several hundred yards before fading. Cunningham recollected, "I was running alone after that." The layout of the track, however, was not conducive to pace-setting. Someone also had opened a window on the north side, causing a freezing wind to hit his legs on that turn each lap. Nevertheless, he ran a paced indoor mile in a world-record time of four minutes, 4.4 seconds, two seconds faster than that distance had ever been covered inside. "The boy who was not supposed to walk had become the fastest miler, anywhere, indoors or out."[30] The *New York Times* reported his time on its front page. If that race had been held at Madison Square Garden, Cunningham predicted that he would have become the first runner to complete the mile in under four minutes. Nevertheless, Cunningham's performance made the one-mile race the "glamour event at indoor races."[31] Track authorities, however, did not accept Cunningham's record officially because the race was not sanctioned. His mark, however, was not surpassed until 1955.

Cunningham performed very impressively on the indoor circuit, making the mile the most popular track and field event. At Madison Square Garden, he set six world records. His best time there came on March 12, 1938, with an official record-setting four minutes, 7.4 second clocking in the Columbia Mile.[32] He engaged in thrilling races against Bonthron, Lovelock, Venzke, Sam Romini, Don Lash, and Chuck Fernley. In 1939, Cunningham captured the Baxter Mile for the fifth time, the Wanamaker Mile for the sixth time, and the BAA Mile for the ninth time, and even bested renowned two-milers Lash and Greg Rice in nine minutes, 11.8 seconds.

Cunningham, who raced competitively until 1940, wanted to win his final 1500-meter race at Fresno, California. In that race, Cunningham faced Walter Mehl, an impressive two-miler who had won the 1939 Big Ten Conference title in the mile, and other young runners. He established the pace at the outset, cheered on by 14,000 spectators, and surged ahead of the competitors. "The crowd of 14,000 fully expected to see him win, and cheered him on." "This was the master at his peak for his last race, running with the grace and power of old, setting a pace as stiff as any he had ever run except for his 'freak' 4:04," Cordner Nelson wrote. "Actually the spectators were surprised to see anyone staying close behind."[33] Mehl strode past Cunningham down the stretch. Cunningham ran his career-fastest 1500 meters in three minutes, 48 seconds, but finished second to Mehl, who clocked three minutes, 47.9 seconds. He retired from competitive racing partly because the 1940 Summer Olympic Games were canceled, and also because he was finishing his doctorate.

In 1979, Madison Square Garden named Cunningham its most outstanding track and field performer of its first 100 years. Cunningham had won 21 of 30 races and set world records there, and had recorded his best indoor mile there in 1938. Nicknamed the "Iron Horse of Kansas," he was inducted into the Kansas Sports Hall of Fame in 1961, the National Track and Field Hall of Fame in 1974, the U.S. Track and Field Hall of Fame in 1979, and the Kansas State High School Athletic Association Hall of Fame in 1983.

Track and field molded and shaped Cunningham as an excellent role model and developer of youth. Cunningham could have parlayed his athletic fame into a small fortune, but declined a $100,000 a year offer to do public speaking. "He was more interested in helping others than in making a fortune."[34] After being director of athletics, health, and physical education at Cornell College in Iowa from 1940 to 1944, he served two years in the U.S. Navy as a physical training officer in San Diego and at the Great Lakes Naval Training Base.

Cunningham wed Margaret Speir in August 1934. They had two daughters before their 1946 divorce. Cunningham married his second wife, Ruth Sheffield, a Cornell College student, in the summer of 1947. Ruth, a strongly religious woman, gave his life additional meaning. They had ten children, six daughters and four sons, and housed nearly 10,000 troubled children from 1947 to 1978 at their 840-acre Cedar Ranch near Wichita, Kansas. Both loved children with their freshness and limitless vitality, taught discipline and persistence, and handled the youth with patience, firmness, tolerance, and love. They often struggled financially, going without a car for five years, but eventually got monetary assistance from the nonprofit group, the Glenn Cunningham Youth Ranch. Cunningham toured as a lay preacher to raise money and later donated land for the Glenhaven Youth Ranch near Little Rock, Arkansas. "With virtually no outside help, the couple handled the youngsters with old-fashioned patience and tolerance."[35] He died in Menifee, Arkansas, on March 10, 1988, at age 78.

Cunningham recorded remarkable collegiate and amateur track and field achievements, but his ability to overcome challenges proved even more inspirational. He continually overcame obstacles from the fire to college track meets and from difficult Olympic races to youth work. Cunningham inherited discipline, hard work, and stubbornness from his father. He demonstrated courage and persistence to achieve many accomplishments, but acknowledged his dependence upon God, who fulfilled and enriched him beyond his wildest dreams. Besides being an outstanding athlete, Cunningham held high principles and convictions. His status as a role model and contribution to the development of youth rank among his finest achievements and were made possible by his remarkable running skills.

# BILL TOOMEY

"Man can do virtually anything he wants to do if he wills it"[1] encapsulates the saga of Bill Toomey, who overcame a devastating play accident to achieve track and field stardom. Toomey's right hand was shriveled when a piece of glass shattered. Enormous willpower enabled him to conquer that seemingly insurmountable hurdle to become an Olympic gold medalist in the grueling decathlon competition.

Toomey, in contrast to most other athletes featured in this book, was reared in affluence. William Anthony Toomey was born January 10, 1939, in Philadelphia. His father worked for Italian Swiss Colony Wine and owned at least five sports cars, including three Mercedes-Benzes and a Porsche. Toomey spent his childhood in New York, Connecticut, and Massachusetts and loved basketball, which honed his jumping abilities. He began running while participating in basketball in Long Island in the fourth grade, learning discipline and receiving excellent instruction. Toomey spent idle time jumping over aisles of folding chairs at church and fences and built a high jump in his yard.[2] His newfound love for track and field coincided with the rise of the sport's popularity. The 1950s featured the first sub-four-minute mile, 60-foot shot put, and seven-foot high jump.

Toomey suffered a major hand problem, stemming from his youth. A childhood accident left his right hand shriveled, partially paralyzed, and almost completely without feeling. According to sportscaster Howard Cosell, "When Bill was 12 years old, he was playing with a piece of ceramics that shattered the nerves in his right wrist were severed, paralyzing the hand." Cosell wrote, "Doctors said he'd never be able to use the hand again, and to this day his right hand is shriveled." Toomey recalled, "A kid threw a dish under the door as I was bending over, and it tore into my wrist." The dish severed his median nerve. Five operations from junior high school through graduate school enabled him to recover 75 percent of his hand's use.[3] Toomey remembered working as a youth with a wood-burning tool, gripping it so low that it began to sizzle. He never felt the pain, but the smell of frying fingers alerted him.

Toomey epitomized the true scholar-athlete. After graduating from Worcester Academy in Worcester, Massachusetts, in 1958, he earned a B.A. degree in advertising from the University of Colorado in 1962 and a master's degree in education from

Stanford University. Colorado in 1961 gave him the Alumni "C" Award for academic and scholastic excellence. John Underwood of *Sports Illustrated* described the verbose Toomey as "an engaging conversationalist with a voice or an accent to fit any occasion and a terribly swift wit. He is Jonathan Winters playing Grandma Frickert, and in the next breath he is explaining Adler's theories on adequacy, relating them to the decathlon."[4]

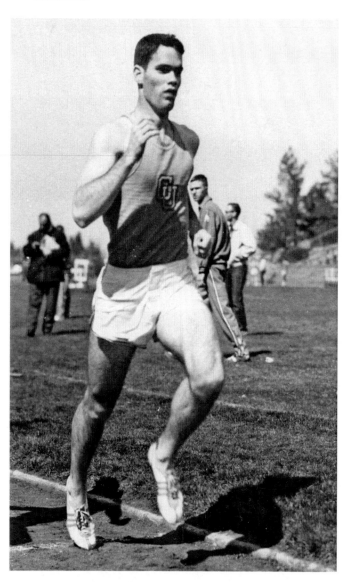

Bill Toomey competed in the pentathlon, long jump, and 400-meter hurdles at the University of Colorado from 1959 to 1962, earning All-America honors in the pentathlon in 1961 and 1962 (courtesy CU Athletics).

Toomey competed on the Colorado track and field team, long-jumping 24 feet, 8½ inches and running the 400-meter hurdles in 51.7 seconds. At Colorado, he ranked among the nation's best intermediate hurdlers. Toomey never placed in the NCAA Track and Field Championships, but earned All-America honors in the pentathlon in 1960 and 1961. Toomey's promising long jump, running, and hurdling skills did not presage his future greatness. "I was not a great athlete," Toomey admitted, but he gradually improved his performance in training and competition. "If you keep adding information, and you're always flexible, and always examine what you're setting out to do, you'll be successful,"[5] he insisted.

Toomey initially hoped to set a world record in the 400 meters, but found there were many who could run that distance in a faster time and never liked finishing in the middle of the pack. Toomey realized, "I was just another quarter-miler in a world of stinking quarter-milers." He found the six years of continual running boring.[6]

At an evening bull session, Toomey started exploring alternative events and decided he would be happier with 10 rather than one. The decathlon involves 10 events, including the 100-, 400-, and 1500-meter races, the 110-meter hurdles competition, and the high jump, long jump, shot put, discus, javelin, and pole vault. "You have 10 mistresses instead of one," Toomey related, "all keeping you busy." He discovered the decathlon's "more work — but more fun, too."[7]

Toomey already had begun competing in the pentathlon in 1959, placing sixth in the Amateur Athletic Union (AAU) Track and Field Championships. His childhood hand injury handicapped him in the shot put, discus, javelin, and pole vault because those events required him to grip an implement. Before the javelin throw, Toomey went through extensive trance-linked mental and physical visualizations of the movements that were to follow. Aided by this technique Toomey won a still-record five consecutive national AAU pentathlon titles from 1960 through 1964, setting American records in 1961 and 1964.

Toomey credits much of his track and field success in the 1960s to his injury, tenacity, and persistence. "I never told anyone I had a paralyzed right hand," Toomey noted. "To tell someone would have provided me with an excuse to fail."[8] He ascended "from the dips to the top of the mountain," recognizing "that I was in control of my own destiny." Toomey believed, "If you have your mental equipment functioning at a high level, and you've got some resources behind you, you will make it out of those tough times."[9]

Toomey, who taught English literature at La Colina Junior High School in Santa Barbara, California, in the 1960s, began serious training in the decathlon full-time in 1963. Some questioned his decision because of his wrist injury. Toomey read extensively about the ingredients for good execution. "I began to understand the psychology of performance," he explained. Toomey learned to think positively. He lacked the natural talent of decathletes Bob Mathias, Milt Campbell, and Rafer Johnson, but eventually outscored them through hard work. To become a decathlete, he discerned, "it takes the upper body of a weight man, the lower body of a sprinter, and the brain of an idiot."[10]

Although a skilled long jumper and 400-meter runner, the undaunted Toomey worked diligently on improving his field events. Despite his shriveled right hand, he threw the shot, discus, and javelin right-handed. Sportscaster Cosell marveled, "Somehow he made that hand work so that he could put the shot, carry the pole for the vault, throw the discus and heave a javelin. Toomey always dreamed of becoming an Olympic champion."[11]

Toomey prepared himself mentally before each decathlon event by playing make-believe. Toomey visualized the role he was going to play, convincing himself that he was "the World's Fastest 400-Meter Man" or "the World's Longest Broad Jumper." He successively thought like a hurdler, javelin thrower, and pole vaulter, assuring himself, "I can fly!" Toomey pointed out, "You're running from this to that, moving, always moving. More work, but more fun too."

Toomey quickly realized the myriad problems facing decathletes, competing in 10 events over two days. He quickly learned that the decathlete not only has few opportunities to set records, but has "to contend with nature, your own physiology and the facilities." The lack of media attention devoted to the decathlon dismayed him. Toomey remarked, "A decathlon man sets a world record, and immediately it's the best kept secret in the world."[12]

After finishing fifth in the decathlon at the national AAU Track and Field Championships, Toomey took fourth place in the decathlon at the 1964 Olympic Trials in Los Angeles, and missed making the U.S. Olympic track and field squad by only 109 points. According to Cosell, Toomey paid his own expenses to witness the 1964 Summer Olympic Games in Tokyo. American athletes had won six consecutive gold medals in the decathlon between 1932 and 1960, but did not medal at the 1964 Olympic Games. Toomey, who vowed to rectify the situation, honed his decathlon skills and became especially proficient at the long jump and 400 meters.[13]

Toomey's dedication to physical and psychological improvement paid dividends. He studied under multi-event coach Pete Peterson because of the latter's all-around excellence. Toomey lauded Peterson as "a healer, and a trainer — a human being who understood frailties, but knew how to develop strengths."[14]

During the next four years, Toomey built his body from 158 pounds to 195 pounds and perfected his decathlon techniques. Underwood pictured him as "a 195-pound strong boy, marvelously proportioned, with a powerful upper torso and sprinter's legs — thin ankles and big calves. Only his hands are disproportionate." By 1965, Toomey began placing in the decathlon at international track meets and "seemed to be getting somewhere."[15]

Toomey's first major decathlon triumph came in 1965, when he won the first of his record five straight AAU decathlon titles with 7,764 points and was ranked third globally. His victory incredibly came less than one month after he required 35 stitches for tearing his right calf while pole vaulting.

Toomey spent six months in West Germany, coached by renowned decathlon mentor Friedel Schirmer. He contracted mononucleosis and caught infectious hepatitis there and was hospitalized four months, clinging "close to death."[16] According to Toomey, "That was a rough time," being bedridden so long. He experienced considerable atrophy and wondered if he would ever compete again.

Toomey resumed decathlon training in April 1966, created a good program, and soon set world decathlon records. "Doubts are only doubts," he discovered. "If you really want something, you can erase them."[17] In July 1966, Toomey established a world decathlon record of 8,234 points at the national AAU Track and Field Championships in Salina, Kansas, although the mark was not ratified. He set personal records in the first four events, recording 10.3 seconds in the 100-meter dash; 25 feet, six inches in the long jump; 45 feet, 8¾ inches in the shot put; and six feet, four inches in the high jump. On the second day, Toomey ran his fastest ever 110-meter hurdles at 14.8 seconds and set a personal record of 147 feet, five inches in the discus. After pole vaulting 13 feet, he threw the javelin 198 feet, 11 inches and clocked four minutes, 30 seconds in the 1500 meters. Toomey battled with Russ Hodge at the Salina meet. According to decathlete Dave Thoreson, Hodge, who had never broad jumped 24 feet, leapt 25 feet, two inches in his final jump. "It was incredible." Toomey "came down the runway like a truck" and jumped 25 feet, six inches. "I loved it," Toomey beamed. His performance earned him national 1966 Amateur Athlete of the Year honors.[18]

By 1967, Toomey had improved in those events he had specialized in before competing in the pentathlon and decathlon. "You get better in the events you were primarily interested in by doing the decathlon," he learned. " I'm a better runner now than I ever was when all I did was run." Psychologically, he trained his body for the decathlon by strengthening it "for throwing things, running, jumping. It's a beautiful thing, like religion."[19]

One of Toomey's kneecaps was shattered in a motorcycle accident, but he rebounded again. In 1967, Toomey won the decathlon at the national AAU Track and Field Championships with 7,880 points and at the Pan-American Games with 8,044 points, becoming the nation's best Olympic decathlon hope. He "had conquered the techniques of the throwing events to be competitive, although the pole vault was still capable of mastering him."[20] A subsequent loss to Kurt Bendlin dropped him to second place in the world rankings.

In 1968, the 6-foot, 1½-inch, 195-pound Toomey enjoyed even greater success. He won his first and only Mt. San Antonio decathlon title with 7,800 points and the national AAU decathlon championship with 8,037 points. Illness contributed to his loss to Bendlin and Hans-Joachim Walde in Germany, but he regained his momentum way taking the decathlon at the British AAA Championships in London with 7,985 points and at the Olympic Trials in South Lake Tahoe, California, with 8,222 points.[21]

At the 1968 Mexico City Summer Olympic Games, Toomey became the ninth American to capture the decathlon since 1912. "It took the 29-year-old California schoolteacher, Bill Toomey, 24 hours to win the decathlon. 12 hours a day for two days." Toomey set a record first-day score of 4,499 points on October 18, gulping many aspirin to alleviate "his tension headaches." His chief competitors were Bendlin and Walde. Toomey seized the lead by clocking 10.41 seconds in the 100 meters and won the long jump with a career-best distance of 25 feet, 9¾ inches. His marks of 45 feet, 1 3/4 inches for the shot put and six feet, 4¾ inches for the high jump kept him ahead, but he suffered a hip strain in the rain. Toomey attained a seemingly insurmountable lead with a sensational 45.6-second time in the 400 meters. He utilized his quarter-miler's speed to record an amazing time in the 400 meters, a world-class clocking for a 400-meter specialist, an astounding time for a decathlete, and his best clocking ever in that event. He shattered Olympic decathlon records for the 400 meters and total first-day score.[22]

A thumb injury, however, troubled Toomey the second day. During the unbearably hot day, Toomey drank gallons of water and suffered diarrhea. Shortly before the pole vault, the Mexican officials misplaced his pole. The pole soon was found, but its temporary loss unnerved Toomey. The pole vault had always posed problems for him. The pole misplacement so unsettled him that he sprained his thumb vaulting and missed his first two vaults at the warm-up height of 11 feet, 9¾ inches. Toomey faced disqualification if he missed that height for the third time. The decathlete recalled, "Everything was closing in on me — the people in that huge arena, the people watching on television back home, my whole life, all those years of working and waiting for this moment. If I missed, it would be like dying."[23] Toomey's parents, his two brothers, and thousands of American rooters watched nervously, as he prepared for his final attempt.

Toomey started his approach, hit full stride, and then inexplicably stopped, "prolonging the agony." Only 30 seconds remained for him to jump. Toomey said, "'The heck with it,' and started again." He sped down the runway again, planted the pole, and sailed upward. The ensuing cheer told Toomey's mother that he had succeeded. She took her hands away from her eyes. Jim raced back into the stands. With years of work and sacrifice at stake, Toomey cleared the height on his third try and eventually vaulted a career-best 13 feet, 9¾ inches. He reflected on what would have happened if he had missed the third jump. "My name would have been mud!"[24]

World record holder Bendlin uncorked a gigantic javelin throw, bringing the contest down to the final 1500-meter event. An hour before that race, "Toomey lay prostrate on a rubbing table, out cold from utter exhaustion." The race began in darkness, with a cool wind that was followed by a steady drizzle that bathed the runners. But gradually Toomey pulled away from Bendlin with a strong finishing kick. "As I stood next to the cinder path watching him stride to victory," Cosell recollected, "I just felt exultant for the whole human race." Cosell termed Toomey's Olympic victory, "the essence of what is great in sports, a complete manifestation of the sheer magnificence of the human spirit."[25] Toomey crossed the finish line, flashing victory signs with both hands, holding off the late-charging Walde to win that race in four minutes, 57.1 seconds and prevail by 82 points. He captured the grueling 10-event decathlon, winning the gold medal with an Olympic record of 8,193 points for his sixth decathlon score over 8,000 points. The stadium was less than half filled upon completion of the 1500-meter event. Walde won the silver medal, while Bendlin took the bronze.[26]

Toomey, who was older at age 29 than most decathlon gold medalists and who had surpassed Johnson's career best by over 100 points, told the media why he competed in the decathlon. "Ten's my favorite number," he explained. "Ten letters in my name, born on January 10, always wore number 10 as a ball player. It had to be the decathlon." The ecstatic Toomey acknowledged, "I never felt I belonged but around the edges until now. Not anymore, though. After 24 hours I earned that son of a gun." Christopher Hosford wrote, "His victory was the triumph of an enormous will to succeed."[27] *Time* magazine lauded Toomey, the sole Colorado Buffalo athlete to win an individual Olympic gold medal, as "the finest athlete in the world."[28]

During 1969, Toomey broke world decathlon and pentathlon records. He not only won his fifth straight AAU decathlon title in June, but scored 4,123 points in a pentathlon event in London in October, the best score in history. His pentathlon records remain unbroken. Toomey entered 10 decathlons, surpassing 8,000 points seven times and regaining his world record with 8,309 points. He averaged 8,321 points in his final three decathlons, "a feat that is still unmatched." Toomey set an official world record of 8,417 points on December 11–12, 1969, at Los Angeles, the twelfth time he scored more than 8,000 points as a decathlete and the thirty-eighth time he had competed in the decathlon. The world record lasted for three years.[29]

Toomey won the 1969 James E. Sullivan Award as the year's outstanding American amateur athlete, outpointing Olympians Jim Ryun, Bob Beamon, and Dick Fosbury. During that year, he had just broken the American decathlon record, been undefeated in world competition, and been named Associated Press California Athlete of the Year. His other honors included being named *Track & Field News* Athlete of the Year, ABC Wide World of Sports Athlete of the Year, and Helms World Trophy winner.[30]

Toomey still does not have his Sullivan Award trophy. The AAU originally left his name off the list of 1969 award nominees. Jesse Pardue, then-AAU president, wrote Frank Dolson of the *Philadelphia Inquirer*, "Toomey hadn't done enough to deserve it." When Dolson notified Pardue what Toomey had accomplished in 1969, the AAU added Toomey's name to the list and named him trophy winner. Toomey did not receive his trophy until May 1970. The AAU presented him with the award at a track meet at the Los Angeles Coliseum about an hour before his airplane flight to Africa. "Nobody in the stadium knew what was happening," Toomey observed. "For all practical purposes, I got the fastest awarding of the Sullivan Trophy in history."[31] He unfortunately left the trophy there with an official to catch a plane flight overseas and has never gotten it back.

Toomey retired after his world-record performance, having won six pentathlons and 23 of 38 decathlons and recorded eight of the 12 best scores in decathlon history. The Olympic medalist, who never considered the decathlon grueling, acknowledged, "I've always enjoyed the decathlon and I think this might have been the key to my success."[32]

Toomey would have relished competing against decathletes Johnson and Bruce

Jenner, claiming, "I would have scared the hell out of them." He did not predict who would have won, but said, "I was a good competitor. I didn't lose. I was faster than they were, and was as good a jumper. I was a little down in the throwing events. But it would have been fun."[33]

In December 1969, Toomey married Mary Rand, Great Britain's 1964 Olympic gold medalist and world record holder in the long jump. She had been married to Sydney Rand, an English businessman. The Toomeys had two daughters, Samantha and Sarah, before their 1991 divorce.

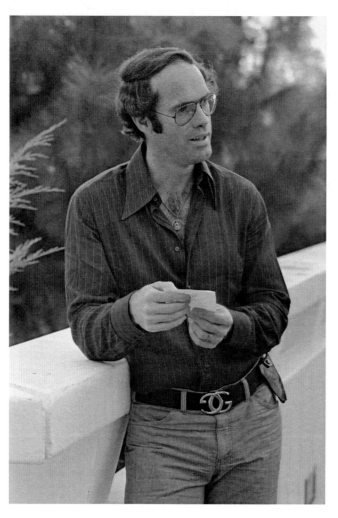

Bill Toomey, circa 1974, outside the Department of Intercollegiate Athletics in Crawford Hall at the University of California, Irvine, where he coached track and field (Special Collections and Archives, University of California, Irvine Libraries, University Communications Photographs, AS-061, Box 42, A74-043).

In April 1970, Toomey became an advertising executive with the Drackett Company and handled radio commercials for Nutrament. The deal enabled Toomey to provide greater financial support for his family, but terminated his amateur career. The AAU judged him a professional, labeling him "Joe Commercial." Toomey complained that the AAU overprotected the amateur athlete "from what happens in real life that he becomes unprepared for anything that isn't measured in time or distance. So now I'm a man without a country in sports." William Reed of *Sports Illustrated* empathized with Toomey's AAU problem, which denied "the best decathlete in the world"[34] from further amateur competition.

During the early 1970s, Toomey still engaged in irregular workouts at the University of California, Santa Barbara, calling himself "the 'workout king' and 'the best-trained spectator in Santa Barbara.'" "I'm not sure why I keep working out," he admitted, "unless I'm following through the neurosis that pushed me to an Olympic victory." If the AAU had rescinded its decision, Toomey claimed that he could have tallied at least 8,000 points with only three weeks of hard practice. He contended, "This country hasn't really produced anybody who can beat me. So how can I go out on the track and knock off some good times and not wish I were still eligible?" The AAU temporarily revived Toomey's hopes of regaining amateur eligibility when it allowed him to run a 300-meter race in San Francisco in December 1970. Toomey easily defeated "three other Olympic gold medalists, all over 30,"[35] in 32.8 seconds. But the AAU never restored Toomey's amateur status, preventing him from competing in the 1972 Munich Summer Olympic Games.

Toomey enjoyed a successful career as a television commentator for ABC, NBC, and CBS and covered the 1972 Olympic Games for ABC. He served as a radio talk show host and competed in masters track and field meets. Toomey gave motivational speeches and appeared in three films, *Fists for Freedom* (1968), *The World's Greatest Athlete* (1973), and *Summer Games* (1999). He coached track and field at the University of California-Irvine in the early 1970s and participated on the President's Council on Physical Fitness.[36]

Toomey remained a leader in the modern Olympic movement. He served on the Board of Directors of the U.S. Olympic Committee from 1968 to 1976 and represented President Richard Nixon at the 1972 Munich Summer Olympic Games. Toomey belonged to the President's Commission on Olympic Sports from 1976 to 1978, contributing to the restructuring of the movement in the United States, and was a consultant for the Los Angeles Olympic Organizing Committee. He and Barry King co-authored *The Olympic Challenge, 1988*, examining the athlete's quest for perfection from the 1968 to 1988 Olympic Games. Toomey co-founded the World Olympian Association, promoting Olympic ideals and strengthening the movement throughout the world. The fundraising director drove development of the Olympic training center in San Diego and facilitated record-setting corporate contributions to U.S. Olympic programs, helping raise $65 million for the U.S. Olympic Committee.[37] Lisa Lareau, a co-worker at the Olympic training center, remarked, "He has opened doors for us that no one else in the world could get their foot into." Toomey also developed sports programs in over 20 countries while conducting clinics for the Peace Corps.[38]

Numerous awards were bestowed on Toomey. Toomey was elected to the Colorado Sports Hall of Fame in 1971, the U.S. Olympic Hall of Fame in 1984, the National Track and Field Hall of Fame in 1985, and the Colorado University Athletic Hall of Fame in 2004, and was selected among the 2000 CNN/*Sports Illustrated* "Top 50 Athletes of the 20th Century." In 2000, the United States Sports Academy presented him with the Distinguished Service Award. The University of Colorado named him its Alumnus of the Century.[39]

Toomey, though, experienced several problems, too. He suffered professional setbacks and personal depression. Toomey's sports management company failed by the mid–1980s. His 22-year marriage to Rand ended in divorce in 1991. Toomey underwent back surgery in 1991 and for a ruptured disk in 1995. He lost his superb physical conditioning, exercised less, ignored proper nutrition, and acquired smoking and drinking habits. His weight rose from 195 pounds to 215 pounds. "I had bad sleep patterns, and I didn't eat right," he acknowledged. In March 2008, Toomey pleaded no contest to driving under the influence of alcohol and drugs after crashing his Mercedes-Benz into two parked cars in San Luis Obispo County, California. Christopher Casciola, his attorney, explained, "He had used a sleeping aid and some painkillers for aches stemming from his athletic career."[40]

Toomey's daughters, Samantha and Sarah, inspired him to set a better example and become a health advocate. Life Extension Foundation helped him restore his physical condition. Toomey married Trish Nelson in 1995 and resides in El Macero, California. He has owned Sports Directors Unlimited for over two decades and has worked extensively with underprivileged children.

# THREE-FINGER BROWN

"A man who would stick and fight to the very end" capsulizes the career of Three-Finger Brown, whose two major childhood accidents did not stop him from becoming a stellar major league baseball player. Brown suffered severe hand injuries in the moving blades of a corn shredder and from falling while chasing a pig. He developed a devastating curveball with the three fingers, making him one of the premier hurlers in major league history.

Brown came from a working-class socioeconomic background. Mordecai Peter Centennial Brown was born on October 16, 1876, in Nyesville, Indiana, the son of Peter Brown, a miner, and Jane Brown, and was named for his uncle, his father, and the nation's one hundredth anniversary. He grew up in the tiny farming and coal community near Terre Haute. His crisis came when he was only five years old. "Mordecai's natural boyhood inquisitiveness altered his life's course."[1] Brown put his right hand under the moving blades of a corn shredder on his uncle's farm. His index finger was so badly damaged that it was amputated just below the knuckle and left only a small, one-inch stump. The accident also severed part of his little finger and mangled his middle finger. Brown exhibited enormous bravery following the mishap. Dr. Gillum, an experienced Civil War surgeon, operated on Brown's hand and splinted the other fingers. "My brother used to cut feed for the horses in a patent box fitted with circular knives," Brown remembered. "One day I was feeding the knives and my hand slipped in among the knives. Every finger was chopped to ribbons, but the doctor managed to sew them together."[2]

Five weeks later, Brown injured his right hand again. With a cast still covering his injured hand, he fell while chasing a pig and broke the third and fourth fingers. Brown and his sister were playing with a pet rabbit in a tub partially filled with water. "I was making it swim," he recollected. "Suddenly I lost my balance and tumbled into the tub, my right hand smashing against the bottom, breaking six bones." Dr. Gillum considered re-breaking Brown's misaligned fingers to straighten them again when removing the splints, but figured, "The boy had already undergone enough trauma."[3] During the healing process, Brown's fingers bent and twisted unnaturally. The mishaps left him without an index finger and with a paralyzed pinky and severely misshapen third and fourth digits. Although prospects looked bleak, Brown nobly battled adversity.

Brown, whose injuries probably precluded an agricultural career, began keeping daily records in the Parke County coal mines at age 14. Most southwestern Indiana communities fielded baseball teams. Brown, who demonstrated a "unique aptitude" for the sport, constantly threw rocks at outbuildings, developing uncanny accuracy. He learned to throw a ball with his deformity and played third base for semi-professional teams in Clinton, Shelburn, Nyesville, and Coxville. Clayton, star Coxville Reds pitcher, fell and hurt his shoulder before the July 22, 1898, game. Manager Johnny Buckley pitched the 21-year-old Brown instead against Brazil. Brown possessed accuracy, good control, and a fair fastball, quickly turning his disability into an advantage. "That day transformed him, an obscure mining team ballplayer, into a celebrity." Brown hurled seven innings without allowing a baserunner and realized, "Right then and there I began to be a pitcher."[4] Only one Brazil batter even made contact with his unorthodox pitch. Brown performed so well that Buckley converted him to a full-time pitcher.

The 5-foot 10-inch Brown, a 175-pound right-hander, threw a remarkable downward curve that snapped off his awkward middle finger. Since his index finger was barely a stub, he was forced to exert extra pressure on the ball with his middle finger. His unique grip caused his curve to drop as if it had rolled off a table, like a modern forkball, and it broke in toward right-handed batters. The stump imparted an odd spin on the ball, causing unusual motion on his pitches. His gnarled hand enhanced his pitching effectiveness.[5] Brown's fastball dropped right at the plate, similar to a modern split finger fastball. His hand was not very flexible, making throwing a ball very painful. "With fingers that gave Mordecai a grip that couldn't be duplicated, the ball likely tailed in such a fashion that batters had never seen before." Batters usually struck out or hit ground balls. When asked if pitching with such a misshapen hand was a disadvantage, Brown did not know. "I've never done it the other way," he explained. He always considered this handicap an advantage because "it imparted a sharper break on his curveball."[6]

In 1901, Frank Pfirman, a Terre Haute semi-pro player, recommended Brown to the Terre Haute Hottentots of the newly-formed Three I League (TIL). Brown never signed a contract, but received $60 a month. He won 23 games in 1901 and paced Terre Haute to the inaugural TIL pennant. Brown learned how to pitch by studying the styles of other pitchers. He won 27 of 42 games for Omaha of the Western League in 1902, hurling 352 innings, pitching three consecutive doubleheaders, and completing every game he started.[7]

St. Louis Cardinals manager Patsy Donovan, upon learning of Brown's unique fastball, signed him in 1903. In his major league debut on April 19, Brown defeated the Chicago Cubs. In 1903, he won only nine of 22 decisions with 83 strikeouts and a 2.60 earned run average (ERA) for a last-place squad. He shared the club lead in pitching victories and boasted the lowest ERA among St. Louis hurlers.[8]

In December 1903, the Cubs traded 21-game winner Jack Taylor and rookie catcher Larry McLean to the Cardinals for Brown and catcher Jack O'Neill. The *Chicago Tribune* noted Brown's "misfortune to lose one of the fingers of his pitching hand," but observed, "That does not seem to militate against his ability as a twirler." Chicago first baseman Frank Chance, impressed with Brown's pitching skills, persuaded Cubs manager Frank Selee to acquire Brown, "a man of undying nerve — a man who would stick and fight until the very end."[9]

Brown surrendered 12 runs on 13 hits to the Cincinnati Reds in his first start and lost his next two decisions before blanking the Philadelphia Phillies, 4–0, at West Side Grounds. Nicknamed "Three-Finger" by the fans and "Brownie" by his teammates, he steadily improved and soon became the mainstay of the Cubs' pitching staff and a team leader. Brown posted a 15–10 record with a club-best 1.86 ERA for second-place Chicago in 1904.[10]

Brown in 1905 joined Jake Weimer and Ed Reulbach as 18-game winners and lost only 12 for the third-place Cubs. He completed every start and ranked fifth in the National League (NL) with a 2.17 ERA. On June 13, Brown and Christy Mathewson of the New York Giants both hurled no-hitters for eight innings before the Giants scored once on two ninth-inning safeties for a 1–0 victory. Mathewson completed the no-hitter. The *Chicago Tribune* commented, "Brown pitched well enough to have won twelve games out of a baker's dozen."[11] Brown performed much better the second half of 1905, defeating Mathewson, 8–1, on a two-hitter on July 12, winning his next four starts, and triumphing in eight of his last nine starts.

Chicago fielded one of major league baseball's greatest dynasties between 1906 and 1910, winning four NL pennants and two World Series crowns. The Cubs boasted the famed double-play combination of Joe Tinker, Johnny Evers, and Chance, while Brown led the Cubs' pitching staff with 127 victories.

In 1906, the Cubs set an all-time major league record with 116 victories and only 36 losses, finishing 20 games ahead of New York. Chicago compiled the best road record ever (60–15), winning 50 of 58 games the last two months. The staff, which also included Jack Pfiester, Carl Lundgren, and Reulbach, produced 30 shutouts and limited opponents to one run 37 times. Brown, who exercised rigorously and improved his fielding agility in spring training at West Baden, Indiana, emerged as the Cubs' ace in 1906 with one of the best major league seasons ever. He and Lefty Leifield of the Pittsburgh Pirates both hurled one-hitters on July 4, with Chicago prevailing, 1–0. Brown out-dueled Mathewson, 6–2, on July 17 and surrendered a lone single to Tommy Sheehan of Pittsburgh in a 2–0 victory on September 1. "It was Mordecai's best year. He was the indisputable ace."[12] He topped the Cubs' staff with a 26–6 record, led the NL with nine shutouts and a brilliant 1.04 ERA, and struck out 144 batters. His ERA was the lowest in the senior circuit in the twentieth century and third lowest in major league history.

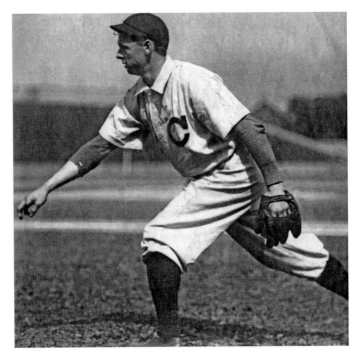

Three-Finger Brown led the Chicago Cubs pitching staff with 127 victories from 1906 to 1910, appearing in four different World Series (courtesy National Baseball Hall of Fame Library, Cooperstown, N.Y.).

Brown, however, did not fare well in the 1906 World Series against the underdog Chicago White Sox, "the Hitless Wonders." Although Brown held the cross-town rivals to four hits in the October 9 opener, Nick Altrock out-dueled him, 2–1, at West Side Park. Brown struck out seven batters, including five in the first three innings. The Pale Hose scored on George Rohe's fifth-inning triple and when Frank Isbell's sixth-inning single plated Fielder Jones. Brown's sixth-inning single contributed to the Cubs' sole run.[13]

Three days later, Brown blanked the White Sox, 1–0, on two hits in just 96 minutes in Game Four, using his forkball to best Altrock. In the seventh frame, Chance singled and scored on Evers's single over third base. Isbell's sharp line drive struck Brown's bare right hand in the ninth inning, knocking him back a couple of feet. Brown threw out Isbell, but temporarily lost feeling in his hand. "That was the nearest thing to a cannonball I was ever compelled to stop,"[14] he revealed.

The White Sox took Game 5 and led the series, three games to two, entering decisive Game 6 at South Side Park. The Cubs needed to win the contest to stay alive. "The crowd was huge and even more disorderly than on the day before."[15]

Chance, who had become manager in 1905, started Brown on only one day's rest and told him, "We're all relying on you." The Pale Hose, sparked by Jiggs Donahue and George Davis, pounded the fatigued Brown for three first-inning runs and four second-inning runs before Orval Overall relieved him with two outs. The White Sox demonstrated superior pitching and dashed the Cubs' hopes with an 8–3 victory, recording among the greatest upsets in World Series history. Brown suffered just one bad performance, striking out 12 batters in 19.2 innings.

Brown enjoyed another remarkable season in 1907, boasting a 20–6 record and 1.39 ERA. The Cubs, paced by Overall's 23 victories, won 107 games and finished 17 games ahead of Pittsburgh. Brown extended his domination over Giants legend Mathewson to five games, triumphing 3–2 on May 21 and 8–2 on June 5.[16]

Chicago swept the Detroit Tigers, 4–0, in the 1907 World Series. After Game 1 ended in a 3–3, 12-inning tie because of darkness, Pfiester, Reulbach, and Overall won the next three contests for the Cubs. The well-rested Brown, who did not start until Game 5, vowed, "I'll finish 'em off today." He won the clinching contest, blanking Detroit, 2–0, on seven hits at Navin Field. Chicago held on after tallying single runs in the first two innings. Brown ensured "the Cubs' position as the best in the world."[17]

Brown's role changed in 1908, which featured one of the most dramatic pennant races in baseball history. Brown recorded 29 victories as the staff ace, hurling 27 complete games and nine shutouts. His triumphs and shutouts remain single-season franchise records. Many of his victories were decided by just one run. Brown also closed games for other starters, leading NL relievers with four victories and five saves. He walked only 49 batters in a career-high 312 innings and handled 108 defensive chances flawlessly.

Brown pitched several masterpieces in 1908, not suffering a setback until July 15. He blanked the Philadelphia Phillies on June 13, allowing just two hits to Sherwood Magee. After hurling a second consecutive shutout two days later against the Cincinnati Reds, he defeated Pittsburgh 3–0 on July 2 and 2–0 on July 4 to accomplish a rare feat of four straight shutouts.

The Cubs repeated as National League champions in 1908, but faced stiff challenges from New York and Pittsburgh. In mid–September, New York led Pittsburgh by two games and Chicago by three games. The Giants and Cubs met in a doubleheader on September 22 at the Polo Grounds. Brown relieved Overall in the seventh inning of the first game and preserved a 4–3 win. "The excitement of rescuing his teammates warmed Brown from crown to toe." He triumphed, 3–1, in the second game to move Chicago into a first-place tie with New York. The *New York World* wrote, "The only thing for [Giants manager John] McGraw to do to beat Chicago is to dig up a pitcher with only two fingers."[18]

Brown pitched superbly in September. starting seven games and appearing in 14 of their last 19 contests. He hurled three games in six days, eliminating Pittsburgh,

5–2, on just two days' rest in the home season finale on October 4 before a record-setting home crowd of 30,427. Brown singled sharply to right field to score Tinker and Johnny Kling with the go-ahead runs in the sixth frame. He was "supreme and superb. His curves never broke sharper and his control never seemed better."[19]

The Giants, meanwhile, won the last three regular season games against the Boston Doves and were tied with the Cubs for first place with 98 victories and 55 losses. The two clubs played on October 8 to determine the NL pennant winner. "The Polo Grounds were filled to the brim, outflowing, bursting at the seams." Nearly 40,000 attended the contest, "including an overflow inside the park and thousands gathered on the grandstand roof, the cliffs behind, and the 'L' viaduct beyond left field." From the crowd, "there was a steady roar of abuse," Brown remembered. "I had a half-dozen 'black hand' letters in my coat pocket. 'We'll kill you,' these letters said, 'if you pitch and beat the Giants.'" He begged manager Chance to let him pitch "just to show those so-and-sos they can't win with threats."[20]

Chance, however, started Pfiester, probably because Brown had been over-worked. The Cubs had not played for three days, giving the physically and emotionally exhausted Brown much-needed rest. Mike Donlin doubled to score Fred Tenney in the first inning, giving the Giants a 1–0 lead. With a deafening crowd roar, Brown relieved Pfiester with two men on and two men out and struck out Art Devlin to end the inning. The Cubs, capitalizing on a triple by Tinker and doubles by Frank Schulte and Chance, scored four runs off Mathewson in the third frame. Brown allowed only one run and four hits in eight and one thirds innings pitched. "I was about as good that day as I ever was in my life,"[21] Brown remembered. The tally came on Tenney's eighth-inning sacrifice fly after Brown gave up singles to Devlin and Moose McCormick and a walk with no one out. Mathewson struggled, yielding four runs in seven innings. Brown disposed of Devlin, McCormick, and Al Bridwell on four ninth-inning pitches to clinch the NL pennant. Brown recorded his twenty-ninth victory of 1908 and his ninth straight win over Mathewson, dating back to July 12, 1905. Three of those triumphs came in 1908.

Chicago thus won its third straight NL pennant in 1908. When the game ended, the Cubs crossed the field "through swarms of angry New Yorkers to get to the club-house." Brown recalled, "We all ran for our lives, straight for the clubhouse with the pack at our heels." Jimmy Sheckard, Tinker, Pfiester, and Chance all suffered physical abuse. "It was as near a lunatic asylum as I ever saw,"[22] he observed. After the Cubs dressed, "the team was ushered out of the stadium by police, herded into paddy wagons, and delivered to their hotel." Brown refused the police escort and instead walked to Chicago's hotel, yelling, "Those uniforms will surely tip me off."[23]

In an anticlimactic World Series, Chicago again bested Detroit in five games. Brown won twice, relieving the final two innings in Game 1 on October 10 at Detroit. He replaced Overall in the eighth frame with the score tied, 5–5, and yielded an unearned run. The Cubs countered with five runs in the top of ninth inning off Ed

Summers. Although allowing a walk and single, Brown blanked the Tigers in the bottom of the ninth frame to preserve the 10–6 victory and was credited with the win.

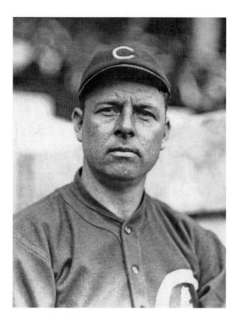

Three-Finger Brown posted four World Series victories, including three shutouts, for the Chicago Cubs between 1906 and 1910. He blanked the Detroit Tigers, 3–0, in Game 4 of the 1908 World Series, the last Fall Classic that franchise has won (courtesy National Baseball Hall of Fame Library, Cooperstown, N.Y.).

Brown started in Game 4 on October 13 in Detroit and blanked the Tigers, 3–0, on a four-hitter, in just one hour, 35 minutes. Noted for his remarkable fielding, he made a superb defensive play. Tiger star Ty Cobb acknowledged, "Brown performed the greatest play I ever saw." With Charley O'Leary on second base and Germany Schaefer on first base, Brown quickly fielded Cobb's bunt and rifled the ball to third base to nail O'Leary. Evers termed Brown's move "a seemingly impossible play, executed chiefly because Brown knew exactly what Cobb would do."[24] Brown became the first major league pitcher to hurl a shutout in three consecutive World Series. Cobb, who won 12 American League (AL) batting titles, rated Brown's curve ball "the most devastating curve ball I have ever faced." Overall defeated Detroit, 2–0, and struck out 10 Tigers in the World Series finale the next day at Detroit.[25] Chicago became the first major league team to win consecutive World Series, with Brown and Overall each recording two victories.

Brown's 1909 season did not begin well, as he suffered heartbreaking 1–0 losses to Pittsburgh in 12 innings on April 18 and in 11 innings a few days later. Brown gained revenge, defeating the first-place Pirates, 8–3, in 11 innings on May 29. Brown squandered a 3–1 lead in the ninth frame to the Cincinnati Reds on June 1, but the Cubs tallied six tenth-inning runs for a 9–3 win. "Although he continues to win with pleasing regularity," Ring Lardner wrote," he manages it so that one is forced to sit on the anxious seat all the time and stay at the ball yard much longer than is absolutely necessary." Mathewson out-dueled Brown, 3–2, on June 8, ending the latter's 10-game winning streak against the Giants legend,[26] and again bested him on August 12. Brown, however, retaliated, blanking New York 9–0 three days later, winning 6–1 on August 28, and shutting out the Giants 2–0 on August 31.

Brown pitched brilliantly for the second-place Cubs in 1909. He led the NL with 27 victories, 32 complete games in 34 starts, 342.2 innings pitched, 50 appearances, and seven saves. Brown suffered only nine losses, his fourth straight season with single digit setbacks. He ranked second in shutouts with eight, trailing only Overall. His 1.31 ERA ranked second to Mathewson's 1.14. Pittsburgh, however, won 110 games and finished six games ahead of Chicago for the NL pennant, marking the first time the Cubs had not led the league since 1905.

Chicago captured another NL pennant in 1910, recording 104 victories and finishing 13 games ahead of New York. Brown defeated St. Louis, 6–1, on May 30 at West Side Grounds, giving the Cubs 11 straight victories. Despite surrendering 11 hits, he triumphed over the Brooklyn Superbas, 14–0, on August 15.

Brown paced Chicago with 25 victories, trailing NL leader Mathewson by only two. He shared the league best in complete games (27) and paced the senior circuit in shutouts and saves (7). His 1.86 ERA placed second to King Cole.

The underdog Philadelphia Athletics assaulted the Cubs' pitching while taking the 1910 World Series in five games, defeating Brown in Games 2 and 5. In Game 2, Brown allowed nine runs in seven innings in a 9–3 loss on October 18 at Shibe Park. Neither he nor Philadelphia starter Jack Coombs hurled very well. Chicago trailed only 3–2 entering the seventh inning when the Athletics plated six runs. After Eddie Collins walked and Frank Baker singled, Harry Davis and Danny Murphy doubled to spark the six-run outburst. "Bitter tears coursed down Mordecai's weather-beaten cheeks as he trudged dejectedly to the clubhouse."[27]

Brown relieved Cole in the eighth inning of Game 4 on October 22 at West Side Grounds, with Chicago trailing 3–2, and hurled two scoreless innings. Schulte and Chance tripled off Chief Bender in the bottom of the ninth inning, knotting the score, 4–4. After Brown held Philadelphia scoreless in the top of the tenth frame, Jimmy Archer doubled down the left field line and Sheckard singled him home for the winning run. This marked Brown's fourth and last World Series triumph. Brown remarked, "I was glad of a chance to go in and do what I could, but it was our pinch hitting that won for us."[28]

Brown suffered the Game 5 loss on October 23, as Philadelphia clinched the World Series before 27,731 home fans. "It was the greatest crowd to see Chance's Cubs play in four Series, and sadly it beheld the death struggle of a great team." Coombs out-dueled Brown for seven innings, leading 2–1. "Brown's Waterloo inning was the eighth. It was a Cub nightmare as five rampaging White Elephants trampled over the plate." Four hits, two stolen bases, an error, and a wild pitch triggered the Athletics' five-run outburst. After Topsy Hartsel and Collins stole bases, Heinie Zimmerman dropped a fly ball to let two runs score, and Brown wild-pitched in another run. Chicago tallied one run in the ninth inning, losing 7–2. Brown, who never appeared in another World Series, lacked his usual command. "His glory years were behind him."[29] Brown had boasted a 5–4 record with a 2.81 ERA in four World Series. Only Mathewson exceeded his three World Series shutouts.

Although Brown won at least 20 games for the sixth consecutive season in 1911, advancing age and overwork began to reduce his effectiveness. Brown defeated St.

Louis, 6–1, on April 21 for his initial season victory. He started two consecutive games against first-place New York on June 3 and 4, besting Hooks Wiltse in the second. Brown again hurled back-to-back contests on June 9 and 10, being victorious in the latter. He won all of his July starts, helping lift the Cubs into first place, and defeated Mathewson on August 7. Chicago finished in second place, however, seven games back of the streaking Giants. Brown won 21 games and lost just 11 decisions in 1911, leading the NL with 53 appearances (including 27 starts) and setting a major league record with 13 saves. Five of his victories came in relief. Brown's ERA rose over 2.00 for the first time in six years.

In March 1912, Chicago signed Brown to a three-year, $21,000 contract. After Brown lost his first two starts in April, a sore arm sidelined him until mid–May. Brown did not win his first game that season until May 28 against Cincinnati. His last start that season came on July 9 in a 5–2 loss to Mathewson. Brown hurt his knee trying to steal second base in the tenth inning on July 15 against Boston. Catcher Kling did not throw the ball to second base. Brown abruptly attempted to abandon his slide, making "probably the biggest mistake of his career." The Cubs' ace "wrenched his knee so badly that he had to be helped off the field."[30] The injury terminated his season with an uncharacteristic 5–6 record in 15 appearances.

In October 1912, the Cubs sold Brown to Louisville (American Association). Cincinnati acquired Brown and offered him a $4,000 contract. Brown made 37 appearances, including just 16 starts. Brown defeated the Chicago Cubs on June 26 and on July 4, but lost his only confrontation with Mathewson, 4–2, on July 15. The *New York Times* observed that Brown "made it intensely interesting for the Giants all the way."[31] Brown, who saved both games of a July 22 doubleheader against Boston, finished the season 11–12 with six saves and a 2.91 ERA.

On December 27, 1913, the St. Louis Terriers of the Federal League (FL) signed Brown to a three-year contract as player-manager for $7,500 a season, the highest salary of his career. The FL started play in 1914, raiding 81 AL and NL players. Although 38 years old, Brown compiled an impressive 12–6 mark with a 3.29 ERA. The Terriers, however, languished in seventh place with a 50–63 mark when Jones replaced Brown as manager in August. St. Louis club executives, claiming that Brown lacked "fighting spirit" and was "too lenient with his men,"[32] traded him to the Brooklyn Tip-Tops (FL). In nine appearances with Brooklyn, Brown won only two of seven decisions.

On April 10, 1915, Brown joined the Chicago Whales (FL). "Brown regained much of his former effectiveness," blanking the Buffalo Buffeds on one hit on June 18. After missing a month with nephritis, he won his last six starts. Brown led Chicago to the 1915 FL pennant by one percentage point over St. Louis, boasting a 17–8 record in 236 innings, a team-best 2.09 ERA in 35 games, three shutouts, and four saves. He made "St. Louis once again regret trading him away."[33]

When the FL folded in December 1915, Brown rejoined the Chicago Cubs. He started only four games in 1916, winning one, and relieved eight times, with a combined 2–3 record and 3.94 ERA. His final major league victory, 8–3, came on July 23 over New York. The 39-year-old's last start occurred on September 4 against Mathewson, now with Cincinnati. Mathewson prevailed, 10–8, in this final confrontation between two major league pitching legends, cutting Brown's career advantage to 12–11. Mathewson surrendered 15 hits, while Brown allowed 19.[34]

During his major league career, Brown won 239 games while losing only 130. His career 2.06 ERA was the third lowest of any hurler logging 3,000 innings. Although never recording a no-hitter, he posted 55 shutouts. Brown hurled four consecutive shutouts in 1908 and won at least 20 games for six straight seasons. He finished 29–19 in relief and retired as the all-time saves leader with 49, a figure unsurpassed until 1924 by Firpo Marberry. His five World Series victories rank eighth, while his three World Series shutouts rank second. He masterfully kept hitters off balance. "If the batter crowded the plate, Brown pitched him tightly; if he stood far away, he worked him outside. If the batter crouched, the pitch would be high; if he stood up straight, it would be low."[35]

On December 4, the Cubs released Brown. Brown hurled the next two seasons for the Columbus Senators of the American Association (AA), posting a 10–12 mark and 2.77 ERA in 30 contests in 1917. He appeared in only 12 games in 1918 and replaced Joe Tinker as manager in June, guiding Columbus to second place. Brown served as player-manager with the Terre Haute Browns (TIL) in 1919, compiling a 16–6 mark with a 2.88 ERA. Terre Haute, however, languished in fifth place, 20 games under .500. Brown pitched briefly for Indianapolis (AA) in September, losing all three decisions, and rejoined Terre Haute as player-manager in 1920 for his final season.

Brown served as fire safety inspector for the Indiana Refining Company in Lawrenceville from 1921 to 1935 and operated a Texaco service station in Terre Haute from 1935 to 1946. In 1941, he bought stock in the Terre Haute baseball club. Brown participated in Old Timers' games and spent many hours at the Elks Club, sharing baseball lore. In November 1944, Brown, a Republican, lost a State Senate race in a predominantly Democratic party district.[36] He suffered a stroke in 1945 and struggled with diabetes until his death in Terre Haute on February 14, 1948, at age 71. On May 5, 1949, the Veterans Committee elected him to the National Baseball Hall of Fame.[37] In 1952, seven Chicago sportswriters voted Brown to an all-time, all-star Cubs team. In July 1979, Brown was elected a charter member of the Indiana Baseball Hall of Fame. On July 9, 1994, a monument was dedicated in his memory near his Nyesville birthplace. In 1999, a special panel of Major League Baseball executives, media, and historians selected Brown among the greatest 100 players of the twentieth century. Brown and his wife, Sara Burgham, left no children. Brown's disability made him determined to overcome the odds, making his story truly an inspiration to anyone who considers a dream.

# MIKE BURTON

Mike Burton, whose life was synonymous with hard work and perseverance, recovered from a tragic childhood vehicular accident to become "the man who revolutionized swimming." Burton suffered serious injuries as a junior high student when a truck struck his bicycle. After giving up contact sports, he set several freestyle swimming records and earned three Olympic gold medals.

Burton was brought up in a working-class environment. Michael Jay Burton was born on July 3, 1947, in Des Moines, Iowa, and moved to a Sacramento suburb when he was 10 months old. His father, Jay, worked as a truck driver, while his mother, Bernice, was a homemaker. Burton led a normal childhood with his brother, Randy, and sister, Barbara, and especially enjoyed playing basketball and football.

Burton was severely injured at age 12 while in eighth grade. He was riding home with a friend on a bicycle after playing basketball one afternoon. Burton was sitting on the handlebars of the bicycle, which his friend was pedaling. He recalled, "We crossed a two-lane highway heading toward a frontage road. Then all of a sudden, we ran into a furniture truck."[1] His friend emerged from the crash unscathed, but an ambulance rushed Burton to the hospital. Burton suffered from torn ligaments under his right kneecap and a dislocated hip. He spent six weeks in traction and was laid up another four weeks because of a knee operation. "Mike was lucky to be alive but it was believed that sports were not in his future." The injuries compelled him to quit contact sports. A doctor told him, "No contact sports for the rest of your life." The doctor's order, Burton acknowledged, "hurt a lot because I really loved all the sports."[2]

Swimming remained the only sport Burton could pursue. The 5-foot 9-inch, 155-pound Burton, therefore, concentrated on swimming as "a therapy for his injured leg" and was determined to become the best swimmer he could. About one year after the bicycle accident, he began swimming at the Arden Hills Swim and Tennis Club in Carmichael, California, under renowned coach Sherm Chavoor. During the late 1960s and early 1970s, Burton, Mark Spitz, Debbie Meyer, and other swimming champions benefited from Chavoor's instruction. Chavoor's swimmers established around 100 world and American records. In addition, "Chavoor revolutionized the sport with a training program in which he pushed his students to swim twice as far, twice as long as anyone else."[3]

Chavoor soon realized that Burton possessed unusual focus and determination. Burton did not live in a very wealthy neighborhood and competed against privileged youngsters, who defeated him soundly at first. "He wasn't about to be embarrassed by any rich kid," Chavoor remembered, "so he made up his mind that he was going to be better than them. Eventually he started to beat his teammates at Arden Hills and he ended up beating swimmers all around the world. Now if that isn't determination, I don't know what it is."

Burton was invited to the 1964 Olympic Trials at Astoria, New York, as a 17-year-old, but did not qualify for the U.S. Olympic swimming team. "I should have made the team," he claimed. "I was very close, so close that it really hit home that there was no way they were going to keep me off the 1968 team." A 1965 graduate of El Camino Fundamental High School, Burton won the Sac-Joaquin Section championships in the 200-meter freestyle and 100-meter butterfly. He entered the University of California at Los Angeles (UCLA) in September 1965.[4]

Chavoor, meanwhile, persuaded Burton to change the strategy for swimming the distance freestyle events. Distance freestylers previously had set a relatively slow pace and turned the event into a kicker's contest at the

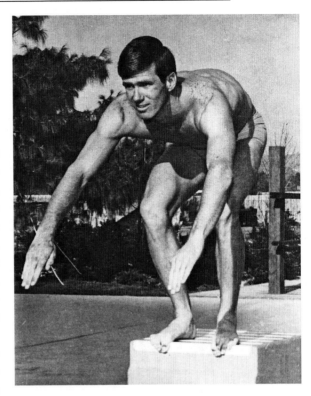

Mike Burton competed for UCLA from 1965 to 1969, establishing world records in the 800-meter freestyle and the 1500-meter freestyle events (courtesy International Swimming Hall of Fame; ASUCLA photograph).

end. Burton, however, always started hard and dared the other swimmers to match his pace throughout the race. He also pioneered the now standard training regimen of mega-mileage, swimming 4,000 meters daily to strengthen his endurance. Burton became the first swimmer to repeat twenty 200-meters with five seconds of rest between them. "All this mileage you see these kids doing today," Chavoor said, "Burton was the first to do it. He proved the human body could survive the punishment."[5]

Burton, nicknamed "Mr. Machine" or "perpetual motion," became one of the great long-distance freestylers, setting seven world records and 16 U.S. records, Between September 1965 and August 1969 at UCLA, he established world records in the 800-meter freestyle and 1500-meter freestyle events. Burton improved his 800-meter freestyle record twice and his 1500-meter freestyle records four times. He became the first swimmer to break 16 minutes for the 1,650-yard freestyle and eight minutes, 30 seconds for the 800-meter freestyle.[6]

Burton won 12 national Amateur Athletic Union (AAU) titles, including six outdoor and six indoor crowns. He captured the 1500-meter freestyle at the national Outdoor AAU Championships from 1966 through 1969 and in 1971, recording a 16-

minute, 4.5-second clocking in 1969, and took the 200-yard butterfly title at the national Outdoor AAU Championships in 1969. Burton won the 500-yard freestyle crown at the national Indoor AAU Championships in 1967 and the 200-yard butterfly title at the national Indoor AAU Championships in 1969. He also captured 1,650-yard freestyle titles at the national Indoor AAU Championships from 1966 through 1969, establishing the American record with a 16-minute, 27.3-second clocking in 1966 at Brandon, Florida, and producing "the outstanding individual performance" in 1967 at Dallas. The UCLA sophomore surged ahead in the first 300 yards of the 1,650-yard freestyle, "swimming's equivalent of the mile run," and covered the entire distance in 16 minutes, eight seconds. His 1967 AAU clocking bested his 1967 NCAA winning time by 9.5 seconds and his 1966 AAU performance by 19.3 seconds. "Talk about Jim Ryun winning the Sullivan Award," one swimming coach remarked. "Look at what this guy's done."[7] Burton broke the 16-minute barrier in the 1,650-yard freestyle at the 1969 AAU meet, clocking 15 minutes, 40.1 seconds.

Burton's first significant international success came in 1966, when he broke the 1500-meter freestyle world record. Burton swam the 1500 meters in "an unbelievable 16:41.6," shattering Steve Krause's former record by 17 seconds. During that race, Burton covered the first 800 meters in eight minutes, 48.8 seconds, "the second fastest clocking ever achieved." His 800-meter time fell merely six-tenths of a second shy of the world record, held by Belits Geiman of the Soviet Union. *Swimming World* named Burton World Swimmer of the Year. Burton also won a gold medal in the 1500-meter freestyle at the 1967 Pan-American Games in Winnipeg.[8]

Burton also won five NCAA Championships, taking the 1500-meter freestyle in 1967 and 1968. At the March 1968 NCAA meet, he broke the 16-minute barrier with a 15-minute, 59.4-second clocking. After missing the 1969 NCAA competition, Burton performed superlatively in his final NCAA Championship in March 1970 at Salt Lake City, winning the 1500-meter freestyle, 500-yard freestyle, and 200-yard butterfly titles. Despite swimming in the rarefied air at 4,200 feet above sea level and in an imperfect pool that slowed down times, he surfaced "as the star of the meet." Burton regained his 1,650-yard freestyle title in 16 minutes, 10.6 seconds, defeating Ralph Hutton by over 13 seconds. He also prevailed in the 500-yard freestyle in four minutes, 37.3 seconds, over two seconds better than Hutton, and completed the trifecta by taking the 200-yard butterfly in one minute, 51.7 seconds, edging John Ferris by .12 seconds. *Sports Illustrated* wrote, "UCLA's tireless Mike Burton" finished his collegiate career "in fine style" as "the meet's only triple winner." The spectators gave him a standing ovation after his 1,650-yard freestyle victory.[9]

Burton's most memorable impact on swimming, however, came in Olympic competition. At the 1968 Olympic Trials in Lincoln, Nebraska, Burton qualified for the U.S. Olympic swimming team in the 400-meter freestyle and 1500-meter freestyle. He and Hutton both lowered the existing world 400-meter freestyle record by over a second.[10]

Burton spent 40 days at the U.S. Air Force Academy in Colorado Springs, training for the 1968 Mexico City Summer Olympic Games. The U.S. Olympic swimming team trained at Colorado Springs because its high altitude better prepared the squad for the 7,349-foot elevation of Mexico City. Burton and Olympic coach George Haines both attributed his later success at the games to those 40 days of training. "There's no question it helped our distance guys," Haines affirmed. Physiological and psychological elements both helped the American swimmers. Burton claimed, "The chief value lay in the psychological component."[11]

Three problems confronted the U.S. Olympic swimmers at Mexico City. First, the swimmers needed to adjust to the higher elevation. The rarefied Mexico City air contained 30 percent less oxygen than at sea level, affecting all races exceeding three minutes. Some Mexico City times resembled those dating back to the 1948 or 1952 Olympics. Second, stomach problems hampered the performances of many athletes. Lastly, the swimmers performed in a relatively slow pool. The water level was "just far enough below the gutters to create everything but whitecaps whenever swimmers competed." The rigorous training regimen, however, helped the U.S. Olympic swimming team win 21 gold, 14 silver, and 16 bronze medals.[12]

A stomach ailment nearly sidelined Burton from the Olympic competition. According to Burton, "A buddy and I went to a pizza parlor after watching the marathon." Although he really enjoyed the pizza, Burton unfortunately woke up at 3 o'clock the next morning fully nauseated and spent around 12 hours in the infirmary. He was sent back to his room, but "got real sick again" on the elevator. "I started to spin around," Burton recalled, "and all of a sudden I passed out." Coach Haines recollected, "We had to carry Mike Burton down four flights of stairs, and take him to an infirmary where they fed him intravenously for about three days. Then he snapped out of it,"[13] before the qualifying heat for the 400-meter freestyle. During the ordeal, Burton's weight dropped from 155 pounds to 140 pounds. "I didn't think there was much of a chance that I'd be able to make it," Burton admitted. "But I gutted it out and swam just well enough to qualify." He needed to finish among the top eight to make the finals and came in sixth. Burton "just barely made it in," Haines said, noting "5/10ths of a second more, and he would have been a spectator."[14]

Burton ultimately won a gold medal in the 400-meter freestyle event. Just before the finals, he asked Haines to predict the winning time for that race. When Haines replied, "Hutton [of Canada] says he's going to go 4:11.0," Burton snapped back, "I'm going 4:09.0 tonight." Burton indeed took control of the race before the halfway marker and pulled away to win by 2.7 seconds, setting an Olympic record with the exact four minute, nine-second time he had predicted. Burton moved "with the power of a pocket battleship" in an event that was "just a warmup for his [1500-meter] specialty." Hutton finished second in four minutes, 11.7 seconds, while Alain Mosconi of France came in third at four minutes, 13.3 seconds.[15]

Three days later, "in the climactic event of a watery week," Burton, now fully recovered, captured the gold medal in the 1500-meter freestyle with a 16-minute, 38.9-second clocking. "He destroyed his top rival, Mexico's Guillermo Echeverria, who finished a stunned sixth." Burton prevailed by nearly 20 seconds, setting another Olympic record. His victory margin was the largest in that event's Olympic history. Teammate John Kinsella took the silver medal in 16 minutes, 57.3 seconds, while Greg Brough of Australia won the bronze medal in 17 minutes, 4.7 seconds.[16] "The thing to do," Burton told the press afterwards, "is go out fast and hang on." Chavoor, the U.S. women's team coach, beamed, "Look at Mike Burton. Kids like this make America great." The U.S. Olympic swim-

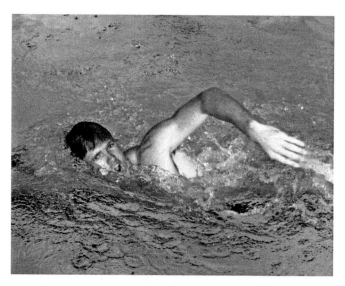

Mike Burton won gold medals in the 400-meter freestyle and 1500-meter freestyle at the 1968 Summer Olympic Games in Mexico City and in the 1500-meter freestyle at the 1972 Summer Olympic Games in Munich (courtesy International Swimming Hall of Fame; ASUCLA photograph).

ming team had swept five events, established four world and 17 Olympic records, and won 58 of the 99 available medals.[17]

Burton and his first wife, Linda, likewise a UCLA swimmer, were married in 1969. He graduated with a bachelor's degree from UCLA in 1970, the same year doctors repeated the surgery on the tendons near his right knee. Burton did not compete in any swimming events in 1971 and was diagnosed with a vitamin deficiency in the spring of 1972, but still hoped to participate in the 1972 Munich Summer Olympic Games. Linda provided the family's sole means of financial support while he trained for the Olympics. "I held three part-time jobs because there were no full-time jobs that would pay enough," she recollected. "While Mike trained, I coached and taught to keep us in hamburgers and French fries."[18]

Burton struggled to qualify in the 1500-meter freestyle for the 1972 U.S. Olympic swimming team. During the semifinals at the 1972 Olympic Trials in Chicago, he swam in the outside lane. Haines recalled, "There were about 20 or 30 people, coaches, swimmers and parents running along the pool deck, yelling for Mike Burton to qualify." Spurred on by his fans, Burton finished eighth and became the last qualifier for the final. "All but discounted before the race," Burton conceded, "These boys are passing me up."[19]

The 1500-meter freestyle finals saw Burton finish third to barely make the 1972 U.S. Olympic swimming team. Rick DeMont won the finals in a world-record time of 15 minutes, 52.91 seconds, overtaking Burton and John Kinsella. He was "powered by a slow but efficient stroke and a deep kick that enabled him to accelerate late in a race." Burton "wept joyfully at having grabbed the third spot." Jerry Kirshenbaum of *Sports Illustrated* wrote, Burton "has swum in pain throughout his career" and affirmed, "His courage was never more evident than now."[20]

At the 1972 Munich Olympic Games, DeMont, the 400-meter freestyle gold medalist, was favored to win the 1500-meter freestyle race. The International Olympic Committee (IOC), however, disqualified him about two minutes before the 1500-meter event for using an illegal drug. DeMont, who suffered from asthma, had taken Marax, an over-the-counter medication. Although Marax likely was more a medicinal drug than performance-enhancing one, the IOC had banned it. Ephedrine, a Marax component, was a stimulant that could trigger heart palpitations and insomnia. The IOC stripped DeMont of his gold medal in the 400-meter freestyle and awarded it to Bradford Cooper of Australia.[21]

Burton had not been swimming well in Munich, and, despite DeMont's disqualification, was not favored to repeat in the 1500-meter freestyle. "Burton," however, "got himself together and swam one of his great races." He paced for the first 750 meters, but Graham Windeatt of Australia assumed the lead for the next 600 meters. According to Haines, Burton "got on the guy's hip. The other swimmer didn't move over, and so Burton stayed right there with the guy until about the last 150."[22] Burton surged ahead of Windeatt at the 1,350-meter mark and retained it for the last 150 meters to secure his third Olympic gold medal. He "tumbled and got away from him and won the race." Burton became the first Olympic male swimmer ever to capture a 1500-meter freestyle title twice or retain it at two consecutive Olympic Games. He covered the distance in a world-record time of 15 minutes, 52.58 seconds, over 46 seconds faster than his 1968 clocking. Windeatt took the silver medal in 15 minutes, 58.48 seconds, while Doug Northway of the United States earned the bronze medal at 16 minutes, 9.25 seconds. Burton, considered an old-timer by the 1972 Munich Games, reflected, "The second Olympic games was probably my most triumphant simply because I was 25 years old. Nobody thought I was even going to win a medal. So, that was really, really fun."[23]

The 1972 Munich Summer Olympics featured Mark Spitz's magnificent performance of seven gold medals in swimming. Spitz accomplished arguably the greatest overall swimming feat in Olympic history until Michael Phelps won eight gold medals at the 2008 Summer Olympic Games. Burton's world-record comeback win in the 1500 meters, however, was the greatest individual feat of those games.[24]

The murder of 11 Israelis by Arab terrorists, the day after Burton's 1500-meter race, overshadowed the athletic events at the 1972 Olympic Summer Games. Eight Arab guerrillas, members of the Black September terrorist group, invaded the Israeli dormitory at the Olympic village in Munich on September 5, killing two members of the Israeli squad and taking nine other hostages. Five of the terrorists, all nine hostages, and a German policeman were later killed in a shootout at a nearby airport.[25]

The terrorist attack occurred hours after Burton had won his third gold medal. After celebrating that night at two bars, Burton did not return to the Olympic village and did not find out until the next morning what had happened. "I stayed that night in an apartment with Linda and my parents," Burton recollected, "and didn't know until the next morning" when he picked up his clothes "what was going on in the village." "There were police all over the place," he remembered. "I didn't stick around too long, but I did see one of the terrorists." Burton remains passionate about separating the Olympics from politics.

Burton had revolutionized the sport by swimming very long distances daily at the Arden Hills Swim Club until he was exhausted. He earned three gold medals by training extremely hard under Chavoor, setting a work ethic hitherto unheard of in practice, and even swimming well when experiencing stomach problems. Top swimming coaches across the world wondered why Burton swam so well. According to Chavoor, "He did it by over distance swimming. Instead of swimming one mile, I'd have him swim 12. And he'd do that until he was totally worn out. Then he'd come back the next day and do the same thing." Chavoor explained, "The top swimmers in the world couldn't believe what we were doing. They said there was no way a human being could take all of that beating. But he proved it to them when he stood on that victory stand."[26]

After the 1972 Olympic Games, Burton retired from swimming competition and became a swimming coach. Coaching assignments followed at Multnomah Athletic Club in Portland, Oregon; Brigham Young University in Provo, Utah; and then in Philadelphia and in Arizona. In the late 1970s, Burton became a technical director for FINA, the body governing international competition in aquatic sports, in Des Moines. He started the Des Moines Aquatic Club in 1980 and coached the Des Moines Swim Federation Team until July 1986, developing Craig Oppel, Jennifer Linder, and Mike Johnson.[27]

Burton and his first wife, Linda, had two children, Eric and Loni. Loni, who competed for a Division II school, remains one of two swimmers in NCAA history to win 12 individual titles in just three years. Burton and his present wife, Carol, married in 1987 and resided in Washington State before moving to Billings, Montana, in the late 1990s. Burton coached the Seahawks at the Billings YMCA and delivers supplies for the Billings Clinic, while Carol serves as president and CEO of United Way of Yellowstone County.

Burton was elected to the International Swimming Hall of Fame in 1977, the UCLA Sports Hall of Fame in 1984, the Iowa Sports Hall of Fame in 1984, and the *Sacramento Bee's* Sac-Joaquin Section inaugural High School Hall of Fame in 2010.

He observed that winning three Olympic gold medals spurred him to strive for greatness daily. Burton enjoys seeing how swimming has progressed each decade and especially watching the sport's young stars, including 14-time gold medalist Phelps. "Phelps was born to swim," Burton reflected. "The way his body is put together; he has a 30-inch inseam but he's 6' 4"; that's amazing."

Although major injuries suffered in the bicycle accident ended his involvement in contact sports, Burton transformed swimming through his relentless work ethic and exhibited the courage, determination, and persistence to become one of the greatest distance freestylers in American history. "You can talk about [swimming greats] Don Schollander and Mark Spitz all you want," Chavoor concluded, "but it was Mike Burton who revolutionized swimming."[28]

# BEN HOGAN

"Concentration and determination — unbroken" marked the courageous life of Ben Hogan, who survived a horrendous automobile accident to resume his great golfing career. Hogan already had achieved golf stardom before being involved in a nearly fatal car crash. After enduring an agonizing rehabilitation, he amazed the golf world by soaring to even loftier heights than before.

Hogan experienced poverty and tragedy as a child. William Benjamin Hogan was born on August 13, 1912, in Stephenville, Texas, and grew up in Dublin, Texas, where his father, Chester, was a village blacksmith. He moved to Fort Worth in June 1921 because his father needed medical treatment for manic depression. His father committed suicide eight months later. To help support his mother, Clara, a seamstress, Hogan sold newspapers two years at the Texas and Pacific Railroad Station.[1]

In 1924, Hogan began his golf career as a caddie at the Glen Garden Country Club in Fort Worth. Although undersized, he became a caddie by winning a fistfight with another youngster. "I got the golf bug," Hogan recalled. He liked the sport's fairness, solitude, and competitiveness. The sport fit his taciturn personality. At age 15, Hogan tied Byron Nelson for the Christmas Day caddie tournament crown. He astonished onlookers, shooting a 39 over nine holes.[2] Nelson sunk a 30-foot birdie on the final hole to force a tie. Hogan ignored the advice of others and quit Central High School in Fort Worth after his sophomore year to play golf. He turned professional at age 19 in February 1930, but shot erratically in the Texas Open. "A chronic tendency to hook cut into his consistency." He quickly learned, "I shouldn't even be out there,"[3] and returned home. He tried the pro golf tour again briefly in 1933.

Hogan attracted little national attention and struggled financially for nearly a decade. "No athlete ever worked harder, or waited longer, to become a champion." Difficult times continued following his marriage to Valerie Fox in April 1935. "It's now or never," Hogan told Valerie before a July 1937 tournament. He nearly abandoned the golf circuit for financial reasons at the end of 1937, but professional Henry Picard persuaded him to continue.[4] Before the Oakland Open in California, Hogan told Valerie, "We've got less than $100 left." He earned $285 for finishing third in that tournament, calling it "the turning point in my golf life."[5] Hogan soon became an assistant professional at the Century Country Club in Purchase, New York. "Hope gained through hard work, vindication achieved from never giving up," he concluded. Hogan practiced long hours, driving every ball as far as possible and improving his putting. He began placing higher and winning tournament money, earning $4,150 in 1938 and $5,600 in 1939.

Hogan captured his first tournament, the North and South Open, at Pinehurst, North Carolina, with a record 277 score in March 1940 and quickly became the most consistent low scorer on the circuit. "The long wait was over. Vindication was his, a victory so sweet it almost ached." Hogan that year won three other tournaments, including the Greater Greensboro Open and Asheville Open the next two weeks. He captured his first three professional golf tournaments in just 10 days, "something no player had ever done so quickly before," and "possibly the most sensational stretch of tournament golf anyone had ever played."[6] He ended 1940 as golf's leading money winner with $10,056, "ripping through everything else but 'the big ones.'" Five more tournament victories followed in 1941, when he shared third in the U.S. Open at the Colonial Club in Fort Worth. Nelson edged him in a playoff in 1942 at the Masters Tournament. Hogan earned the Vardon Trophy for lowest average score in 1940 and 1941 and led the Professional Golfers Association (PGA) tour in earnings again with $18,358 in 1941 and $13,143 in 1942. Sportswriter Grantland Rice termed Hogan "the greatest of all 'concentrators,'" and observed, "He plays with more lasting determination than anyone."[7]

After serving three years in the U.S. Army Air Corps from March 1943 to August 1945, Hogan returned to the PGA circuit in 1945 and rejoined Nelson and Sam Snead as the nation's best golfers. He won the Portland (Oregon) Open in August 1945, setting a record with a remarkable 27-under-par 261 for the lowest 72-hole score in PGA tour history. Golf writer Fred Corcoran boasted, "It was an incredible, unbelievable performance."[8]

Hogan again paced golfers in earnings and snagged his first major tournament, the 1946 PGA Championship, in August at the Portland Golf Club in Oregon, defeating Ed "Porky" Oliver, six-and-four, in the 36-hole final of the match play. His first major title came "years behind schedule."[9] Club member Peter Walsh observed, "Hogan just devoured the field," while historian Herbert Warren Wind added, "He played like a killer in the afternoon of the final." Wind described the intense Hogan as "a volcano always on the brink of eruption," overly determined, controlled, inflexible, and purposeful.

In 1946, Hogan amassed 13 victories and $42,556 and barely missed taking the

Masters and U.S. Open. Although again conquering no majors in 1947, he captured
seven more tournaments and earned $23,000. His thought and execution improved.
Wind wrote that no contemporary golfer "generated the clubhead speed and unleashed
a shot like Hogan did just before he learned how to win."[10]

Hogan soared to greater heights in 1948 with 11 victories. "No other golfer ever
dedicated himself so totally to the game," Wind claimed. Hogan prevailed in five
consecutive tournaments: the U.S. Open at Riviera Country Club in Los Angeles;
his second PGA Championship at Northwood Hills Country Club in St. Louis, Missouri; the Motor City Open; the Reading Open; and his second Western Open. He
tied the U.S. Open mark with a 69 in the final round, shattering the tournament
record by five strokes with 276. Hogan played the U.S. Open "coldly, methodically,"
resembling "a heart surgeon in the closing stages of a life-and-death operation."[11]
Runner-up Jimmy Demaret noted that the Texan seemed unbeatable, calling Riviera
"Hogan's Alley." Despite back pain, Hogan rallied to garner the PGA Championship.
Besides finishing among the top three in 17 of 25 events, he paced competitors in
earnings for the fifth time and snared his third Vardon Trophy. "I love the competition,"[12] he affirmed.

Hogan won the Bing Crosby Pro-Am and Long Beach Open in January 1949,
giving him a record 37 victories since 1946. After Hogan placed second at the Phoenix
Open, he and his wife, Valerie, began driving on February 1 to their Fort Worth
home. After staying overnight in Van Horn, Texas, Hogan started driving on Highway
10 the next morning, in extremely foggy conditions.[13]

Hogan's career took a tragic turn that morning, when he was seriously injured
in a traffic accident on the narrow two-lane highway. Hogan had slowed his Cadillac
to 30 miles per hour when his vehicle confronted "a lumbering, skidding transcon-
tinental bus." Alvin Logan, a substitute Greyhound Bus driver, crossed the center
line and attempted to pass a truck on a bridge in a valley. An eighth of a mile away,
Hogan "suddenly saw two sets of headlights bearing down" on his vehicle. "The concrete bridge abutments left no room to bail out." Valerie, petrified, immobile, and
speechless, thought, "It was the end. We had no chance."[14]

An instant before the collision, Hogan "dove headlong to his right, hurling his
body protectively over Valerie's terrified ninety-eight-pound frame." Instantly, the
rural setting "resounded with shrieking brakes and a sickening crash." The bus
smashed directly into the Hogans' Cadillac. Hogan's car skidded sideways and slid
down the culvert grade, "engulfed in steam and smoke,"[15] and was "a mass of twisted
metal. The impact drove the steering wheel through the driver's seat, like a javelin
from an angry hand." Valerie escaped with only minor injuries. Hogan, though, suffered a double-ring fracture of the pelvis, broken left collarbone, fractured left ankle,
broken rib, and deep cuts and contusions around his left eye. He experienced shock,
a weak, rapid pulse, falling blood pressure, and a lack of consciousness. "A dozen
times he woke and a dozen times breathtaking pain stabbed and throbbed through

his body."[16] An ambulance did not arrive from El Paso for over 90 minutes. After being rushed to Hotel Dieu Hospital in El Paso, Hogan commenced his lengthy, painful battle to survive and then regain his form as America's premier professional golfer. The accident made him realize, "It was important to let his growing legions of fans and admirers see occasional glimpses of the real man within, not just the golf machine that won tournaments with intimidating mechanical precision."[17]

Hogan seemingly weathered the crisis until February 18, when doctors detected three large life-threatening blood clots traveling up his damaged left leg to his chest. "The clots were floating time bombs in his circulatory system, large enough to block a key artery to the legs and possibly kill him." His condition deteriorated quickly. "Time was running out." Dr. Alton Ochsner of Tulane University performed two-hour, emergency abdominal surgery, binding the principal veins in Hogan's legs. The operation kept Hogan alive, but physicians predicted he would struggle "to walk normally again, let alone resume the toil of tournament golf."[18] Doctors, though, underestimated his "flaming determination" and "fierce competitive fire."[19]

After being hospitalized 58 days until April 1, Hogan convalesced at his Fort Worth home. He gradually learned to walk again by doing laps around a room, but his bad left knee and shoulder never fully recovered and his weight dropped by 18 pounds to 120 pounds. Hogan did not go outdoors for two months, but began taking afternoon hikes by the summer. On December 10, he played an 18-hole round for the first time in nearly a year at the Colonial Club in Fort Worth. Heavily bandaged from thighs to ankles, he did not complete some holes and walked with assistance from an electric cart. The round exhausted and depressed him, making him think that he might never compete again in tournament golf.[20]

In mid–January 1950, Hogan amazingly resumed the PGA golf circuit at the Los Angeles Open at Riviera Country Club and uncharacteristically became the sentimental crowd favorite. The 72-hole, four-day tournament tested his endurance and faltering legs. His tour appearance astonished sportswriters and fans. Demaret observed that Hogan looked frail, but added, "His golf shots zinged with all the startling force and accuracy they had before the accident."[21]

Despite the long layoff, Hogan played brilliantly with a 73 on the first round and 69s on the next two rounds, stunning the golf world. "Ben is a walking miracle," Dr. Cary Middlecoff, fellow golfer, remarked. "Bennie has more heart than anybody I've ever known."[22] Hogan, fatigued, led Snead by four strokes with only four holes left, but the latter recorded birdies on the last four holes to tie him at 280 and force a playoff. Snead captured the anticlimactic 18-hole playoff with a 72, prevailing by four strokes. Grantland Rice claimed Hogan "didn't lose, his legs simply were not strong enough to carry his heart around." Sportswriter Will Grimsley penned, "He had written one of the most dramatic stories in sports."[23]

The public followed Hogan's incredible comeback, altering their perception of him. Instead of being "the lion among the Christians," Hogan was considered "an

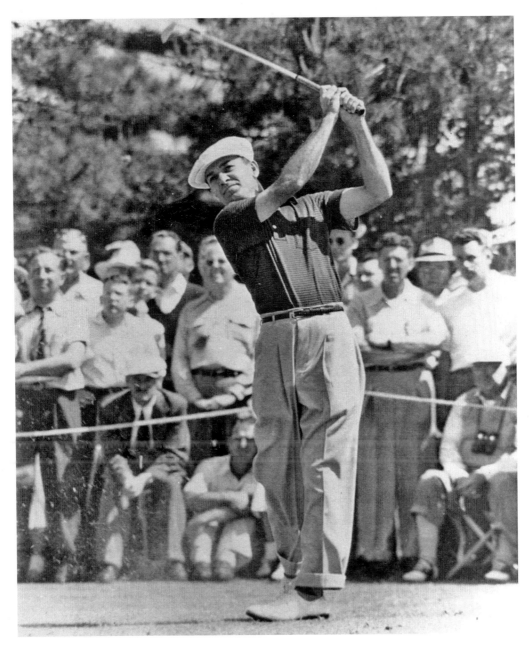

Ben Hogan won nine major tournaments, including four U.S. Opens, two Masters, two PGAs, and one British Open. In 1953, he captured the Masters, U.S. Open, and British Open, but did not compete in the PGA (courtesy World Golf Hall of Fame).

appealing underdog." Hogan gradually gained 40 pounds, but endured chronic back and shoulder pain, inflamed tendons, and fatigue. His annual tournament appearances dropped from 30 to five. After Hogan's score ballooned in the final Masters round, he captured the Spring Festival of Golf at White Sulphur Springs, West Virginia. He skipped the PGA and British Open, however.

In June 1950, Hogan won the U.S. Open at Merion Golf Club in Ardmore, Pennsylvania. After shooting a two-over-par 72 in the first round, he recorded a 69 in the next round and trailed Dutch Harrison by just two shots. Hogan was fatigued and limped badly on his left leg. His round nearly ended on the eleventh hole of the second round because of "constant pain that alternately throbbed and stabbed." The final day demanded a taxing 36 holes, something Hogan had not attempted since the accident. Severe cramps struck him on the thirteenth hole. "That's it. I just can't make it," Hogan told his caddie. "No, Mr. Hogan, you can't quit," the caddie replied, "because I don't work for quitters."[24]

Hogan struggled to a 72 in the third round, behind Lloyd Mangrum by two strokes. He seized the lead with a 39 on the front nine of the final round and widened his advantage to three shots over George Fazio after 11 holes. Since Hogan's sharp leg pains worsened, however, Middlecoff lifted the ball from the eleventh hole for him. After driving from the twelfth tee, Hogan "staggered as if he had been hit with a knockout punch"[25] and bogeyed that hole. He also bogeyed the fifteenth and seventeenth holes, knotting him with Mangrum and Fazio. He barely missed a 40-foot birdie on the final hole, having squandered a three-stroke lead on the final six holes.

Hogan shot a 69 in the playoff, defeating Mangrum by four strokes and Fazio by six strokes. Mangrum briefly led after the second hole, but Hogan never trailed thereafter. The Texan led Mangrum by one stroke after 15 holes and both parred the sixteenth hole. Tournament referee Ike Grainger, however, penalized Mangrum two strokes for lifting the ball to remove a ladybug. Hogan miraculously converted a mammoth uphill 50-foot birdie on the seventeenth hole, easing the pain for Mangrum. "He was not only back, he was back on top." Hogan's "'miraculous' comeback was complete."[26] Hogan had captured one of golf's most prestigious tournaments just sixteen months after his accident. "The 1950 Open was my biggest win," he affirmed. "It proved I could still play." Sportswriter Dan Jenkins classified it "the most incredible comeback in the history of sports." Hogan's brilliant final round "dispelled all questions of whether he would be able to reclaim his old throne."[27]

In 1951, Hogan continued his remarkable comeback with two major titles. Hogan's dramatic film, *Following the Sun*, was released March 23, profiling his compelling story and portraying his heroic, miraculous return to golf and subsequent triumphs. Since Hogan had never won the Masters, he practiced thoroughly on the Augusta golf course for 10 days before the tournament. The Texan gave "one of his most memorable demonstrations of how to win a golf tournament by using your head as well as your hands," shrewdly gauging the probable performance of his rivals and calculating the score he needed to win. He insisted course management accounted for 80 percent of his success, talent only 20 percent. Hogan shot rounds of 70 and 72 and trailed Skee Riegel by one stroke after two rounds. "I couldn't be playing better,"[28] he remarked. Riegel and Snead shared the lead at 211 after the third round, with Hogan one stroke behind.

Snead struggled with an eight on the eleventh hole and an 80 for the final round, while Riegel recorded a 71. Hogan, who needed a 69 to prevail, traversed the front nine holes in three-under 33 and conquered the perilous back nine in one-under 35. He played so skillfully "you wondered why that back nine had given anyone the least bit of trouble." Hogan birdied the thirteenth and fifteenth holes and was two strokes ahead of Riegel entering the final hole. Before a record gallery of 8,000 fans, the Texan parred the last hole to capture his first Masters title, scoring 68 on the final round. The disappointed gallery witnessed Hogan eschew spectacular shots, "but they will probably never see a finer exhibition of how to play solid, heady, sticking-with-par golf." The green jacket ceremony with legend Bobby Jones followed. "If I never win another, I'll be satisfied,"[29] Hogan sighed.

Hogan captured his third U.S. Open crown at challenging Oakland Hills Country Club in Birmingham, Michigan. The course, designed by Robert Trent Jones and nicknamed "The Monster," was the most challenging ever confronted by U.S. Open golfers. Although Hogan preferred to attack, he played the first two rounds conservatively and trailed Bobby Locke by five strokes. No player bested par during the first two rounds. A record 18,000 spectators witnessed the final two rounds. Hogan shot three-under-par through the first 13 holes of the morning round and seemed headed toward "a round so dazzling that it would have had the effect of taking the heart out of the opposition."[30] Hogan tallied 71, the tournament's second best score, to pull within two strokes of the lead. Demaret caught Locke for the lead after three rounds.

Hogan's finest round of his stellar career came that afternoon. "Something in the moment — the buzz from the crowd, his anger at himself or at this Civil War battlefield of a golf course — allowed Hogan to find the perfect balance between fury and control." Hogan made the turn at even-par 35 and covered the back nine in 32, birdieing the tenth, thirteenth, and fifteenth holes to record a 67. "He finished with a flourish" on the final hole, converting a 15-foot birdie. Hogan's three-under-par 67 came on a day that the field averaged 75. "His final round was already being hailed as a masterpiece of discipline and execution." Hogan, "the finest final-round player of his era,"[31] bested Clayton Heafner by two strokes and termed that round "the finest" of his distinguished golf career. He boasted, "I brought the beast to her knees." Hogan and Heafner were the only players to break 70 over the four rounds "on perhaps the severest layout on which the open has been played." Hogan captured five consecutive tournaments, including the World's (Tam O'Shanter) Championship, netting golf's largest purse at $12,500.

Hogan thereafter concentrated on the major tour events. According to Hogan, "The most important factor in playing a championship is to be fully prepared."[32] He appeared in only three 1952 tournaments, taking the Colonial National Invitation at Fort Worth. He performed poorly in the final Masters round and relinquished the lead in the third round of the U.S. Open at the Northwood Club in Dallas, losing to Julius Boros by five strokes. His legs and stamina abandoned him. He did not compete between the U.S. Open and the PGA, citing declining eyesight and diminished putting ability.[33]

Hogan's premier season came in 1953. Hogan prepared two weeks for the Masters Tournament at Augusta. He shot a 70 in the first round and, despite missing three short putts, catapulted to first in the second round with a 69. He extended his lead with a third-round 66, converting a 50-footer on the ninth hole and a downhill 25-foot putt on the tenth. His 205 shattered Nelson's 54-hole Masters scoring record by two strokes. In the final round, Hogan nearly converted long shots on three holes, recording birdies on the thirteenth, fifteenth, and eighteenth holes. The huge gallery leapt to its feet when Hogan birdied the final hole, tallying a final round of 69.

Hogan's 274 brought his second Masters title, besting Oliver by five strokes and shattering the previous tournament best of Ralph Guldahl and Claude Harmon by five strokes. His new tournament record 14-under-par "blew away the old mark."[34] The Texan played "four consecutive rounds of comparable errorless character," and "literally was on the pin with just about every shot." Golfer Gene Sarazen lauded Hogan's performance as "the greatest four scoring rounds anyone had ever put together in golf," while Wind boasted, his play was "about as forceful and as flawless as golf can be." An ecstatic Hogan agreed it was "the best I've ever played for seventy-two holes."[35]

Hogan won five of seven 1953 tournaments, nearly equaling Jones' 1930 Grand Slam. After taking the Pan-American Open in Mexico City and Colonial Open in Fort Worth, he captured his fourth U.S. Open at Oakmont Country Club in Pennsylvania. Hogan shot a brilliant 67 in the first round, missing the course record by one stroke and catapulting him to a three-stroke lead. He led Snead by two strokes after two rounds, but the latter halved the margin in the third round Saturday morning. Both tallied 38 over the front nine in the Saturday afternoon finale. Snead recorded a disastrous six on the twelfth hole. Although bogeying the fifteenth hole, Hogan "unleashed one of his most irresistible finishes," birdieing the seventeenth and eighteenth holes. He tallied 33 over the back nine for a round of 71 and 283 overall score, routing Snead by six strokes. His superlative 71, "capped off by the boldest finish in Open history,"[36] obliterated the course tournament record by 11 strokes. Hogan joined Willie Anderson and Jones as the only four-time U.S. Open champions.

No subsequent golfer has matched Jones' Grand Slam. Hogan and Tiger Woods remain the only golfers to snag even three major championships the same year. Woods competed in all four majors in 2000, but Hogan was denied that opportunity in 1953 because the PGA tournament occurred the week following the U.S. Open and involved match play. "You had to play something like seven matches to make it over 36 holes. That would have been too much,"[37] he recalled.

Hogan had attained every major American championship, but he had not played in the prestigious British Open. Hogan competed against the world's finest golfers

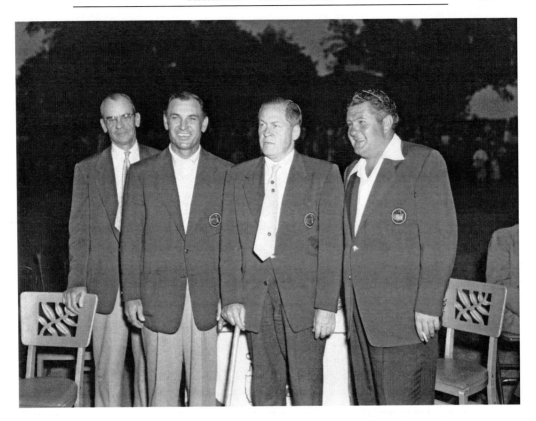

Ben Hogan, second from left, pictured here with Bobby Jones, second from right, at the Augusta National Golf Club in Augusta, Georgia, won the Masters Tournament there in 1951 and 1953 (courtesy Kenan Research Center at the Atlanta History Center).

under far more challenging conditions than he had experienced. Nevertheless, he captured the British Open at Carnoustie, Scotland, in July 1953, in his only attempt. His victory had "the aura of a romantic novel about it, it was so utterly triumphant."[38] The British Open long had stood "as a measure of the greatness of the great golfers before him." To learn the difficult course, he had studied its natural features and the problems it posed. The perfectionist Hogan "calculated the precise coordinates of movement required, like a violin virtuoso playing a sonata."[39]

Hogan delivered a 73 in the first round of the British Open, three strokes behind Frank Stranahan. He followed with a 71 in the second round, trailing Eric Brown and Dai Rees by two strokes. Six birdie putts just skimmed the hole. The final 36 holes transpired the last day. Hogan, whose "body temperature had soared to 103," three-putted on the seventeenth hole and tallied 70 in the morning round to share the lead with Roberto DeVincenzo at 224. He seized the sole British Open lead for the first time with a dramatic 35-foot birdie on the fifth hole that afternoon. His ball "landed nicely up the slope, started to run fast for the hole, kept running, hit the back of the cup, jumped three inches in the air, and came down in the hole."[40] Hogan navigated the first nine holes in 34, two under par. He birdied the thirteenth and final holes for a 282 overall score, four strokes better than Antonio Cerda, Peter Thomson, Stranahan, and Rees. On the final hole, the large gallery "cheered the 'Wee Ice Mon,' expressionless as ever, on to his epochal triumph." Hogan set course records for a single round with 68 and for a tournament "by a whopping eight strokes" with 282, He also authored the best 72-hole score for a British Open Championship.

Adoring Scots christened Hogan the "Wee Ice Mon" because of his steely demeanor. After accepting the Claret Jug, Hogan lauded the Scottish fans as "the greatest galleries I've ever seen." He revealed, "The British Open gave me my greatest pleasure."[41] According to Wind, "Hogan's immensely popular victory inspired a spate of accolades, written and verbal, saluting his capability, temperament, and courage, and pronouncing him the peer of any golfer who ever lived."[42]

Hogan had achieved an epic feat, scoring "progressively better over the toughest links in Scotland." He had missed just one fairway in 108 holes of golf. His "Carnoustie triumph matched any championship in Open history for drama and courage." Hogan's sweep of the three 1953 major titles rivaled Jones's historic Grand Slam of 1930, a trifecta that "endeared the rugged Texan to his Scottish hosts" and "made his name a household word back in America."[43] New York City gave Hogan a ticker tape parade up Broadway, the first for a golfer since Jones in 1930.

Millions of Americans followed Hogan's daily exploits, viewing Hogan's win "as a national triumph." Wind wrote, "You might have thought that the whole story was the concoction of a garret-bound author of inspiration books for children who had dreamed up a golfing hero and a golfing tale he hoped might catch on as had the exploits of Frank Merriwell." The Texan remained "a consummate strategist, shot-maker and competitor."[44]

Hogan played in the Masters and U.S. Opens the next three years. He struggled with a 75 in the final round of the 1954 Masters, blowing a three-stroke lead over Snead in the last 90 minutes in "a collapse that would chew at him like an ulcer for years." Snead birdied the thirteenth hole, defeating Hogan by one stroke in the Masters playoff. Hogan coveted an unprecedented fifth U.S. Open title to "set him apart even from the immortal Jones."[45] In the 1955 U.S. Open at the Olympic Country Club in San Francisco, Hogan shot a 70 on the final round to finish with a 287 and seemingly clinch that title. Jack Fleck started the final round three strokes behind Hogan and trailed him by one stroke after 15 holes. He just missed birdies on the sixteenth and seventeenth holes and sank an eight-foot putt for a birdie on the eighteenth hole, shooting a sizzling three-under-par 67 to force a playoff the next day. "I was wishing it was over — all over,"[46] Hogan rued.

Hogan trailed Fleck by three strokes after 10 holes of the U.S. Open playoff the next day, but sliced the margin to one over the next seven holes. Fleck, meanwhile, shot a par-four on the eighteenth hole to finish the round with a 69 and captured the playoff by three strokes. By contrast, Hogan struggled with a double-bogey six on the final hole to record a 71. Fleck, "the angular 32-year-old Iowan who accomplished miracles two days and running," played "crisp, precise shots from tee to green" and putted "like a man in a trance" to stop Hogan's bid for an unprecedented fifth U.S. Open title. The Texan's knee bothered him. "The more I walked, the more it hurt,"[47] he disclosed. Hogan vowed never to work that hard to win another tournament. "This one doggone near killed me."[48]

Hogan provided a formidable challenge at the 1956 U.S. Open at Oak Hill Country Club in Rochester, New York. He needed merely to par the final two holes to tie Middlecoff, but lost by one stroke, missing a short, 30-inch putt on the seventeenth hole. His last PGA triumph came at the 1959 Colonial Invitational in Fort Worth. At the 1967 Masters, he set a record by shooting the back nine in 30 strokes in one of his most dramatic, heartwarming career performances.

Hogan constantly ranked among the finest strokers in golf history. He prevailed in 63 tournaments, including nine majors between 1940 and 1956 and six after his accident. Hogan finished among the top five in 27 majors, including five U.S. Opens. His majors titles included the 1951 and 1953 Masters; the 1948, 1950, 1951, and 1953 U.S. Opens; the 1946 and 1948 PGAs; and the 1953 British Open. Besides setting the Masters Tournament low-scoring record in 1953, Hogan placed second in four Masters and among the top seven from 1941 through 1956. He came within two strokes of a fifth U.S. Open crown six times. Hogan participated in four Ryder Cups, captaining the squad three times, and won the PGA Player of the Year Award in 1948, 1950, 1951, and 1953. "He became the fairway Goliath of the Fifties, the one man able to awe and consistently overpower the tough precisionists."[49]

Hogan ranks with Harry Vardon, Jones, Jack Nicklaus, and Woods as the five greatest players in golf history. Only Nicklaus, Woods, Jones, and Walter Hagen captured more majors. Hogan symbolized "a man of fortitude who fashioned an almost unbelievable comeback" and "one of the great all-time champions of the game." The postwar era became "The Age of Hogan." Wind wrote, future generations "will be struck by awe and disbelief that any one man could have played so well so regularly."[50] Hogan approached golf and life with the same determination. The key ingredients for his success included hard work, a drive for excellence, analytical devotion to practice, and dedication. Hogan possessed a natural swing and constantly improved his game as the era's greatest shotmaker. He golfed daily into his seventies and claimed, "There is not enough daylight in a day to practice all the shots you ought to be practicing." Hogan epitomized mental toughness, self-control, and focus, blending mood with performance. "His name alone defined concentration, determination, even perfection." Grimsley attributed Hogan's success to his "seemingly insatiable — almost fanatical — urge to keep proving something to the world, and to himself." Grimsley pointed out, "Hogan was a sullen tailor methodically stitching a dark cloak of defeat for his rivals."[51]

The author of *Power Golf* (1948) and *Five Lessons: The Modern Fundamentals of*

*Golf* (1957), Hogan later operated a golf equipment company and supervised construction of a new golf course. Hogan's company made high quality golf balls, clubs, and bags, becoming the world's largest golf equipment manufacturer. His Ben Hogan tour sponsored 30 tournaments for PGA tour aspirants. Hogan, who underwent colon cancer surgery in 1995 and suffered from Alzheimer's disease, died on July 25, 1997, of a stroke in Fort Worth at age 84.[52] He had made a truly remarkable comeback in the golfing world, overcoming incredible odds after a nearly fatal automobile accident.

# GREG LEMOND

"Never give up. You push yourself to where you think you can't go. The key is to endure psychologically," reflected cyclist Greg LeMond, who made a remarkable comeback from a near fatal hunting accident. LeMond already had won the Tour de France, the world's most difficult, glamorous bicycle race, when he received major shotgun wounds. Through determination and hard work, he gradually restored his endurance and captured two more Tour de France races.

LeMond was brought up in a middle-class family. Gregory James LeMond was born in Lakewood, California, on June 26, 1961, the son of Robert LeMond, a real estate broker, and Bertha LeMond. His family moved to Lake Tahoe, California, in 1968, and Washoe County in northwestern Nevada in 1970. LeMond began skiing at age seven and took up the sport more seriously two years later.

LeMond started cycling near Reno, Nevada, in 1975 to strengthen his legs for skiing competitions. He rode considerable distances with his father several times a week. "I was so tired I wanted to cry,"[1] he recalled. The 1975 Nevada State Cycling Championship went past LeMond's home, shifting his interest from skiing to cycling. LeMond continued cycling that winter and joined the local Reno Wheelmen Cycling Club. He enjoyed reading European cycling magazines and began competitive racing in 1976. LeMond, who quit high school to concentrate on cycling, won 11 races against 12-to-15-year-olds and began competing against more seasoned 16-to-19-year-olds. In 1977, he won two of three events at the U.S. Junior World Cycling team trials and the U.S. Junior Road Racing Championship. He finished ninth in the 1978 World Junior Road Race Championship.

In 1979, the 5-foot 10-inch, 160-pound LeMond "ascended in his sport at a dizzying pace,"[2] becoming the first road racer to earn three medals in a world meet. At the World Junior Men's Road Race Championships in Buenos Aires, Argentina, he amazed spectators by capturing the gold medal in the 120-kilometer road race, a silver in the 3,000-meter individual pursuit race, and a bronze in the team 70-kilometer time trial.

LeMond trained in Europe with the U.S. national cycling team for the Moscow 1980 Summer Olympic Games, the youngest captain at age 18. He won the grueling 346-mile Circuit de la Sarthe bike race in Brittany, becoming the first American to take a major stage race. The United States, however, boycotted the 1980 Olympics in protest of the Soviet invasion of Afghanistan. LeMond, who turned professional, married Kathy Morrison in December 1980 and has three children, Geoffrey, Scott, and Simone.

Cyrille Guimard, Renault-Elf-Gitane professional cycling team coach, liked LeMond's drive and character and urged him to join the European peloton racing with the Paris-based Union Sportive de Creteil. In 1981, LeMond signed a professional contract with Guimard's team to develop further as a cyclist. French cyclist Bernard Hinault, legendary team captain and brilliant strategist, taught him racing tactics and predicted LeMond would succeed him as world champion. Although soft-spoken, the determined LeMond soon ranked among the elite European cyclists "when the U.S. was decidedly a Third World country in that sport."[3] He possessed the requisite physical qualities, including a large lung capacity, the speed required in the time trials of the long races, and the muscle power needed for torturous climbs up steep mountain roads.

The 1981 season saw LeMond triumph in five races, including the Coor's Classic in Colorado, the biggest American race, record two stage wins, and finish third in the prestigious Dauphiné Libéré week-long stage race. In 1982, LeMond captured the 12-day, 837-mile Tour de l'Avenir by a record-setting 10-minute margin and took three stage wins. His dramatic sprint enabled him to finish second in the 170-mile World Road Racing Championship in Goodwood, England.

In 1983, LeMond secured his first major victory, a 169-mile race in Switzerland. In May 1983, he finished fourth in the Tour of Switzerland, capturing the Dauphiné Libéré stage race over mountainous stretches. At Altenrhein, Switzerland, LeMond became the first American to win the World Professional Road Racing Championships, the sport's most prestigious one-day event. The 170-mile course consisted of laps, each including a 600-foot climb, followed by two miles of steep, steady climbing. LeMond labeled the course "a bear" and added, "Each time up, my lungs were on fire." His gold-medal-winning roller coaster ride took slightly over seven hours. He was awarded the Super Prestige Pernod Trophy as the year's best all-around cyclist.

In his 1984 debut at the prestigious Tour de France, LeMond placed third in the grueling, 24-day, 2,600-mile race. He likened the race to "running a marathon a day for three weeks."[4] Bronchitis impeded his progress the first two weeks. After reaching the French Alps, LeMond, a strong climber, ascended to third place. The second American entrant ever, he became the first non-European to finish among the top three. LeMond mounted the winner's podium for earning the white jersey as the best young rider and finished third in the Stage 3 Team Time Trial. He also placed third in the Liège-Bastogne-Liège and Dauphiné Libéré, winning one stage.

At Hinault's urging, LeMond signed a four-year, $1.4 million contract with new French La Vie Claire cycling team in 1985. He placed second in the UCI World Road Racing Championships and captured the Coors Classic, taking Stage 5. LeMond and his teammates were asked to help Hinault win his record-tying fifth Tour de France instead of trying to win that race. Hinault led the race until being injured in a crash and falling behind three minutes. LeMond, who did not realize that Hinault trailed by that much, dutifully followed team instructions, letting the Frenchman regain the lead and win the race. He sacrificed an opportunity for victory, finishing second instead, the best showing ever for an American there. He later finished third in the Giro d'Italia and second in the Vuelta al País Vasco.

In 1986, LeMond co-captained the La Vie Claire team with Hinault and was favored to win the Tour de France. Hinault publicly promised to support LeMond this time in gratitude for the American's sacrifice in 1985. It soon became apparent, however, that Hinault did not intend to fulfill his promise. The French crowds also wanted Hinault to capture an unprecedented sixth crown. Hinault, who aspired to seal his immortality as a cyclist, suddenly took a commanding five-minute, 25-second lead on the first day in the Pyrenees in Stage 12. LeMond, who dropped to third place, realized, "Everything he said was designed to take the pressure off him" and "put him in a no-lose situation." Hinault led for most of Stage 13, but his endurance faltered on the last steep 1,100-meter climb up to Superbagnères in 80-degree heat. LeMond swept by Hinault to take Stage 13 and slice four minutes, 39 seconds of the Frenchman's overall lead. Hinault attempted another breakaway to "crush Greg, put him away,"[5] two days later. LeMond, however, pursued and caught Hinault. Although the two crested the Alpe d'Huez together to win the stage in a show of unity, Hinault continued competing aggressively against him. LeMond contemplated quitting the race.

The persistent LeMond regained the overall lead, surging ahead of Hinault on a dangerous downhill in the Alps during Stage 17 and taking over the prized yellow jersey. During the next stage, LeMond and Hinault broke away from the pack and collaborated for 80 miles to withstand a determined challenge from Switzerland's Urs Zimmermann. They took turns breaking the headwind. "Like birds in flight, they whirred through the turns, locked back wheel to front wheel, fast and free." In a public display of camaraderie, LeMond, who still held a 2-minute, 47-second overall lead, decelerated so Hinault could cross the finish line first. Hinault won Stage 20 by 25 seconds and trailed LeMond by two minutes, 18 seconds overall. LeMond, though, really had wanted to win that stage, the meet's final time trial, to prove he had the panache needed to win the race and felt Hinault betrayed him. "I just wish he had said at the start it's each one for himself," he remarked, because "I would have ridden a different race."[6]

During the final three stages, LeMond continued exhibiting immense willpower to overcome Hinault and the partisan French crowd. He rode into Paris for the final

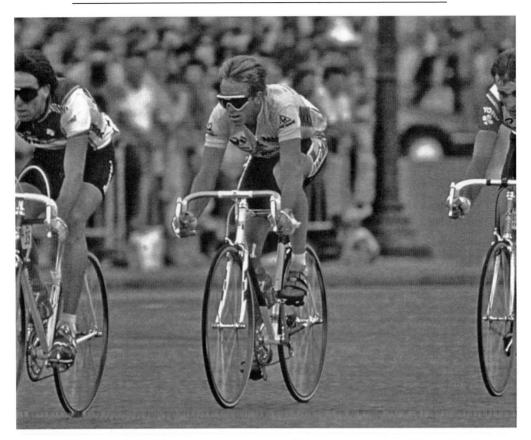

Greg LeMond won the yellow jersey on the Champs Élysées during the final stage of the 1986 Tour de France. He was the first American and non–European Tour de France winner, defeating Bernard Hinault of France by more than three minutes (courtesy Leo Mason/Action Plus/Icon SMI).

six laps up and down the Champs Élysées and claimed his victory in 100 hours, 35 minutes, 19 seconds. The first American and non-European Tour de France winner, LeMond defeated Hinault by three minutes, 10 seconds to take the grueling, 23-day, 2,000-mile event, the world's longest, biggest, richest, and most prestigious cycling race. After the race, Hinault stressed, "I pushed him to go to his every limit. He knows now to which point he can go."[7] LeMond took second in the Milan–San Remo and Coor's Classic races, third in the Tour de Suisse and Paris-Nice events, and seventh in the World Professional Road Racing Championships at Colorado Springs. In 1987, he shifted to the powerful Dutch team PDM.

Disastrous injuries forced LeMond to miss both the 1987 and 1988 Tour de France races. After LeMond broke his left wrist and collarbone in an Italian crash in March 1987, he planned to rejoin the European tour in late April. LeMond was scheduled to have his doctor remove the hard cast off his hand on April 20, but nearly died that morning during a wild turkey hunting expedition on his uncle Rod's farm in

Lincoln, California. The hunting party split off and lost track of each other. LeMond had just settled behind a bush when Patrick Blades, his brother-in-law, whistled from close range to locate where the others were. LeMond did not respond verbally, but moved. Blades accidentally shot LeMond in the back, mistaking him for a bird in the bushes. When LeMond asked, "Who shot?"[8] Blades fired over 60 pellets in the biker's back and side.

The pellets lodged in LeMond's body, breaking two ribs, penetrating his liver and kidney, and piercing his right lung. Two even struck the lining of his heart. LeMond saw blood in the ring finger of his left hand and experienced numbness. He nearly passed out when trying to stand up. "I tried talking," he recollected, "but my right lung had collapsed and I could barely breathe." As he lay in the field, LeMond feared that he might die and not see his wife, Kathy, and children again. Although severely injured, he discovered, "Your body takes over and you really don't realize how much it hurts."[9]

LeMond's uncle soon dialed 911 for an ambulance. A police helicopter from nearby Roseville saved LeMond's life, rushing him to the trauma center at the University of California, Davis Medical Center. One physician told LeMond he came "within twenty minutes of bleeding to death. It was very, very close." Kathy recollected, "We didn't know if he'd ever ride his bike again, if he was even going to live." Medics rushed LeMond to the emergency room. "I could barely talk because my punctured lung hurt so much,"[10] LeMond disclosed. Surgeons inserted a chest tube in his punctured lung and conducted surgery for five hours, removing over 30 pellets from his liver, kidney, intestines, and arm. Thirty pellets remained, mostly in his back and legs.

LeMond started having spasms the next day. Without using anesthesia, doctors inserted a tube in his chest to draw blood out of his collapsed lung. LeMond later noted, "The suffering you feel on your bike is nothing compared to real pain." His shoulder especially throbbed, while his right arm was numb. The tip of his left ring finger was shattered and broken. During the slow recovery, LeMond took several morphine shots daily to relieve the pain. Hospitalization lasted only six days, but the pain persisted after he returned home. LeMond revealed, "I'd just cry and cry because it hurt so much."[11] The accident made him realize the importance of being healthy and reorganizing his priorities to spend more time with his family.

The recovery tested LeMond both physically and psychologically, leaving him weak and 15 pounds lighter. "The shooting covered such a large part of my body," LeMond recollected, that it sapped his energy for five weeks.[12] LeMond began walking short distances within three weeks and fly fished in five weeks, eventually regaining his strength. In July, he embarked on an intensive training program to recover racing form. LeMond started riding a mountain bike for 15 to 20 minutes daily and gradually increased the time to two hours a day. An emergency appendectomy in mid–July delayed his recovery.

After a long convalescence, LeMond gradually returned to training and racing. During his recovery, he displayed extraordinary determination, motivation, and mental strength to augment his natural talent. "He always seemed to be able to last a little bit longer than anybody else."[13] LeMond utilized his energy well, possessed better heart and lung capacity than most people, and conditioned himself well. He regained his body weight and muscle tone, but took it longer to recoup his leg strength.

Despite these qualities, LeMond initially struggled upon returning to the racing circuit in September 1987, aware that he could not sprint. "I'd reach anaerobic," he noticed. "I'd go very quickly into oxygen debt."[14] LeMond trailed in races and even was pushed up some hills by a teammate. That fall, he fared poorly in the Tour of Ireland and the Créteil-Chaville race in France. LeMond dropped out of the Tour of Mexico in November because the mountains were too demanding. In February 1988, he struggled in the Ruta del Sol race in Spain.

LeMond moved to Wayata, Minnesota, and anticipated competing in the 1988 Tour de France. "His yearning to win it again had become an obsession." He finished second in the Tour of the Americas in late February, faring well on a 20-kilometer climb. LeMond considered himself "on the verge of a triumphant comeback." The following month, he won the Tirreno-Adriatico race in Italy. LeMond competed in several other European races and vowed to return to the victory podium in Paris as the world's premier bicycle racer. "I'm on track," he explained.

During the spring of 1988, LeMond started returning to form. He unfortunately crashed in a Belgian race. "All I remember is doing a flip, rolling on the ground, doing another flip, and landing on my back," he recalled. "I slid about thirty meters and landed on my head and shoulder."[15] LeMond developed tendinitis and an inflamed right shin infection when he tried resuming training too quickly. He did not finish another race because of the pain and conditioning loss, canceling plans to compete in the Tour of Italy and Tour de France. In July 1988, doctors operated on LeMond's tendinitis in Minnesota. LeMond dropped from number two to three-hundred forty-fifth in the professional rankings.

LeMond slowly rebuilt his endurance by 1989, but had missed two consecutive Tour de Frances and was given little chance of regaining his former glory. He still hoped to win his second Tour de France, but doubted if he could do it in 1989. PDM lost confidence in LeMond and asked him to take a $120,000 pay cut, prompting him to switch to the Belgium-based ADR (All-Drie Renting) team. Despite his dedication and rigorous work ethic, LeMond needed time to regain top form. "It's impossible to go straight there," he noted. His new ADR teammates were less skilled than those he had ridden with at PDM. LeMond conceded, "There's no way it could help me win a race, let alone the Tour."[16] He finished sixth in the Tirreno-Adriatco race in March 1989 and fourth at the Critérium International in France, being edged by Marc Madiot of Toshiba at the tape in the time trial.

LeMond fared poorly in several one-day races in the spring of 1989. In May, he competed in the circuitous Tour de Trump from Albany to Atlantic City. Donald Trump designed the race to promote cycling in the United States. The race drew a huge crowd, but LeMond ended a disappointing twenty-sixth. Reporters interviewed just the top racers and considered him a has-been. "The Tour de Trump was the low point of my season, maybe of my career," he recalled. ADR began fearing it assumed "too much for damaged goods" with LeMond. LeMond even described the last two years as "the most humiliating of my life. Riders and team managers thought I was through."[17]

LeMond also struggled in the mountain stages of the Tour of Italy in mid–June, dropping eight minutes in the first climb to Mount Etna and nearly quitting the race. "I had no strength at all," he revealed. After taking iron injections in the latter stages, LeMond started feeling better. He stood forty-seventh, more than 55 minutes behind, with only the time trial left. He finished second in the time trial behind Lech Piasecki. "The Giro time trial," he claimed, "was the race that turned things around. It gave me a lot more confidence." LeMond finished thirty-ninth overall and was treated for a severe iron deficiency, increasing the supply of oxygen to working muscles.

In the 1989 Tour de France, LeMond rode for the ADR team. The difficult course wound for 2,000 miles from Luxembourg around France, with four difficult stages in the Alps. Twenty-two teams of nine men each competed for $2.1 million, the biggest cycling purse. Spaniard Pedro Delgado, the defending champion, was favored. LeMond, who hoped to place among the top 15, declared, "I'd really like to win a stage, especially a time trial." He finished fourth in the prologue.

LeMond performed well in the time trials and maintained his position on the climbs. In a rainstorm five days later, he won a 45-minute time trial by 24 seconds and took the overall lead by five seconds from Laurent Fignon, two-time Tour winner, who had been LeMond's teammate at Renault. "It was like winning a world championship," he exulted. LeMond acknowledged, "This is the most wonderful day of my life. It's almost a miracle." He accepted the yellow jersey as the Tour leader for the first time in three years. "You can't imagine what I've gone through the last few years," he stressed. LeMond attributed his time trial victory to his aerodynamic helmet and Scott triathlon extension handlebars that improved his speed. Historian Samuel Abt, though, insisted, "His willpower, returning form, and zest for victory meant more than the handlebars." Abt maintained, "When he had his body under control he was one of the best cyclists of his time."[18]

The last two weeks featured a classic duel between LeMond and Fignon. For the next week, they retained their respective positions on the flat terrain. Fignon assumed the lead by seven seconds in Stage 10 on the second day in the Pyrenees Mountains, gaining 12 seconds in the final 500 meters. LeMond retook the lead in Stage 15, a time trial. Fignon dropped to second place, 40 seconds behind. LeMond widened his advantage over Fignon to nearly one minute by Stage 18.

During the dizzying, steep climb to Alpe d'Huez in oppressively hot weather, the weary LeMond relinquished the lead in Stage 19 to Fignon in the final four kilometers and trailed by 26 seconds. "Maybe I put too much effort into yesterday's stage," he speculated. Fignon won the next stage on a short climb to Villard de Lans and led LeMond by 50 seconds. Undaunted, LeMond attacked and captured the next stage to Aix-les-Bains in a sprint finish with Fignon. Fignon, however, retained his sizable, 50-second overall lead. Since the next stage was on flat terrain, the pair rode the 70-mile penultimate phase in a "party atmosphere."[19]

The short 15.2-mile (24.5 kilometer) time trial from Versailles to Paris remained LeMond's only opportunity to pass Fignon. Despite having bested Fignon in two previous time trials, "LeMond wasn't given much of a chance of catching Fignon on the last day."[20] The Frenchman held a nearly insurmountable lead. The distance was considered too short, the slightly downhill course too easy, and the time differential too great.

For the final dash to Paris, the riders started singly, two minutes apart and in reverse order of their position in the standings. A huge crowd watched the time trial begin on the Avenue de Paris in Versailles. In order to win, LeMond needed to make up a lot of time. Not since 1975 had the Tour de France ended in a time trial. LeMond, the next-to-last-rider, left two minutes before Fignon. "I started extremely fast," he recalled. "I didn't think. I just rode." LeMond blitzed the whole time trial, "gaining precious seconds with each kilometer"[21] and having "nothing to lose." He wore his aerodynamic helmet and leaned on his Scott extension handlebars. LeMond approached Paris "like a lone soldier on a heroic mission." Upon passing the Arc de Triomphe and turning down the Champs-Élysées, he found strength for one more long kick. "I rode as if my whole career depended on it,"[22] he emphasized. LeMond, who finished very strong, claimed that he even could have ridden at the same pace for another 10 miles.

Despite blustery conditions, LeMond covered the final 15.2-mile stage in 26 minutes, 57 seconds, averaging 34 miles per hour, the fastest time trial of the day by 33 seconds and in the event's history. He won that stage, outpacing Fignon by 21 seconds after 11.5 kilometers, 45 seconds after 20 kilometers, and 58 seconds at the finish, and gaining over two seconds per kilometer. After crossing the finish line, Fignon fell from his bike and collapsed from exhaustion. Kathy, LeMond's wife, realized that her husband had dramatically overcome Fignon's huge lead, and shouted, "Eight seconds, Greg. You've got eight seconds less than Fignon." LeMond pumped the air with his fists and grinned. "The last thing I wanted to do," he remarked, "was race twenty-one days and 2,000 miles and lose the Tour de France by one or two seconds."[23]

LeMond had captured his second Tour de France, edging Fignon by merely eight seconds, the closest winning margin in the race's 86-year history. The smallest margin previously was the 38-second victory by Jan Janssen of the Netherlands over Herman Van Springerl of Belgium in 1968. The race signified "the most stunning victory of LeMond's remarkable career." LeMond prevailed "not so much on talent as on sheer force of will." In savoring the victory, he enthused, "Nothing compares to this,"[24] and exulted, "It was unbelievable, just unbelievable." Around 500,000 people cheered him on the victory stand. LeMond, who nearly had quit bicycling in May, learned from the race always to battle relentlessly.[25]

LeMond certified his status as the world's premier cyclist, garnering his second World Professional Road Racing Championship in a late August downpour in Chamberry, France. The race consisted of traveling a 12.3-kilometer course 21 times. Dmitri Konyshev of the Soviet Union and Sean Kelly of Ireland led LeMond by several seconds entering the bell lap. "I was ready to quit," LeMond disclosed, "but I figured a lot can happen in the last two laps." LeMond started sprinting with 200 meters remaining and "just went all out at the finish."[26] He won by half a wheel over Konyshev and raised his right arm triumphantly, as he crossed the finish line in six hours, 40 minutes, and 59 seconds.

LeMond became just the fifth cyclist to conquer the Tour de France and World Championship Road Race the same year, joining Eddy Merckx, Stephen Roche, Louison Bobet, and Hinault. The French sports newspaper, *L'Equipe*, nicknamed him "Superman!" "It's really a great year," LeMond reminisced. "I never would have believed this."[27] Kelly nipped Steven Rooks of the Netherlands for third, with Fignon ending sixth. LeMond's exceptional year was capped off with the birth of his daughter, Simone, in October.

LeMond's stellar 1989 performance earned him *Sports Illustrated's* Sportsman of the Year honors as one of America's greatest athletes in perhaps its most grueling sport. "With his prime competitive years now upon him," LeMond was "back on top of the heap," *Sports Illustrated* wrote. *L'Equipe* designated him as its "Champion of Champions" among world athletes. LeMond, who has promoted the growth of American cycling, signed a three-year, $5.5 million contract for the strong France-based Z team in 1990. *Forbes* magazine ranked him twenty-sixth among the world's richest athletes, with an estimated $4.2 million annual income.

LeMond began the 1990 Tour in questionable condition. After being sidelined nearly all April with a lingering virus, he struggled to finish seventy-eighth in the Tour de Triumph and one-hundred-fifth in the Tour of Italy. "I couldn't get out of my own way for four weeks,"[28] he moaned. LeMond began silencing critics in late June with a tenth-place finish in the Tour of Switzerland.

LeMond in July captured his second consecutive Tour de France, although being the first overall titlist since 1969 not to win any of its 21 stages. Novice Claudio Chiappucci of Italy assumed a commanding lead of 10 minutes, 35 seconds in Stage 1. LeMond sliced the advantage through the mountain stages, making his biggest charge on the descent of the Col du Tourmalet in Stage 16. He came "ripping down the twirling road, pedaling hard to the next summit as if he were a kid late for a big test at school," and "took the big step toward winning his third Tour." Chiappucci, however, remained ahead by five seconds before the final individual time trial. LeMond placed fifth in the time trial, beating Chiappucci by two minutes, 16 seconds, to vault into the overall lead. He turned the final stage into Paris into a triumphal procession. This victory, giving LeMond triumphs in all three Tour de Frances he had entered between 1986 and 1990, cemented his rank among cycling's all-time greats. *L'Equipe* called him "ROI-SOLEIL [The Sun King] as he wore regal raiment (the yellow jersey) for the second consecutive year. *Sports Illustrated* wrote that the "improbable" LeMond "is MADE IN AMERICA" and "captures French minds, if not necessarily French hearts. He takes the biggest bike race in the world and folds it in his pocket and makes it his own."[29]

LeMond placed a disappointing fourth in the 1990 World Professional Road Racing Championships in Maebishi, Japan, in August, never making a serious challenge and finishing eight seconds behind Rudy Dhaenen of Belgium.

In 1991, LeMond aspired to join Jacques Anquetil, Merckx, and Hinault as the only cyclists to win four Tour de Frances. He signed lucrative endorsement deals and racing contracts, but quit the Tour of Italy six days from the finish, struggled at twenty-fourth in the Tour of Switzerland, and ended a disappointing seventh in the Tour de France. LeMond "fought sickness and adversity" during the mountain stages, suffering from a white blood cell count that rose to nearly double normal levels because of a foot infection. After one mountain stage, he collided with an ABC cameraman and landed atop an automobile hood. Following the final stage, LeMond pointed out, "It's harder to get to the same level of conditioning."[30] He received the 1991 Jesse Owens International Trophy as the athlete best personifying and promoting cooperation and understanding among peoples.

LeMond's final major victory came in the 1992 Tour Du Pont, a stage race in the United States. He became the first American to win that race, patterned after the Tour de France. LeMond won the prologue in record time while securing his first American triumph since the mid–1980s. The same year, he received USA Cycling's Korbel Lifetime Achievement Award.

In 1994, LeMond retired from professional cycling. He attributed his declining performance to mitochondrial myopathy, an impairment of muscle proteins that prevents the intense power delivery needed by a world-class cyclist. LeMond ultimately blamed overtraining for that condition.[31] He was inducted into the U.S. Bicycling Hall of Fame in 1996 and was ranked by Fox Sports Network among the "50 Greatest Athletes of the Century" in 1999. Cyclinghalloffame.com ranked LeMond tenth among the all-time top 100 riders.

LeMond founded a bicycle company that bore his name in 1990, but the business floundered because of undercapitalization and poor management. In 1992, he struck a deal with Trek, which would license his name for bicycles it would build, distribute and help design, and sell them under LeMond's name. Trek built bicycles for LeMond until 2008.

LeMond, who authored *Greg LeMond's Complete Book of Cycling* (1988), launched

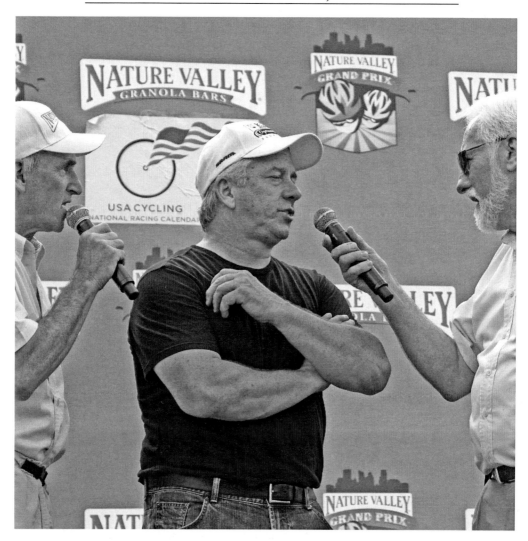

Greg LeMond (center) spoke with announcers Michael Aisner (left) and Jeff Blake before kicking off the Stillwater Criterium at the Nature Valley Grand Prix on June 19, 2011, in Stillwater, Minnesota (courtesy Joe Ferrer/Shutterstock.com).

an incredible comeback from a near-fatal accident to make a major impact on the cycling world. His three Tour de France titles and two World Road Race Championships rank him among cycling legends. LeMond, the pioneer U.S. cyclist and first cyclist to wear a hard-shell helmet while competing in the Tour de France, opened the doors in what previously had been a sport only of European champions and paved the way for Lance Armstrong and other U.S. cyclists to test themselves at the sport's highest level. "He was both a path and a light, extending the popularity of cycling beyond its European borders and inspiring fellow countrymen to emulate him."[32]

# *Injuries*

## LOU BRISSIE

"If someone tells you that you cannot climb the mountain, you set out and find a way to do it," explained Lou Brissie, who fulfilled his aspiration of playing major league baseball after being severely wounded in World War II. Brissie valiantly endured countless operations and hardships to pitch in the major leagues for seven seasons. Few major leaguers have faced greater tribulations than Brissie.

Brissie came from a working-class family. Leland Lou Brissie Jr. was born on June 5, 1924, in Anderson, South Carolina, and grew up in Greenville, South Carolina, the son of a motorcycle shop owner. In January 1936, his father, Leland Sr., moved to Ware Shoals, South Carolina, to work in the maintenance department at the Riegel Textile Corporation. Brissie, who overcame rheumatic fever at age 10, dreamt about becoming a major league pitcher after meeting South Carolina baseball legend Joe Jackson.

Although his high school did not field a baseball team, the 14-year-old left-hander pitched for Riegel as a ninth-grader in the textile league against ex-professionals. "Our heroes were the guys that played in the textile leagues,"[1] Brissie recalled. Chick Galway, baseball coach at Presbyterian College in Clinton, South Carolina, wrote Connie Mack, long-time Philadelphia Athletics manager-owner, about Brissie's baseball skills. After Brissie graduated from Ware Shoals High School in May 1941, Galway took him to Philadelphia for a tryout with Mack. At Shibe Park, Brissie's sizzling fastball, sharp breaking pitches, poise, and smooth delivery impressed Mack. Mack paid for Brissie to attend Presbyterian College, where he won five of seven games as a pitcher and batted .350 as a first baseman in 1942. The 6-foot 4½-inch, 205-pound Brissie twice wanted to sign up for the U.S. Army, but was rejected because he was too young and his parents did not approve.[2] After enlisting in the U.S. Army in December 1942, he entered military service in April 1943. Brissie married Dorothy Morgan in April 1944 at Spartanburg, South Carolina.

During World War II, Brissie served with the 88th Infantry Division at Camp Croft, South Carolina. The 20-year-old corporal was shipped to Italy in mid–1944 and led his G Company unit into battle in the Apennine Mountains near Bologna in northern Italy. He was aboard one of seven canvas-covered trucks in the convoy on December 7 when a powerful German mortar shell exploded amidst the infantry detachment. "This shell burst with a shriek, the noise shattering to the ear, the earth erupting as if it had been dynamited." The impact knocked Brissie to the ground and tore his clothes and boots. "His entire body felt as if it had just been struck with a bolt of electricity." More artillery shells exploded. His immobile left leg "had been nearly shredded from the knee to the ankle."[3]

Brissie dragged his body along the snow-covered ground about 20 yards to a creek and forced it down the bank and through most of the stream. He lay in a muddy creek bed for eight hours, often blacking out and hallucinating, "one foot severely damaged and the other seeming to be missing."[4] Brissie and only three other platoon members survived. Eight enlisted men from the company and three of their four officers were killed or wounded.

Medics rescued Brissie several hours later, but a German mortar strike detonated at the front of the jeep. The driver swerved off the road, ejecting him from the stretcher into a snowbank. Brissie hit the back of his head on a rock, bruised his neck, fractured a vertebra, and suffered more shrapnel wounds in the right shoulder. Besides breaking his left leg, ankle, and foot and his right foot, he suffered contusions in both thigh bones, wounds in each hand, and a shoulder concussion. The muscles and tendons in his left leg were gone. Brissie was treated at two hospitals near Florence, receiving the Purple Heart for his wounds. Since his left leg had become infected, doctors warned him that gangrene would likely occur and that they would have to amputate his leg if he wanted to survive. "You can't take my leg off," he replied. "I'm going to need it to play baseball."[5] The doctors yielded to Brissie's pleas to save his left leg and gave him several blood transfusions instead.

Brissie was flown on December 10 to 300th General Hospital in Naples. Doctors calmed his infection with penicillin. Dr. Wilbur Brubaker operated the next morning and did not amputate the leg. He wired back the torn bone and stitched together the ripped muscles and severed tendons. "I wanted to shout with joy," Brissie exulted. His left leg was three-quarters of an inch shorter than his right leg. Brissie, who remained bedridden, vowed to play baseball again. After the operation, he affirmed, "I didn't wonder if I could make it back to pitch, but how I could do it."[6] Dr. Brubaker considered Brissie's aspiration of pitching for the Athletics remote, although admiring his ambition, will, and courage.

Despite Brissie's optimism, the recovery progressed very slowly, with 23 major operations and 40 blood transfusions in two years to enable him to walk. Brissie was very fortunate to have survived. "Few would have considered the notion of him playing baseball again anything but folly."[7] Doctors removed 17 fragments from his body. During his three months in Italian hospitals, Brissie underwent operations on his right shoulder, left hand, right hand, right foot, right thigh, left thigh, left knee, left leg, and left ankle. He received a Bronze Star and two Purple Hearts.

Mack wrote Brissie encouraging letters during his recovery. In a December 28 letter, he penned Brissie "to try to get well, and whenever I felt I was ready to play, he would see I got the opportunity." Mack's letter "really put octane in my mind," an ecstatic Brissie remembered. "The idea that I would have the 'opportunity' to be a major league pitcher with the A's really lifted my spirits." On January 31, 1945, the Athletics' manager counseled him, "The main thing now is your health," and predicted, "Everything will turn out as you may desire." Mack told Athletics pitching coach Earle Brucker that Brissie intended to join the club soon. The determined Brissie earnestly sought a way to "pitch with a bum leg," hoping to return "to baseball albeit with a metal plate in his leg."[8] Doctors reconstructed his leg with wire.

After flying in late March 1945 to New York City on a stretcher with both legs in casts, Brissie entered Finney General Hospital in Thomasville, Georgia, in April. He was still bedridden and confined to a wheelchair. "The doctors thought I had a good chance to be on my feet," Brissie wrote, although predicting it would "be a fairly long process." When medics removed his right foot cast in June, Brissie began walking with crutches and hospital aides for the first time in six months. "My first steps were awfully painful," he admitted. Brissie arose early each morning and walked slightly more each day. Physical therapists spent long hours with him. Brissie was fitted with a thick aluminum brace, making his lower leg "look as thick as a fence post." He began throwing baseballs to a hospital aide while balancing himself on one crutch. After spending months in rehabilitation hospitals, he hobbled around at home on crutches and still aspired to pitch in the major leagues.[9]

In June 1945, the doctors told Mack that Brissie soon would be able to play baseball again. Brissie visited the Athletics at Shibe Park in Philadelphia in July for "an unusual tryout." Sympathetic Philadelphia players admired him, as he batted and threw with a crutch. Brissie was transferred to Northington General Hospital in Tuscaloosa, Alabama, for reconstructive surgery to help tighten and strengthen his left leg. Dr. Alfred Suraci completely rebuilt Brissie's left leg, operating on him six times to remove shrapnel from August 1945 to April 1946. Dr. Suraci wanted Brissie to have even more surgery, but the latter demurred. Brissie, who had not played baseball in almost two years, replied, "I had to get to throwing again, and pitching."[10]

Brissie was discharged from the Army in April 1946 and returned to Ware Shoals, South Carolina. He walked more daily with a cumbersome, inhibiting steel brace that covered his left leg from knee to ankle. Brissie developed a sore arm with his awkward, stiff legged delivery while trying to pitch for the Riegel team. A month later, he surrendered eight runs without retiring a batter in the first inning. "It was the most disappointing, deflating, discouraging thing to happen to me in baseball," Brissie recalled. After striking out 30 batters in his next two starts, he notified Mack that he was ready to join the Athletics. Brissie met with Mack in Philadelphia in July and suffered severe leg pain while pitching batting practice for two days. The Athletics' trainer discovered Brissie had contracted a badly infected left leg and sent him to

Valley Forge Hospital in Phoenixville, Pennsylvania. Mack assured Brissie, "This is just a temporary setback."[11]

Philadelphia signed Brissie again in December 1946. Brissie worked hard that winter to prepare for spring training, walking extensively, lifting weights, and altering his pitching motion to improve his velocity. The exposed bones and nerves in his legs still caused him problems. He wore a protective shinguard with heavy foam rubber underneath on his left leg and a brace on his left ankle to keep from getting hit.

During March 1947, Brissie trained with the Athletics at West Palm Beach, Florida, harboring doubts he could still pitch. Mack in February had inquired about how Brissie's left leg felt. When Brissie replied he was "ready for spring training," Mack gave him an opportunity to make the team. Brissie exhibited considerable progress. Art Morrow of *The Sporting News* observed, "The players hardly recognized in the powerfully-built southpaw the anemic invalid they had seen at Shibe Park the previous fall. And he was throwing with plenty of speed."[12] Mack sparingly used Brissie against Class AAA teams.

Mack assigned Brissie to Savannah, Georgia, of the Class A South Atlantic League (SAL). Brissie was sidelined for six weeks because of a leg infection and struggled in his first few appearances. Manager Tom Oliver encouraged him. Brissie gradually found his pitching rhythm, enhancing his confidence. He tied a league record by striking out 17 Macon Peaches on May 29 and won 13 consecutive games. Batters tried to exploit his leg problem by bunting against him, but he converted several into double plays. Brissie anchored Savannah's pitching staff with a 23–5 win-loss mark in 1947, recording a sparkling 1.91 earned run average (ERA) and 278 strikeouts in 254 innings. He led the SAL in victories, ERA, and strikeouts, being selected a unanimous SAL All-Star and helping Savannah capture the pennant.[13] Brissie struck out 107 more batters than his closest competitor and was one of only two pitchers with an ERA below 3.00. "The season was phenomenal,"[14] he remembered.

In September 1947, the Athletics recalled Brissie to pitch the season finale on September 28 against the American League (AL) champion New York Yankees before 25,000 people at Yankee Stadium. Philadelphia lost the contest, 5–3, as Brissie surrendered five runs and nine hits, including a home run by Johnny Lindell, walked five, and threw two wild pitches in seven innings. Babe Ruth, who was being honored that day, Ty Cobb, Tris Speaker, Cy Young, and other National Baseball Hall of Fame legends witnessed his debut. Brissie enthused, "I thought I had gone to heaven. I lost the game, but it was still a great experience." Mack observed, "Brissie had great stuff, a beautiful fast ball and a fine curve," although "nervous and wild."[15] Brissie had made a seemingly insurmountable jump from Class A to the major leagues.

Brissie, determined to make the 1948 Athletics squad, kept in condition during the off-season and attended education classes at Erskine College. Mack sent him a $5,000 contract in January for the 1948 season and instructed him to report to spring training camp at West Palm Beach in March. "Despite struggling with pain," Brissie made the Athletics' roster by pitching well in spring training.

On Opening Day at Fenway Park in Boston on April 19, Brissie started the second game of a doubleheader against the Boston Red Sox. He pitched a complete-game, 4–2 victory and singled with the bases loaded to score Sam Chapman and Buddy Rosar in the fourth inning. Brissie allowed just four hits, striking out seven and walking just one.[16]

Philadelphia led, 4–1, in the sixth inning, when Brissie uncorked a fast ball to Red Sox slugger Ted Williams. Williams lined a drive up the middle off the metal plate in Brissie's left leg. The ball caromed almost to the right field wall. According to Mack, "The ball shot from the end of the bat like a bullet out of a gun" and struck Brissie's injured leg. "Brissie dropped like a felled ox." Mack recalled, "My heart must have stopped beating." He reflected, "That poor boy! That's the end of his baseball career." Williams, who stopped at first base rather than trying for a double,[17] described his liner as "a real shot" that made a sound like "a rifle clap off the aluminum leg." When Brissie fell, Williams experienced "this awful feeling I've really hurt him" and quickly visited the mound to check on the hurler's health. As Williams approached the mound, Brissie yelled, "'Damn it, Ted! Why don't you pull the ball?"[18]

The Athletics' trainer also immediately rushed to the mound. Brissie, who feared his numb left leg was broken, initially lamented, "I'm back in that creek in Italy — all that work and it ends here." The line drive dented his aluminum plate. Mack wanted to summon a reliever, but Brissie demurred. Brissie finished that game, striking out Williams in the ninth inning. The left-hander recorded his first major league victory, allowing only four hits and striking out seven. "That took a lot of courage," Mack told Brissie. "You just pitched a great game." Brissie beamed, "That was a great experience and a great day." He spent overnight at Faulkner Hospital, however, and did not sleep well because of the throbbing pain. The courageous Brissie, however, did not miss his next start. John Griffin, an English professor from Brissie's home state, praised him as "a living symbol of man's will to win against all odds."[19] On May 31, Williams clouted a two-run homer over the right field light tower at Shibe Park off Brissie. Upon rounding the bases, Williams yelled, "I didn't mean to pull it that much!"

Philadelphia battled with the Cleveland Indians, New York, and Boston for the 1948 American League pennant and occupied first place by one-half game in August. Brissie, the lone Athletics left-hander, started and relieved games. He bested Boston, 4–2, on July 5 and front-runner Cleveland, 10–5, on July 16. David Kaiser described the Athletics as a "remarkable aggregation of gutsy pitchers, fine fielders and line-drive hitters" the most remarkable pennant race in the history of major league baseball." On August 15 at Yankee Stadium, Brissie stifled a New York rally after slugger Joe DiMaggio had tripled. Thirteen days later, he hurled all 10 innings to edge the St. Louis Browns, 5–4, notching his thirteenth victory. Brissie, however, triumphed only once in September. Philadelphia lacked the power to compete with the other three teams and faded to fourth place that month, but still finished in the upper division for the first time since 1933. Brissie compiled a 14–10 mark with a 4.13 ERA in 194 innings. His 127 strikeouts ranked fourth behind aces Bob Feller, Bob Lemon, and Hal Newhouser. Brissie finished 10–8 in 25 starts and fared 4–2 in relief with five saves. Although unable to plant his left leg, he batted .237 with 10 runs batted in (RBI). Brissie finished fourth in the Rookie of the Year balloting. Dr. Brubaker lauded "the indomitable raw courage of a most determined young man."[20]

The next season marked Brissie's pinnacle. A sensational catch by center fielder Chapman preserved Brissie's seven-hit, 3–2 victory over Boston, in Philadelphia's home opener at Shibe Park on April 19. After suffering a heartbreaking, 14-inning, 2–1 loss to New York, Brissie defeated Cleveland, 7–3, in the second game of a doubleheader on May 22 to move the Athletics within two games of New York. On June 14, he limited the Detroit Tigers to eight hits, including only one over the last five innings, in a 7–3, complete-game triumph. Brissie prevailed the next three games to elevate his record to 9–3.

Cleveland manager Lou Boudreau selected Brissie for the 1949 AL All-Star team. Brissie hurled three innings at Ebbets Field in Brooklyn and relished being in "this dream world, with all these great ballplayers." He compared sitting on the bench with Williams and Joe DiMaggio to being "like a kid in a candy shop." "To pitch in the game was an added thrill."[21] Brissie relieved in the fourth inning with the AL ahead, 6–5, and pitched two scoreless innings before surrendering a two-run homer to Ralph Kiner in the sixth frame. The AL triumphed, 11–7. He registered three victories in September. In 1949, Philadelphia finished 81–73 in fifth place. Brissie fared 16–13 with a 4.28 ERA, completing 18 of 29 starts, posting three saves, and ranking among AL leaders with 118 strikeouts in 229.1 innings. A .267 batter, he tripled in an 8–7 victory over the Washington Senators on August 10.[22]

Brissie in 1950 lost his first six games, including Opening Day to Boston, twice to New York, and once to Cleveland. On May 27, he hurled a three-hit, 6–1 masterpiece over New York at Shibe Park. Brissie was defeated in a 3–2 heartbreaker to the Yankees on August 18, when DiMaggio clouted "an electrifying shot" deep into the left-field upper deck at Shibe Park.[23] He suffered four straight one-run setbacks, including 1–0 to the Chicago White Sox on August 23 and 2–1 to New York on September 4. Brissie blew a 9–0 lead in his fifth appearance in 13 games, surrendering seven unanswered runs in 5.1 innings to Cleveland on September 17 at Municipal Stadium. "My leg had flared up, and I could hardly walk," he explained. Mack did not start Brissie in Philadelphia's final 10 games. Brissie led the Athletics' staff with a 4.02 ERA in 1950, but dropped 19 of 26 decisions. Ten setbacks came by one run. Brissie completed 15 games, including two shutouts, struck out 101 batters, shared third with 46 pitching appearances, and ranked fifth with eight saves.[24] Philadelphia finished last with a 52–102 record, prompting 87-year-old manager Mack's retirement.

In 1951, Brissie lost his first two starts to the Washington Senators and New York Yankees. First-place Cleveland acquired him from last-place Philadelphia on April 30 in a seven-player trade. Cleveland manager Al Lopez "needed a left-handed pitcher badly." Brissie, who initially balked at leaving Philadelphia, lamented, "It was the most devastating thing in the world to me. I had only wanted to play for the A's." He shared his father's dream to "help Mr. Mack win his last pennant."[25] Cleveland general manager Hank Greenberg persuaded Brissie to join the Indians.

Cleveland fielded among the best AL starting rotations with Feller, Lemon, Early Wynn, Mike Garcia, and Steve Gromek the next three seasons and used Brissie mostly as a reliever. Brissie found the transition difficult because it was much harder to stay in condition as a reliever. In his Indian debut against Boston at Municipal

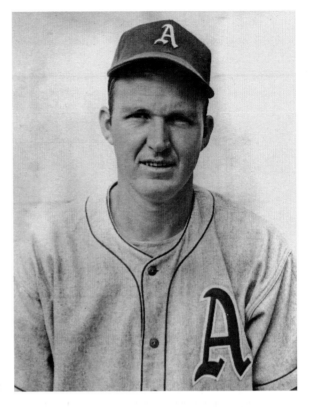

Lou Brissie pitched for the Philadelphia Athletics from 1948 to 1951. He compiled a 14–10 win-loss record his rookie 1948 season, helping his club finish in the first division for the first time since 1933 (courtesy National Baseball Hall of Fame Library, Cooperstown, N.Y.).

Stadium on May 2, he relieved Lemon in the sixth inning and allowed only two hits, including a three-run homer to Boudreau, in the final four innings to preserve a 4–3 victory. Brissie lost two starts to New York, with two saves interspersed. His first Cleveland triumph came on June 7 at Philadelphia, as he permitted only three runs and struck out five over nine innings. "It always feels good to win," he affirmed, "but this one, returning to where I had begun, felt especially good." Brissie also preserved victories for Feller against Philadelphia on June 12 and Detroit on July 6. The Indians finished second behind New York in 1951. Feller, Garcia, and Wynn recorded at least 20 triumphs. Brissie ranked second in the junior circuit with 56 appearances and third with nine saves, making four starts and compiling a 4–3 slate and 3.60 ERA.[26]

Cleveland used Brissie almost exclusively in relief in 1952. His first victory that season came on July 1 in a four hour, 49-minute marathon against St. Louis. Satchel Paige of the Browns relieved Ned Garver in the seventh inning with the score knotted, 2–2, and hurled 10 scoreless innings. Brissie relieved Feller in the ninth frame. St.

Louis scored once off Brissie in the top of the nineteenth inning. Cleveland rallied with two runs in the bottom of that frame off Paige, as Bobby Avila singled, Al Rosen doubled, and Hank Majeski singled. "That was a big thrill,"[27] an exhausted Brissie remembered. At Philadelphia on August 27, Brissie relieved Feller in the ninth inning with the bases loaded, one out, and the score tied, 3–3, and fanned the next two Ath-

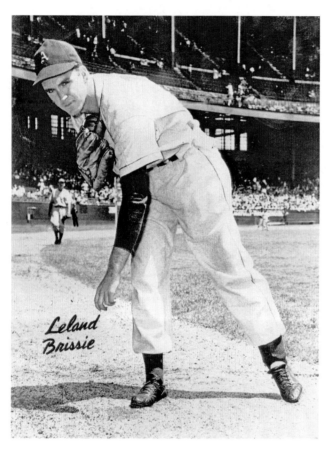

*Leland Brissie*

letics batters. The Indians tallied three runs in the eleventh inning, enabling him to record his third victory. Cleveland remained in the race until the Yankees clinched the AL pennant on September 24. Lopez depended heavily on his starters, with Wynn notching 23 victories and Lemon 22. Brissie ranked fifth in the AL with 42 appearances, compiling a 3–2 record with a 3.48 ERA and two saves.[28]

Brissie saw scant action in 1953. He relieved Feller on April 17 in the ninth inning against Detroit, surrendering the winning run. Brissie needed to pitch more often to remain in condition and be effective, but Lopez seldom summoned him and ignored him altogether in the final 24 games. "It was discouraging, disappointing, disgusting," Brissie acknowledged. During 1953, Brissie pitched just 13 innings with two saves and a 7.62 ERA. He classified the

Lou Brissie in 1949 recorded a career-high 16 victories, ranked among American League leaders with 118 strikeouts, and made the American League All-Star team (courtesy National Baseball Hall of Fame Library, Cooperstown, N.Y.).

season as "miserable" and explained, "When you don't pitch a lot in games, you lose your edge up there against those guys."[29]

During his major league career from 1948 through 1953, Brissie netted 44 victories with 48 losses, 29 saves, and a 4.07 ERA in 234 games, striking out 436 batters and walking 451. Nearly all of his losses with Philadelphia came when the Athletics compiled a losing record. Brissie batted .227 with five doubles and one triple in 295 official at bats. Feller claimed, "Lou Brissie would have been a Hall of Fame pitcher, if it hadn't been for World War II."[30]

In February 1954, Cleveland sold Brissie to Indianapolis of the American Association. Brissie requested to be traded rather than reporting to Indianapolis, stating, "I'd be failing all those guys still in hospitals, guys who follow my games." The Baltimore Orioles, Detroit Tigers, and New York Yankees inquired about Brissie, but the Indians refused to send him to an AL competitor. Brissie declined to report to Indianapolis and retired from professional baseball at age 29. "I believe my leg affected my longevity," he thought. "I was never able to bend it more than 60 percent of normal."[31] The Indians won the AL pennant that year, but were swept by the New York Giants in the World Series. Brissie never played in a World Series.

From 1954 to 1962, Brissie served as commissioner of the American Legion Junior Baseball Program in Indianapolis. He led an American Legion team that played in eight Latin American countries in 1956 and tried to expand youth baseball in Australia in 1957. In June 1957, President Dwight D. Eisenhower appointed him to the Citizens Advisory Committee on the Fitness of American Youth. Brissie also conducted baseball clinics throughout Australia. He left the American Legion program when his wife, Dorothy, was diagnosed with breast cancer. Brissie returned to Greenville, South Carolina, and scouted part-time for the Los Angeles Dodgers in 1962 and 1963. In 1964, he began scouting part-time for the Atlanta Braves.

After Dorothy died in May 1967 at age 42, Brissie worked more than a decade representing the United Merchants and Manufacturers of New York in discussions and negotiations with regulatory agencies in Washington, D.C. He married Diana Smith in December 1975 and lived in North Augusta, South Carolina. Brissie worked 14 years as an industrial consultant for the state of South Carolina, retiring in 2000 after bypass heart surgery. He was elected to the South Carolina Sports Hall of Fame in 1974 and the SAL Hall of Fame in 1994.[32]

The mortar attack still impedes Brissie, who became deaf in his left ear and lost 30 percent of the hearing in his right ear. Brissie still suffers incessant pain in the left leg and has walked with crutches since 1985. His leg started bowing, raising concerns about osteomyelitis. Brissie still requires treatment at Veterans Administration hospitals, visiting regularly every four to six weeks. He admits having endured pain daily for over 60 years and has learned to manage it. But Brissie still considers himself fortunate. "I'm here. Others, friends of mine in the war, never came back."[33] He praises them as the real heroes.

Brissie, who inspired thousands of veterans with his courageous story, reflected, "It made me feel like I did add a little something." Sportswriter Grantland Rice eulogized, "Brissie captured the hearts of baseball fans everywhere by his courageous triumph over a severe leg injury and by his performance on the mound."[34] Playing major league baseball unquestionably marked his biggest triumph. Experiencing pitching success added icing to the cake.

# ROCKY BLEIER

"Be the best you can be" was the inspirational creed of Rocky Bleier, whose name exemplified sacrifice, commitment, and winning. Bleier suffered severe combat wounds in the Vietnam War and battled back to become a star professional football running back with the four-time Super Bowl champion Pittsburgh Steelers of the National Football League (NFL) in the 1970s.

Bleier emanated from a working-class environment. Robert Patrick "Rocky" Bleier was born on March 5, 1946, in Appleton, Wisconsin, and grew up there. His father, Bob, owned a bar and later worked in a clothing store, while his mother, Ellen, was an account clerk, bookkeeper, and seafood wholesaler. They lived in the back section of the bar and eventually moved upstairs. His father nicknamed him "Rocky" because the chubby baby resembled "a little rock"[1] in his crib. Bleier had three younger siblings, Patty, Dan, and Pam.

Bleier tore ligaments in his ankle in fourth grade and was diagnosed in sixth grade with Osgood-Schlatter's disease when his bones grew much more rapidly than his muscles, ligaments, and cartilage. The disease affected his knee, but he returned to basketball in seventh grade and football in eighth grade. Bleier graduated in 1964 from Xavier High School in Appleton, where he starred in football and basketball. Coach Gene Clark developed Bleier's competitiveness and intensity.

Bleier earned All-State honors in football as a running back three times and All-Conference honors at both linebacker and defensive back. He scored 55 touchdowns, including 21 his senior year. Xavier finished 9–0 each season, winning a state title his junior year and ending runner-up his senior year. His Xavier basketball teams finished 25–0 his junior campaign and 24–0 his senior season, as he averaged 12 points per game. He also competed in the 100-yard dash, half-mile relay, shot put, and long jump in track and field, helping his team win three conference titles.

Twenty colleges and universities recruited Bleier, who visited the University of Notre Dame, University of Wisconsin, and Boston College. Notre Dame football coach Hugh Devore offered him a grant-in-aid. "I loved the campus," Bleier recalled. Notre Dame's national reputation impressed him. He especially enjoyed playing under Ara Parseghian, who became head coach in 1964.[2]

Bleier lettered for three years in football, starting on their 9–0–1 1966 National Championship squad. Despite suffering a lacerated kidney, he led the "Fighting Irish" with 57 yards rushing and caught three passes for 16 yards at second-ranked Michigan State University. Football historians often call the classic 10–10 tie "the game of the century." Bleier reflected, "I'll never forget the unbelievable hype."[3] Notre Dame annihilated the University of Southern California, 51–0, in the season finale.

Bleier captained the 1967 Notre Dame squad, which finished 8–2. His finest game came against Navy, as he combined 59 yards and two touchdowns rushing with a 30-yard kickoff return and 27-yard punt return. Two weeks later, Bleier tore ligaments in his left knee while scoring a first-half touchdown. He miraculously played the second half, running, blocking, catching passes, and punting, but underwent season-ending surgery three days later. After the season finale at Miami of Florida, Parseghian gave him the team ball. Bleier recalled, "I didn't stop crying for another twenty minutes."[4] He earned a bachelor's degree in business administration in 1968.

Scouts considered Bleier competent, hard-nosed, and productive, but too small and too slow for professional football. The beleaguered Pittsburgh Steelers, however, drafted Bleier as the four-hundred-seventeenth player on the sixteenth round in 1968. Pro scouts did not consider him an exceptional running back and questioned his speed. Bleier also had suffered a lacerated kidney and ruptured knee ligament.[5] Scouts

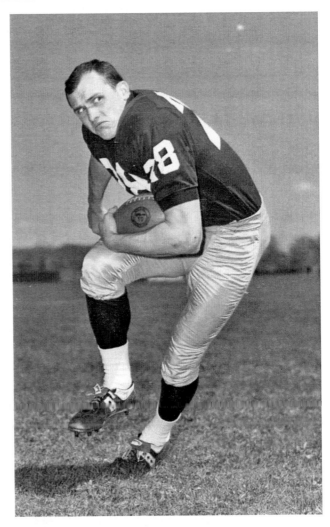

Rocky Bleier captained the 1967 University of Notre Dame football team and enjoyed his best game against the U.S. Naval Academy, combining 59 yards rushing and two touchdowns with a 30-yard kickoff return and 27-yard punt return (courtesy Notre Dame Sports Information).

gave him only six to seven percent odds of making the Steelers.

Pittsburgh backfield coach Don Heinrich, however, liked Bleier's "intangibles" and "heart." Although outgaining the San Diego Charger rushers and scoring a touchdown against the Washington Redskins in exhibition games, he made the final Steeler roster because of his enthusiastic special teams play. "I had become the only thing in life I really wanted to be," Bleier beamed. "I was a professional football player."[6] The Steelers finished a dismal 2–11–1 under head coach Bill Austin. In 1968 Bleier rushed only six times for 39 yards and caught just three passes for 68 yards, averaging 22.7 yards per catch. He also returned six kickoffs for 119 yards and two punts for 13 yards.

In December 1968, the U.S. Army drafted Bleier. His student deferment had expired, and he was classified 1-A. The Steelers arranged for him to join a National Guard unit in Washington, Pennsylvania. Bleier was inducted into the Army on November 28 in Pittsburgh[7] and underwent basic and advanced training at Fort Gordon, Georgia.

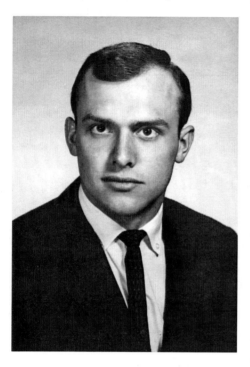

Rocky Bleier earned a bachelor's degree in business administration from the University of Notre Dame in 1968 and later starred as a blocking back for the Pittsburgh Steelers, helping the latter win four Super Bowl championships (courtesy Notre Dame Sports Information).

Bleier served in South Vietnam from May until August 1969. He was shipped with the 196th Light Infantry Brigade to Chu Lai in May 1969 and joined Company C (or Charlie). Bleier was on patrol near Chu Lai on August 20 when the North Vietnamese Army (NVA) ambushed his platoon.[8] Bleier's 25-member platoon suddenly heard an NVA automatic weapon and dove off a dike into a rice paddy. Bleier rolled onto his back and attempted flipping off his pack. After grabbing his launcher and the grenades, he crawled on his stomach 20 yards to the front of the paddy. Bleier spotted an NVA machine gun about 75 yards away in a wooded knoll. He breached a load in his grenade launcher. "A bullet struck his left thigh and shrapnel entered his left leg."[9] Blood gushed through two holes in his pants.

Bleier's platoon disappeared into the nearby jungle. The first ambush killed three from his 25-man platoon. Bleier crawled directly behind a row of hedges, fired three dozen rounds of ammunition, and lay there for 90 minutes while his brigade organized a counteroffensive. "My leg was burning," he recollected. Bleier discovered a deep gash on his thigh. A piece of muscle and flesh was sheared off. Bleier and the platoon doctor crawled down the hedgerow, along a rice paddy, across a road, into an open field. Around 130 NVA troops chased his platoon across the rice paddy and spread themselves over the edge of the woods and began firing. The defenseless Bleier watched the small arms fire.

Two hours later, an NVA grenade deflected off the back of commanding officer Tom Murphy and another platoon member. The grenade bounced toward Bleier and exploded at his feet. Bleier landed on top of Murphy. The grenade sent pieces of shrapnel into Bleier's right leg, destroying part of his right foot. "The pain in my right foot pierced me," Bleier recollected. "I had shrapnel blow up both legs, and several shattered bones in my right foot," His right leg quivered uncontrollably, and his pants were drenched with blood. "It scared me,"[10] he said. The NVA nearly had overrun Bleier's brigade before reinforcements finally arrived from a second platoon. Murphy ordered the platoon to hold their automatic weapons fire and defend against the final assault. "The enemy kept it up," Bleier recollected. Two members from Bleier's platoon were killed in the second confrontation, while most of the remainder were seriously wounded.

When another platoon appeared, four men took turns carrying Bleier on a poncho liner to the medivac helicopter until they could go no further. A black soldier hauled him over his shoulder for 30-yard intervals. "It was an ordeal for both of us," Bleier remembered. After collapsing, he wanted a stretcher to transport him the remaining distance. "That's when it really started to hurt," Bleier remembered. "The agony surged through my right foot." Four platoon members dragged him the final 500 meters to the helicopter on Million Dollar Hill. Bleier feared, "The helicopter would leave without me and never come back."[11]

It took six hours to carry him two miles to the helicopter. Bleier waited two more hours for a third helicopter to take him to the Ninety-fifth Evacuation Hospital in Da Nang. He arrived there at 5 A.M. on August 22 and was given two shots of morphine to help alleviate the pain. He earned a Purple Heart for being wounded and a Bronze Star for heroic or meritorious achievement in 1969.

Bleier underwent minor surgery to clean out over 100 pieces of shrapnel and was transferred on August 25 to Camp Oji Military Hospital in Tokyo. The steel plate in his combat boot saved his foot, but the infection had spread and some shrapnel remained deeply embedded. The grenade had gashed his foot along the instep extending to the ball of the foot, alongside the big toe reaching the bone, and under the second toe, shattering the bone. Dr. Anan Laorr did not close the wounds on his foot because of the infection, but the flesh wound in his left thigh was stitched. The damage to his legs and knees would heal.

Bleier worried whether he would play professional football again. He told Dr. John Baughmann, Dr. Laorr's associate, that he played with the Pittsburgh Steelers and inquired about his chances of playing again. Dr. Baughmann replied, "Rocky, you won't be able to play again. It's impossible."[12] Dr. Baughmann wanted him to concentrate on just walking normally. Bleier, however, remained undaunted, sustained by his belief system, prayers, and hard work.[13]

Bleier was flown on September 14 to Fort Riley, Kansas, for more surgery on his damaged ligaments, tendons and muscles and for months of grueling rehabilitation. Bleier initially found walking quite difficult. "For seven months," he recollected, "there were crutches, and canes, and operations, and leg casts, and physical therapy."

Despite traumatic, painful rehabilitation and pessimistic medical opinions, Bleier was determined to resume playing professional football. He regularly wrote Art

Rooney Sr., the Steelers' owner, from Tokyo and Fort Riley, overstating his medical progress. Rooney privately doubted whether Bleier would ever play again, but never conveyed that pessimism. He wrote, "Rock—the team's not doing well. We need you."[14] Rooney advised, "Take care of yourself and we'll see you when you get back."[15]

In January 1970, Dr. Peter Keblisch and Dr. Phil Taylor removed bone spurs in Bleier's foot and cut some ligaments out of his scar tissue to improve his foot mobility. Physical therapy increased the strength and flexibility in Bleier's legs. Bleier began reflecting on his Vietnam War experience and rehabilitation and how both prepared him for his return to football. Bleier concluded, "Football was not a life-and-death situation," but "there were no guarantees in Vietnam."[16]

After being released from the hospital in April 1970, Bleier remained at Fort Riley and moved to a nearby Manhattan apartment. He arose at 5:30 A.M. to resume workouts and tried to run the first day, but soon learned that he was out of shape. "The first few steps were agony," Bleier disclosed. After running only one quarter of a mile, he fell on the grass, sobbing. "My foot hurt, my heart was pounding, I couldn't breathe." He wondered, "Will I ever play football again?" and admitted, "The doctor might have been right."[17]

Bleier worked out the next three months with Steve Eller of Roland, Iowa, running several miles around the apartment complex in the morning, lifting weights from 6 P.M. to 8 P.M., and running sprints for an hour. Eller tried to build Bleier's confidence. They ran the steps at the Kansas State University Stadium on weekends. The U.S. Army discharged Bleier in July 1970, six months early.

After spending a week in Appleton, Wisconsin, Bleier confounded his doctors by rejoining the Pittsburgh Steelers in training camp just eleven months after being wounded. "I wanted to come back and play," he insisted. "Playing football was the only thing I knew how to do."[18] The Steelers had hired Chuck Noll as head coach and played in new Three Rivers Stadium. Thirty pounds lighter, Bleier "could not walk, let alone run, without pain and a noticeable limp."[19] Although Bleier really believed he could make the Steelers, teammates and club officials wondered why he endured the pain.

Bleier spent two full years trying to regain a spot on the Steelers' active roster. The Steelers waived him twice, but he remained undaunted. A week before the 1970 season opener, Noll advised Bleier to return home and work on body conditioning. "For the first time since fifth grade," Bleier realized, "I wasn't a football player anymore."[20] The Steelers placed him on the injured reserve and wanted him to have another operation. Dr. John Best surgically removed a large piece of shrapnel on the surface of his fourth toe.

Bleier became a field underwriter for Hinsdale Associates outside Chicago, selling Mutual of New York life insurance. He valiantly fought his way back, running two miles daily and lifting weights during his spare time. "The physical pain of those mornings," Bleier recollected, matched "the mental anguish of knowing what lay in wait." He struggled to run 10 laps at the Lyons Township High School track.

Bleier convinced Rooney to let him report to training camp in 1971, but spent that season on the taxi squad. "The only thing that saved me," he confessed, "was the lack of strong competition."[21] Bleier appeared in only three games, returning one kickoff for 21 yards, receiving one punt, and making two tackles. Injuries sidelined him from mid–September until December 1971. Rooney allegedly retained him on the Pittsburgh roster because he was Irish, a Notre Dame graduate, and a war hero. "I was a pretty pitiful-looking football player," Bleier conceded, "limping around with that hamstring" in "another season of torment." He improved his speed and flexibility during the off-season and astonished the Steelers by sprinting 40 yards in 4.6 seconds, two-tenths of a second faster than he had done previously. Noll lauded Bleier's feat as "unbelievable," "phenomenal," and "incredible."[22]

In 1972, Bleier led the Steelers in rushing during pre-season and made the roster, appearing mainly on special teams. Pittsburgh won its first division title in 40 years, while Bleier regained his physical strength. "Slowly, agonizingly, I progressed," he detected. Bleier returned two kickoffs for four yards and rushed once on a draw play up the middle for 17 yards against the Cleveland Browns. "I felt great," Bleier beamed.[23] The Steelers, with quarterback Terry Bradshaw and rookie fullback Franco Harris, finished 11–3.

During the off-season, Bleier worked three hours daily six days a week on improving his leg, back, and shoulder strength, and physique. "I was in the absolute best shape of my life," he recollected. Only two Steeler teammates exhibited greater strength and speed than Bleier. Noll began playing him more. Bleier again paced the Steelers in rushing during the 1973 pre-season, carrying 32 times for 220 yards and averaging seven yards per carry.

Bleier aspired to become the NFL's best special-teams player in 1973. He led teammates downfield and made several tackles. His blocked punt preserved a victory over the Cincinnati Bengals and his fumble recovery against the Houston Oilers helped the Steelers make the playoffs. Bleier returned three kickoffs for 47 yards, rushed the ball three times for no net yards, and made two fair catches in 12 games. He eventually replaced Preston Pearson on third down and short yardage situations because of his blocking ability. Pittsburgh made the playoffs with a 10–4 record, but lost to the Oakland Raiders, 33–14, in the American Football Conference (AFC) Division Playoff Game. The 1973 campaign began "with great expectations," but "finished in dismay."[24]

After the 1973 season, Bleier decided to quit pro football. "I thought I'd be lucky to be the fifth running back in 1974," remarked Bleier, who "saw the handwriting on the wall." The Steelers planned to use Harris and Steve Davis as starting backs, with Pearson and Frenchy Fuqua as reserves.[25] Steeler linebacker Andy Russell, who was attending an NFL Players Association (NFLPA) dinner in Chicago, invited Bleier to come. Bleier told Russell, "I've decided to quit." Russell dissuaded Bleier, insisting, "You can't quit. You've got to come back." Russell's pep talk convinced him to return. "It made some sense to me," Bleier concluded. "I didn't need a lot of arm twisting."[26] Pittsburgh in 1974 may have drafted the best class in NFL history, selecting middle linebacker Jack Lambert, center Mike Webster, and receivers Lynn Swann and John Stallworth.

An off-season weightlifting training regimen restored Bleier's weight to a more realistic 212 pounds. Bob Guida devised a program to maintain Bleier's strength and increase his endurance. Bleier also played paddleball with teammates Jack Ham and Gerry Mullins and ran around Three Rivers Stadium twice weekly in a 12-minute workout with Russell. Bleier's incessant training enabled him to show his courage and determination. When the NFLPA called a strike against the owners, the players boycotted the 1974 training camp. Bleier supported the strike because of the inequities in the pro football establishment.[27]

Bleier's superior blocking ability earned him a starting backfield position in 1974. Bleier topped the Steelers in pre-season rushing for the third straight year, but began the season with special teams again. His first playing opportunity came in the fourth game at the Houston Oilers on October 6, when Harris was sidelined with a leg injury, Fuqua got hurt, and Davis struggled. With just one minute, 51 seconds left in the first half, Noll inserted Bleier at fullback and Pearson at halfback. The Steelers marched 39 yards in less than one minute and kicked a field goal. In the second half, Pearson gained 117 yards and Bleier rushed 37 yards in Pittsburgh's 13–7 victory. "I had one of my greatest days blocking,"[28] Bleier enthused.

Bleier made his initial NFL start at the Kansas City Chiefs on October 13, scoring his first NFL regular-season touchdown in a 34–24 triumph, and became starting fullback alongside Harris. Before a national television audience, the Steelers on October 28 defeated the Atlanta Falcons, 24–17, at home. Bleier, who had not practiced one play at halfback all season, started that contest at left halfback. "I couldn't believe it," he said. Bleier returned to the hotel to get his playbook because "I didn't think I knew the plays."[29] Harris and Bleier recorded career highs rushing with 141 yards and 78 yards, respectively, with the latter blocking very effectively.

The Steelers centered their offense around Harris, using Bleier primarily as his blocker. The solidly built Bleier enjoyed blocking and possessed better leverage because of his shorter stature. "That victory over Atlanta was truly a turning point for our offense," he claimed. "In retrospect, I guess I was in the right place, with the right skills, at the right time."

Two weeks later at the Cincinnati Bengals, Bleier unleashed the most devastating block of his NFL career. He cleared the way for Harris, ripping through the center, driving middle linebacker Ken Avery seven yards backwards, and flipping him on his back. "We found the right combination for a while,"[30] Bleier noted. He exhibited a jerkier, choppier stride than most halfbacks, but his steady, if unspectacular, play and yardage gained gradually earned him more carries. Bleier, however, stretched his Achilles tendon later in the Cincinnati game and was sidelined for three weeks. The Steelers ended the regular season by edging the New England Patriots, 21–17, to clinch their second AFL Central Division crown, and then thrashed Cincinnati, 27–3, to finish 10–3–1.

The Steelers began dominating the NFL that year. Bleier excelled as a blocker and ball carrier, rushing 88 times for 373 yards (4.2-yard average) and two touchdowns, catching seven passes for 87 yards (12.4-yard average), and returning three kickoffs for 67 yards (22.3-yard average).

Pittsburgh trounced the Buffalo Bills, 32–14, at home in the AFC Division Play-off Game on December 22. The Steelers exploded with 26 second-quarter points, highlighted by Bradshaw's 27-yard touchdown aerial to Bleier along the sideline. Bleier was not the intended receiver, but no Bill defender covered him. He told himself, "'Don't drop it. Don't lose it in the sun. Don't fall. Don't do anything. Just catch it.' I did, for a touchdown."[31] Bleier gained 93 yards rushing and receiving, 13 more than the Bills' O.J. Simpson.

The Steelers tallied 24 fourth-quarter points to overcome Oakland, 24–13, on December 29 in the AFC Championship Game. The host Raiders had owned the NFL's best regular season record and had blanked Pittsburgh, 17–0, in September. The Steelers kept Oakland's defense off guard with dives, specials, traps, and reverses. Harris rushed for 111 yards, while Bleier gained 98 yards, barely missing his first 100-yard game since high school. "My biggest play was a fumble recovery," Bleier insisted. With the Steelers ahead, 18–13, Bradshaw fumbled the ball on a bootleg play midway through the fourth quarter. Dan Conners, the Raiders' middle linebacker, appeared best positioned to recover it, "but the ball took a crazy hop into my arms,"[32] Bleier beamed.

On January 12, 1975, the Steelers ended 40 years of frustration for owner Rooney with a 16–6 victory over the Minnesota Vikings in Super Bowl IX at Tulane Stadium in New Orleans, Louisiana. On Pittsburgh's second possession, Bleier exploited an opening on the left side and gained 18 yards. "Boy, I wish I had more speed," he muttered. "A chasm like that, I should have made more of it." The Steelers advanced the ball three times into Minnesota territory in the first quarter, but could not score. With third down and 15 on the Steeler 10-yard line in the second quarter, Bleier exploded through a big hole at right tackle. He appeared to have made a first down when he tried to stiff arm safety Jerry Wright and fumbled the ball. The Vikings recovered the ball on the Steeler 24-yard line.[33] Minnesota only advanced the ball two yards in three plays and did not score. Later that quarter, Pittsburgh's defensive end Dwight White tackled Viking quarterback Fran Tarkenton in the end zone for a safety to give the Steelers a 2–0 halftime lead.

When Minnesota fumbled the second-half kickoff, Pittsburgh's Marv Kellum recovered the ball on the Vikings' 30-yard line. Harris rushed 24 yards to Minnesota's six-yard line. Two plays later, Bleier blocked 275-pound right end Jim Marshall, enabling Harris to score, giving the Steelers a 9–0 lead. Marshall landed on Bleier with a thud. "Nothing is as much fun," Bleier reminisced, "as lying under Jim Marshall, ... looking up at Franco, who is easing into the end zone." Vikings defensive end Carl Eller pummeled Bleier during the Steelers' next offensive series, turning and twisting the latter's ankle. Bleier's painful sore ankle prevented him from pushing or driving off it. The Steelers blanked the Vikings for 48 minutes, forcing two fumbles and two interceptions.

After Minnesota scored a touchdown on a blocked punt, Pittsburgh got the ball at their 34-yard line with 10 minutes, 18 seconds remaining. On third down and two, Bradshaw fired a 30-yard pass to Larry Brown to the Viking 28-yard line. After the Steelers were penalized five yards, Bleier rushed 17 yards through a hole left by Doug Sutherland.[34] Harris gained five yards on the next two plays. Bradshaw passed to Bleier for a first down on the five-yard line and to Brown for a touchdown three plays later for the 16–6 triumph. The Super Bowl victory marked the culmination of six hard years for Bleier, who shook hands and exchanged big smiles with teammates. "Each knows the euphoria I feel now," he beamed. Bleier hugged and thanked a teary-eyed Rooney, who was standing strangely alone against a wall.

For the first time, Bleier revealed his strenuous comeback regimen to the media. He recalled "those first horrifying weeks" when "shots of pain launched up through my legs." Bleier recollected, "Seeing a thousand different sunrises while I ran myself to the brink of exhaustion; of finishing a workout, my skin tingly with perspiration, my legs wobbling unsteadily, my head feeling light and faint, my lungs gulping and gasping." The training paid handsome dividends for Bleier, who forced himself to stick to the regimen. "Ultimately, I did it all for myself,"[35] he acknowledged, in his quest to make the team. The workouts, toil, and pains gave him fulfillment.

The 1975 Steelers, considered one of the greatest in NFL history, compiled a 12–2 record and recorded another Central Division title. Bleier enjoyed one of his best NFL games, gaining 163 yards on October 26 at the Green Bay Packers. During 1975, Bleier rushed 140 times for 528 yards (3.8-yard average) and two touchdowns and caught 15 passes for 65 yards (4.3-yard average). Pittsburgh dominated the Baltimore Colts, 28–10, on December 27 at home in the AFC Divisional Playoff Game. Bleier scored the Steelers' second touchdown with a seven-yard run in the third quarter. Pittsburgh bested Oakland, 16–10, in the AFC Championship Game and repeated as NFL titlists, edging the Dallas Cowboys, 21–17, in Super Bowl X at the Orange Bowl in Miami on January 18, 1976. Bleier rushed 15 times for 51 yards against Dallas.[36]

Bleier's stirring comeback has been recognized. Bleier won the George Halas Award as the NFL's Most Courageous Player in 1974, the Whizzer White Humanitarian Award in 1975, and the Vince Lombardi Award in 1975. He later was named the Most Courageous Athlete of the Decade and one of the U.S. Jaycees' Ten Outstanding Young Men of the Year. The American Sports Art Museum and Archives in

1985 gave Bleier its initial Mildred "Babe" Didrikson Zaharias Courage Award for demonstrating courage, perseverance, grace, and strength in overcoming adversity to excel in sport.

In 1975, Bleier published his autobiography, *Fighting Back: The Rocky Bleier Story*, co-authored with Terry O'Neil. It dramatically recounts his agonizing two-year rehabilitation from Vietnam War wounds and persistent struggle to return to the Pittsburgh Steelers. Bleier's personal courage and strength helped him overcome physical disabilities and insurmountable odds to build a professional football career. *Fighting Back* was made into a 1980 television movie, with Robert Urich starring as Bleier.

In 1976, an injury to Bradshaw forced the Steelers to rely on the ground game. Pittsburgh, bolstered by its Steel Curtain defense, claimed its third straight Central Division title. Bleier enjoyed his best NFL campaign with 1,036 yards rushing in 220 carries (4.7-yard average) and five touchdowns, becoming just the third Steeler to gain over 1,000 yards in a season. He and Harris became only the second NFL backfield duo to rush for over 1,000 yards the same season. Mercury Morris and Larry Csonka had accomplished that feat for the undefeated 1972 Miami Dolphins. Bleier also caught 24 passes for 294 yards (12.3-yard average) and consistently made significant plays in important games with uncanny regularity. The Steelers routed Baltimore, 40–14, in the AFC Divisional Playoff Game, but injuries sidelined Harris and Bleier from the AFC title game. Oakland throttled Pittsburgh's ground game and dethroned the Steelers, 24–7, in the AFC Championship Game.

Pittsburgh repeated as Central Division champions in 1977. Bleier rushed 135 times for 465 yards (3.4-yard average) and four touchdowns and caught 18 passes for 161 yards (8.9-yard average). Denver eliminated the Steelers, 34–21, in the AFC Divisional Playoff Game.

Pittsburgh enjoyed its greatest season in 1978 with a 14–2 mark. The Steelers intensified their passing attack, capitalizing on the NFL's new liberalized pass-blocking rules. Bleier rushed 165 times for 633 yards (3.8-yard average) and five touchdowns and made 17 pass receptions for 168 yards (9.9-yard average) and one touchdown. Bradshaw led Pittsburgh to a 33–10 victory over Denver in the AFC Divisional Playoff Game and a 34–5 triumph over Houston on January 7, 1979, at home in the AFC Championship Game. Bleier tallied the Steelers' second touchdown in the first quarter against the Oilers with a 15-yard run.[37]

Bleier helped Pittsburgh capture a third NFL title, edging the Dallas Cowboys, 35–31, in Super Bowl XIII at Miami on January 21, 1979. The Steelers led, 14–13, in the second quarter. Bradshaw, who threw four touchdown aerials, drove the Steelers to the Dallas seven-yard line, capitalizing on two long passes to Swann. On third down, he called a pass-run option play and moved to his right. The Cowboys seemingly trapped Bradshaw, who finally spotted Bleier in the end zone. Bleier leaped high to catch Bradshaw's pass behind linebacker D.D. Lewis. He jumped "higher than he should have been able to jump." His spectacular catch gave Pittsburgh a 21–13 halftime advantage and landed him on the cover of *Sports Illustrated.*[38]

The Steelers widened the lead to 35–17 in the fourth quarter, scoring two touchdowns in 19 seconds. Dallas tallied two late touchdowns to make the score 35–31 with just 22 seconds left, and then tried an onside kick. Rafael Septien's kick went to Bleier on the Dallas 45-yard line. Bleier, who sealed the victory by recovering an onside kick, remembered getting "hit by at least 20 Cowboys on that play."[39] He also rushed twice for three yards. Pittsburgh became the first NFL team with three Super Bowl victories, while both squads established a Super Bowl record for total points scored.

Noll's team claimed its sixth straight Central Division crown in 1979, pacing the NFL in scoring with 416 points. Bleier rushed 92 times for 434 yards (4.7-yard average) and four touchdowns and snared a career-high 31 passes for 277 yards (8.9-yard average). The host Steelers thrashed Miami, 34–14, on December 30 in the AFC Divisional Playoff Game, with Bleier scoring on a one-yard third-quarter run for Pittsburgh's fourth touchdown. They defeated the Oilers, 27–13, on January 6, 1980, at home in the AFC Championship Game, clinching the contest on Bleier's four-yard touchdown run in the final minute. Pittsburgh earned its fourth Super Bowl crown when Bradshaw rallied the Steelers past the upset-minded Los Angeles Rams, 31–19, in Super Bowl XIV on January 20, 1980, in the Rose Bowl in Pasadena, California. Bleier rushed 10 times for 25 yards in his final Super Bowl appearance.[40]

Bleier, who had started at halfback in four victorious Super Bowl games, reflected, "I loved all four of them," ranking Super Bowl XIII as his favorite.[41] He retired after the 1980 season, having rushed 78 times for 340 yards (4.4-yard average) and one touchdown and caught 21 passes for 174 yards (8.3-yard average) and one touchdown in his final NFL campaign.

During 11 NFL seasons, Bleier rushed 3,865 yards on 928 attempts (4.2-yard average) and 23 touchdowns, and caught 136 passes for 1,294 yards (9.5-yard average) and two touchdowns.[42] Although having only five 100-yard games, he ranked as the fourth leading rusher in Steeler history. In 1982, Pittsburgh fans named Bleier to the All-Time Steeler Team. "I was fortunate," Bleier reminisced. "I had important people in my life who made a difference." Bleier, "The Good Soldier," who blocked for Harris, "did little things well" and "could pick up tough yards in tough times." The reliable, durable Steeler testified, "I'm a breathing example of what you can do if you want to."[43]

Bleier married Aleta Giacobine on September 7, 1975. They had one daughter, Samantha, and one son, Aidri-James, but were divorced in October 1996. Bleier was forced to declare bankruptcy in 1995 and sold off his Super Bowl rings to pay off back taxes. He has two adopted children, Rosie and Elly, with his second wife, Jan Gyurina, and resides in Mt. Lebanon, Pennsylvania.

Bleier worked as investment banker with Russell, Rea, Bleier, and Zappalla in

Pittsburgh and presides over Rocky Bleier Enterprises. He founded RB VetCo, a construction company based in Pittsburgh. Bleier served as a board member of the Vietnam Veterans Memorial Fund, which enabled the erection of the Memorial in Washington, D.C. In October 2007, the football field at Xavier High School in Appleton, Wisconsin was renamed Rocky Bleier Stadium.

Bleier has recouped the money he lost (and has bought back his Super Bowl rings) by earning an estimated $300,000 per year, touring the United States as a motivational speaker. His presentation, "Be the Best You Can Be," inspires audiences to keep on striving for greater accomplishments and stresses the importance of "setting goals" and "overcoming barriers and perceptions." A dynamic speaker, Bleier relates his gripping tale of courage in the Vietnam War and on the gridiron details how ordinary people can become extraordinary achievers. He summed up how the Vietnam experience changed his life. "Sure it was a struggle," but, "if I was an inspiration to somebody, terrific," and "if I was perceived as a hero to someone who was looking for a hero, so much the better."[44]

# TOMMY JOHN

"I can't imagine anyone overcoming the hurdles he did to last as long" describes the medical fairy tale of Tommy John, who suffered a career-threatening arm injury after pitching 13 major league baseball seasons. John tore ligaments in his left elbow and was given a one percent chance of ever pitching again. After undergoing experimental ligament surgery never performed on an athlete before, he became an even better major league pitcher and set a longevity record for pitchers by completing 26 major league seasons.

John grew up in a working-class, athletic-minded family. Thomas Edward John was born in Terre Haute, Indiana, on May 22, 1943. His father, Thomas, was employed in utilities, while his mother, Ruth, was a homemaker. Thomas, who had played semi-professional baseball, spent "many extra hours"[1] honing his son's pitching skills.

John graduated in 1961 from Terre Haute Gerstmeyer High School, where he starred in basketball, baseball, and golf. Besides holding the city single game basketball scoring record, he averaged 20.3 points and 17.5 rebounds per game as a senior in basketball. The University of Kentucky and 49 other colleges offered him basketball scholarships. He compiled a 28–2 win-loss record as a pitcher and interested several major league baseball scouts, but received only one college baseball scholarship offer. Sportswriter Will Grimsley penned, "He might have been another Jack Nicklaus or Larry Bird had he not chosen baseball over golf and basketball."[2] John later studied mathematics at Indiana State University in Terre Haute between baseball seasons.

In June 1961, the Cleveland Indians signed John for $40,000. The 6-foot 3-inch, 203-pound, left-handed John compiled a 10–4 record and 3.17 earned run average (ERA) for Dubuque, Iowa, of the largely rookie Midwest League in 1961. John, just 18 years old, had not yet learned proper pitching mechanics. He split the 1962 and 1963 seasons between Charleston, West Virginia, of the Eastern League and Jacksonville, Florida, of the International League.

John surrendered one unearned run in two relief innings in his major league debut with Cleveland in 1963. Although losing twice in six appearances, he boasted a 2.25 ERA in 20 innings.[3] His first major league victory came against the Baltimore Orioles on May 3, 1964, when he out-dueled Robin Roberts, 3–0, at Memorial Stadium in Baltimore. Roberts, whom John idolized, had starred in basketball and baseball. John hurled a complete game, throwing only 72 pitches. Indian pitching coach Early Wynn wanted John to begin throwing a slider, but the latter encountered wildness and struggled with a 2–9 record for Cleveland in 1964. The Indians optioned him to Portland, Oregon, of the Pacific Coast League, where he regained his control and split 12 decisions. John, whose fastball was clocked at around 85 miles per hour, developed an outstanding sinker ball and good curveball, typically inducing ground balls. Pitcher Nolan Ryan observed John "never threw hard, but he had a deadly, heavy sinker, a decent slider, and exceptional control."[4]

In January 1965, the Chicago White Sox acquired John. John joined the regular starting rotation and experienced mixed success through 1971, triumphing 82 times and losing 80 decisions. He won 14 and lost just seven with a 3.08 ERA for second-place Chicago in 1965 and finished 14–11 with a 2.62 ERA in 1966, leading the American League (AL) with five shutouts. Although prevailing only 10 of 23 times in 1967, John boasted a 2.48 ERA and shared the junior circuit lead with six shutouts. The following year, his record improved to 10 wins and five losses with a career-best 1.98 ERA and an AL All-Star team selection.

In August 1968, however, John was involved in an incident with Dick McAullife of the Detroit Tigers. When John lost his grip on one pitch, the ball sailed over McAuliffe's head. McAullife charged the mound, and John tried to tackle him. McAullife's knee battered John's shoulder.[5] The impact separated John's left shoulder, sidelining him the rest of that season with torn ligaments.

The White Sox began declining in the AL standings and lost confidence in John's pitching skills. John struggled his final three seasons with Chicago, tallying a 9–11 mark and 3.26 ERA in 1969, a 12–17 record and 3.28 ERA in 1970, and a 13–16 slate and 3.61 ERA in 1971. Pitching coach Johnny Sain tried to alter John's pitch selection and mechanics, but the latter was convinced he needed "to depend chiefly on my breaking pitches to win ball games."[6] He married Sally Simmons in July 1970 in Plainfield, Indiana, and had four children, Tami, Tommy, Travis, and Taylor.

On December 2, 1971, the Los Angeles Dodgers obtained John in a trade for first baseman Dick Allen. John beamed, "That was a dream come true," since he considered the Dodgers "a first-class operation!" Pitching coach Dwight "Red" Adams persuaded John that his fastball had considerable movement. John rebounded with an 11–5 win-loss record and 2.89 ERA in 1972 and 16–7 mark and 3.10 ERA in 1973, leading the National League (NL) with a .696 winning percentage in 1973.

John attained greater heights in 1974, pacing the NL with a 13–3 record, and boasted a stellar 2.59 ERA through mid–July. Los Angeles, which had not reached the playoffs since 1966, jumped 10 games ahead of the defending champion Cincinnati Reds. John was perturbed about not making the NL All-Star squad.[7]

In July, however, John encountered a major crisis so formidable that no one expected him to conquer it. "No pitcher had ever faced what John now faced and kept his career alive. John himself compared it to a dead-end prison sentence." Misfortune struck John on July 17 during a twilight game against the Montreal Expos at Dodger Stadium. The Dodgers led, 4–0, after three innings. In the fourth inning, Willie Davis singled and Bob Bailey walked. John tried throwing a sharp sinker ball to pull-hitter Hal Breeden, hoping to induce a double play. Upon releasing the ball, John detected "the strangest sensation I had ever known." His arm suddenly went dead. "The ball just blooped up to the plate," missing the strike zone badly. John, wanting to make sure his arm was still attached, moved it freely without pain. He attempted to throw another sinker ball, which again blooped to the plate. "This time, however, I felt, or heard, a sort of 'thump!' in my forearm as I let the ball go," John recollected. "It still didn't hurt. But I knew I could not pitch." John left the mound and told manager Walt Alston, "You'd better get somebody in there, I've hurt my arm."[8]

Dr. Frank Jobe, the Dodgers' orthopedist, did not know the extent of the injury and told John to ice his arm at home. John recalled, "It felt as if I had left my arm someplace else." He had "no inkling of permanent injury," but found "it was really sore"[9] the next morning. The injury dashed John's chances for his first 20-victory season and possible NL Cy Young Award. That afternoon, Dr. Jobe X-rayed John's forearm at his office. "I don't want to be alarmist," he warned. "But I have to be realistic, too. I think you've torn a ligament." John had placed too much long-term stress on his left arm, causing an inflammation, scar, calcification, degeneration, and rupture of the ligaments. Dr. Herb Stark confirmed Dr. Jobe's diagnosis and told John, "You sure did a job on your arm!"[10]

John's elbow did not improve the next few days, as spasms tightened the muscles on either side of the joint. Dr. Jobe considered an operation "unavoidable," but initially told John to rest it at home. John, who experienced only stiffness, rejoined the Dodgers and tried throwing batting practice in Atlanta three weeks later. His pitches did not even reach home plate and lacked both normal velocity and movement, confirming his need for elbow surgery. "My pitches flew in six different directions and my arm hurt." John's forearm did not feel attached. John tried pitching again two days later with the same results. Alston advised him to forget the 1974 season and concentrate on rehabilitation.[11]

John had nothing to lose undergoing the surgery after exploring all other possible avenues and phoned Dr. Jobe that he wanted the operation right away, "a decision that would forever change his life, his career, and indeed, the sport." He feared even missing the 1975 season otherwise. "At the time," John recalled, "operations on arms

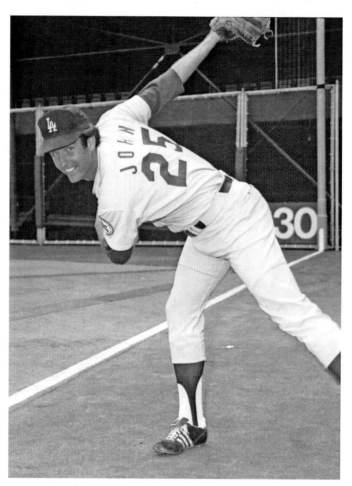

and shoulders weren't that effective, but were dangerous."[12] Dr. Jobe warned John what might happen if he found a slight ligament tear, if the ligament had torn free of the bone, or if the ligament was ruptured. He preferred not to perform the "extremely risky and extremely difficult" surgery and gave John "about one in a hundred" chance of ever pitching again. Doctors had performed the operation on accident victims, but not on athletes. Dr. Jobe advised John to "consider another line of work."[13] When John asked what would happen if he did not have the operation, Dr. Jobe replied, "Zero in a hundred." John was prepared to risk surgery, explaining, "I never would pitch in major league baseball again otherwise." No baseball player, however, had undergone the oper-

Tommy John pitched for the Los Angeles Dodgers from 1972 through 1978, pacing the National League with a 13–3 win-loss record before being sidelined with a career-threatening elbow injury (courtesy National Baseball Hall of Fame Library, Cooperstown, N.Y.).

ation while "still holding out hope that he could recover and eventually be the player he was before the surgery."[14]

The severity of John's ligament tear was revealed when the 31-year-old pitcher underwent three-hour surgery on September 25. Dr. Jobe confirmed that John had ruptured the ulnar collateral ligament in his left pitching arm and "because of the long years of wear, there was nothing left to repair." He employed a radically new technique, replacing John's medial collateral ligament. Dr. Jobe removed eight inches of tendon from John's right wrist and transplanted it to reconstruct his left elbow. Ligament transplant surgery had been done on people's wrists and hands, but not on their elbows. Dr. Jobe also repaired a muscle and ulnar nerve damage. Upon awakening from surgery, John not only noticed his whole left arm was bandaged and difficult to move, but also found his right hand bandaged and knew that he had ruptured a ligament. "I was in real trouble,"[15] he realized.

The doctors, religious faith, and Sally helped him through the operation and recovery. "The doctor got me part of the way and I had to get the rest of the way myself," John recognized. He continually repeated a scripture verse from Luke 1:37: "For with God, nothing shall be impossible." John especially praised Sally, who "has always been there for me and the rest of our family. Sally always puts family interests ahead of her career ambitions." The day after the operation, Sally gave birth to a baby girl, Tami. John, who watched the delivery, rejoiced, "I had forgotten my operation completely."[16]

John's rehabilitation, however, brought greater anxiety than the actual surgery. No moundsman had ever undergone this type of operation or had to come back from it. "No one knew what to expect," John pointed out. "We were making medical history." The days following the operation marked John's nadir. The surgery damaged his ulnar nerve. His left hand resembled "a useless claw, with feeling in several of his fingers lost."[17]

Los Angeles, meanwhile, won the NL West in 1974 and invited John to throw out the first pitch of the NL Championship Series at Dodger Stadium. John tossed that pitch right-handed, believing he had thrown his last left-handed pitch in a major league park. According to team president Peter O'Malley, the Dodgers probably would not have made the playoffs without him.[18]

In December 1974, Dr. Jobe performed another, much shorter operation on John. He rerouted the nerve through fatty tissue on the middle of the elbow, well away from the scarring tissue affecting his hand, because the little finger on his left hand numbed and contracted into a full fist. The doctors had inadvertently put a tiny twist in John's ulnar nerve while moving it during surgery, blocking circulation in his little finger. If that surgery had not been performed, John's elbow would have been permanently deformed. Dr. Jobe had warned him, "You're going to have a crippled hand." John's nerve needed to regenerate. Dr. Jobe anticipated that John would not pitch for at least one year, and in fact the latter's first pitch came just one year and one day later.[19]

John spent the entire 1975 season in rehabilitation. After doctors removed the cast on his arm, he tried to regain the muscle strength and control required to pitch again. John strengthened his arm by working diligently daily on exercises prescribed by Dr. Jobe. "I worked as hard as I possibly could on my rehabilitation," he remembered. John reported to spring training in 1975, performing the same tasks as the other pitchers except for throwing the ball. He devised his own practice procedure, tossing balls against a concrete wall, squeezing Silly Putty, running six miles daily, and golfing. Of the wall exercise, John said, "It took on an almost symbolic aspect, representing the 'wall' that I was trying to break through. I'd take four or five balls, throw them against the wall, pick them up again and continue until I felt tired." His throwing ability improved daily. Chief Dodger scout Ben Wade cautiously observed, "I can see you pitching again within a year." "This lifted my spirits about fifty degrees," John enthused, "and I went back to my exercises with some real zest."[20]

Two of John's fingers still lacked full sensation, preventing him from properly gripping the ball. When driving to the ballpark in June 1975, John suddenly uncurled his two paralyzed fingers. He rushed home to Yorba Linda and slowly stretched his fingers out full-length in Sally's presence. Sally screamed, "Then we hugged each other," John said, "and started dancing around. This was sure IT! This meant that little by little I could get all the fingers back."[21] Sensation returned to his other fingers when he continued squeezing the silly putty.

John's velocity increased during a bullpen session in July. John started throwing batting practice to pitchers and joined the Arizona Instructional League in September, hurling fast balls and curves between three and seven innings under game conditions. He started seven games in 28 days, concentrating on building his arm strength and mastering pitch location rather than throwing hard.

Defying the odds, John rejoined the Dodger roster in 1976. The spring training lockout by the owners, however, afforded John little opportunity to regain pitching shape or demonstrate his soundness.[22] The Dodgers worried that John could not throw above 85 miles per hour, although he had not pitched any faster before his surgery. John's performance was mediocre in his initial start against the Atlanta Braves on April 16, allowing five runs in five innings in a 5–1 loss. Alston told John the Dodgers were prepared to release him if he did not fare well in his next start. John equated Alston's admonition to "sending a guy to the electric chair." He won a reprieve against the Houston Astros, hurling six shutout innings. "I was not hit hard,"[23] he stressed.

Amid much fanfare, John pitched on April 26 against the Pittsburgh Pirates at Dodger Stadium. Los Angeles led throughout the game, winning 7–1. John blanked the Pirates until surrendering consecutive ninth-inning doubles. Reliever Mike Marshall preserved John's first victory in 15 months. The whole crowd applauded, yelled, screamed, and whistled. "What a welcome!" John exulted. "I could feel the chill down my spine."[24] The Dodgers reworked his $78,000 contract, promising another $30,000 if he pitched 30 games. John started 31 contests, blanking the Cincinnati Reds, 9–0, in his season finale.

John split 20 decisions with a respectable 3.09 ERA in 207 innings in 1976. *The Sporting News* named him NL Comeback Player of the Year for overcoming tremendous adversity. He also received the Fred Hutchinson Award for his courageous effort and numerous other awards. John labeled himself "the only right-handed southpaw to ever pitch in the major leagues."[25]

Remarkably, John won at least 20 games three of the next five seasons. In 1977, he compiled a 20–7 record and 2.78 ERA for new manager Tom Lasorda. John hurled 11 complete games, his highest total in five years. Lasorda inspired John's renewed success. "His confidence in me," John reflected, "pulled me through many a tough inning and his willingness to stay with me when I was having a bad moment or two just added to my own confidence."[26] John, whose arm strengthened as the season progressed, won 14 of his last 17 decisions and ranked fifth in the NL with a 2.78 ERA.

The Dodgers unseated the two-time world champion Cincinnati Reds in the NL West. John started twice against the Philadelphia Phillies in the NL Championship Series, winning once, boasting a 0.66 ERA, and striking out 11 batters in 13.2 innings. He faced Steve Carlton in Game 1 at Los Angeles, but both struggled in "a real donnybrook."[27] Philadelphia led, 5–1, in the seventh inning, when Ron Cey's grand slam home run knotted the score. The Phillies triumphed, 7–5.

The Dodgers led the NL Championship Series, two games to one. John pitched the entire clinching Game 4 in a steady downpour at Philadelphia, prevailing 4–1. John's sinker worked to perfection. Dusty Baker clouted a two-run homer in the second inning. John recounted, "My uniform was soaked and my shoes were full of mud."[28] He fanned Bake McBride to clinch the NL pennant. The ecstatic John termed the contest, "the best game of my career in a game that was for everything." It was "certainly the most exciting as well as the most important, for it put us in the World Series."[29]

Los Angeles reached the World Series for the first time since 1974 and split the first two games with the New York Yankees. John faced Mike Torrez in Game 3 at Los Angeles, surrendering four unearned runs in six innings. "The New Yorkers raked Dodger starter Tommy John over the coals in the first inning," staking Mike Torrez to a 3–0 lead. The Dodgers knotted the score on Baker's three-run, third-inning home run. John surrendered two more runs the next two innings. New York triumphed, 5–3. Mickey Rivers proved John's nemesis, doubling twice and singling once. John did not start again in the World Series, which the Yankees won, four games to two. He finished second to Carlton in the NL Cy Young Award voting, indicating, "He was a better pitcher now, at age 34 and after radical elbow surgery."[30]

John continued his remarkable comeback with 17 wins, 10 losses, a 3.30 ERA, and an NL All-Star selection in 1978, helping Los Angeles capture the NL West.[31] He won his lone decision of the 1978 NL Championship Series against Dick Ruthven of Philadelphia in Game 2, blanking the Phillies, 4–0, with "his sinker in high gear." The hard-hitting Phillies recorded only four singles, bouncing into three double plays and hitting 18 ground balls. John's victory gave the Dodgers a two-game advantage.

Los Angeles took the NL Championship Series, three games to one, dramatically winning Game 4, 4–3, in ten innings.[32]

John started twice against the New York Yankees in the World Series, winning his only decision and fanning six batters in 14.2 innings. Ed Figueroa faced him in Game 1 at Los Angeles. The Dodgers jumped to a three-run advantage in the first inning and prevailed, 11–5. "We beat them badly," John exulted. John "kept the Yanks at bay with a low sinker." In Game 4 at New York, John and Figueroa hurled four scoreless innings.[33] Los Angeles tallied three times in the fifth inning, but the Yankees won, 4–3, in 10 innings. John allowed two seventh-inning runs, but did not figure in the decision. New York won the World Series in six games.

John signed a five-year contract exceeding $1 million with the New York Yankees in November 1978 and became the team's most dependable winner. He enjoyed a tremendous 1979 season with 21 victories, just nine losses, and a 2.97 ERA, "finessing hitters with his sinkerball and control." John began 1979 with nine consecutive triumphs and hurled four straight complete games in May. He led Yankee pitchers in wins, games started (36), complete games (17), innings pitched (276), and shutouts (3). His ERA ranked second best in the AL. John became just the eighth pitcher to win 20 games in both leagues, made the AL All-Star team, and trailed only Mike Flanagan in the AL Cy Young Award voting.[34]

In 1980, John posted a career-high 22 victories with only nine losses. He boasted a 3.43 ERA and amassed a league-best six shutouts, helping New York win the AL East title, being named to *The Sporting News* All-Star team, and finishing fourth in the AL Cy Young Award balloting. John led New York pitchers in triumphs, games started (36), complete games (160), innings pitched (265), and shutouts. He allowed two runs in six innings against the Kansas City Royals in Game 3 of the AL Championship Series, but was not involved in the decision in the 4–2 loss.

A two-month baseball strike split 1981 into two separate seasons. John won the opening games of both halves, defeating the Texas Rangers, 10–3, on April 9 and 2–0 on August 10. Bucky Dent's three-run homer and Bobby Murcer's dramatic, pinch-hit grand-slam home run helped the Yankees conquer Texas in the April contest before a record crowd of over 55,000 fans.[35] John fared 5–4 with a 3.19 ERA through mid–June, helping the Yankees win the first-half season championship. In the August rematch, he limited Texas to two hits in seven innings.

Three days later, tragedy struck the Johns. Their 2½-year-old son, Travis, was critically injured when he fell through a screen from a third-story window, bounced off the hood of Sally's car, and struck his skull on the pavement. Sally phoned John in Detroit about the accident. She frantically shouted, "Oh hurry! Hurry! Travis is in critical condition!" John immediately flew that night to Travis's bedside at Point Pleasant Hospital in Monmouth, New Jersey. "Fear, believe me, was thick as soup, in that tiny room,"[36] John reflected.

Travis was transferred that night to New York University Medical Center. Initial tests disclosed no broken neck, bones, or irreversible brain damage. After Travis spent 14 days in a coma, Dr. Fred Epstein rated his chances of recovery without damage at 70 percent. The Johns kept a bedside vigil for weeks, massaging Travis's arms and legs. The Johns received almost 10,000 letters from well-wishers, answering each personally. Travis completely recovered and resumed a normal life after several agonizing weeks.[37] *The Sally and Tommy John Story*, describes how their Christian faith helped them survive the ordeal. The Johns considered Travis's full recovery miraculous.

John pitched home games when it was his turn, but did not accompany the Yankees on road trips. "How can you choose baseball — or any job, or any profession — ahead of your little boy?" he asked. John tried pitching against Chicago at Yankee Stadium a few nights after Travis's accident, but kept picturing "a little boy entrapped in tubes and wires." He found the experience extremely stressful and performed poorly in the Yankees' loss.

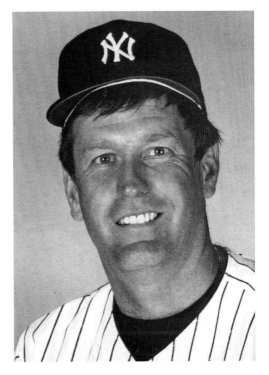

Tommy John pitched for the New York Yankees from 1979 to 1982 and from 1986 to 1989 and was the team's most dependable winner. In 1980, he posted a career-high 22 victories and amassed a league-best six shutouts (courtesy National Baseball Hall of Fame Library, Cooperstown, N.Y.).

"Everything seemed to go wrong that night," John lamented. Yankee owner George Steinbrenner told him afterward, "That was a hell of a gutsy performance you put on out there."[38]

John logged five consecutive complete games in September during Travis's recovery and split eight decisions the latter season. "The games took my mind off Travis's situation," he said. For his courageous display, John received the Lou Gehrig Memorial Award. "Nothing stopped Tommy, which tells you about his faith and dedication,"[39] Ryan observed. John keyed the Yankees' 3–1 triumph over the Oakland Athletics in Game 1 of the AL Championship Series, allowing just one run in six innings and sparking a three-game sweep.

John started twice against triumphant Los Angeles in the 1981 World Series, allowing one run in 13 innings with a stellar 0.69 ERA. He blanked Los Angeles, 3–0, in Game 2 of the 1981 World Series. Larry Milbourne's run-scoring double in the fifth inning keyed the Yankees' victory. John hurled four innings in Game 6. With the score knotted 1–1 in the fourth inning, manager Bob Lemon inexplicably had

Murcer pinch hit for John. "The TV camera caught Tommy's unrestrained anger about the decision."[40] The bullpen imploded, as Los Angeles triumphed, 9–2.

John, who pitched in four World Series, never played on a major league championship team. His pitching skills, however, had dramatically improved since undergoing the radical elbow surgery. Between 1976 and 1981, John had compiled 99 wins and 53 losses with a 3.06 ERA, 14 shutouts, and 64 complete games, and averaged over 235 innings per year.

When John struggled in the first half of 1982, new manager Gene Michael demoted him to the bullpen. John, who requested to be traded, compiled a 10–10 record and 3.66 ERA with New York and hurled a three-hit victory over the Toronto Blue Jays on August 29. Two days later, the Yankees shipped him to the California Angels. John joined the Angels amid a wild AL West race. California won its division with a club-record 93 victories. John finished with a 14–12 composite record and 3.69 ERA in 1982. "That '82 Angels team was probably the best team I ever played on," John reflected. "At least talent-wise, it was the best."[41] California, however, lacked a reliable closer and lost to the Milwaukee Brewers in the AL Championship Series. John's record fell to 11–13 with a 4.33 ERA in 1983 and 7–13 with a 4.52 ERA in 1984. Relievers failed to preserve leads for John in several games. John split two decisions with a 5.11 ERA against the Baltimore Orioles in the 1983 AL Championship Series.

The Angels released John in June 1985. The Oakland A's signed him the following month. John blanked Milwaukee for seven innings and the Seattle Mariners for three frames, but then dislocated his left little finger tagging a runner at first base and pitched ineffectively thereafter. During 1985, John compiled a lackluster 4–10 mark with a 5.53 ERA. "It was a bad year all around,"[42] he confessed. His mother died of cancer and Sally underwent abdominal surgery for removal of benign tumors.

The New York Yankees invited John to spring training in 1986. John hurt his back and remained in Florida. When injuries sidelined starters John Montefusco and Ed Whitson, New York activated him on May 2. John logged a 5–3 record and 2.93 ERA, but missed two months with a strained Achilles tendon and broke his thumb in early September.[43] He briefly became pitching coach at the University of North Carolina, but Steinbrenner talked him out of retirement in December 1986. Thirteen years after his historic surgery, John posted a 13–6 mark and 4.03 ERA in 1987. "The club's workhorse,"[44] he led the Yankees in games started (33) and innings pitched (187). The following year, John won nine of 17 decisions with a 4.49 ERA and again paced New York with 32 starts. The 46-year-old pitched opening day in 1989 and became the then oldest left-handed hurler to win a major league game. After John struggled with a lackluster 2–7 mark and 5.80 ERA, the Yankees released him May 30, short of reaching 300 career victories.[45]

John officially retired in September 1989, maintaining, "I gave it the best I had."[46] Although possessing a good curve and a sinking fastball, he lacked the overpowering stuff of many National Baseball Hall of Famers. John attributed his longevity "to having good genes, knowing what he was good at and sticking with it, and resorting to his strengths at crunch time."[47] "Heart, moxie, perseverance, or just plain guts" sustained his career. John survived many peaks and valleys, overcoming sore arms and injuries and "two critical turning points [his surgery and Travis's accident] that would have ruined just about any other player."[48]

In 26 major league seasons, John appeared in 760 games, compiled 288 wins and 231 losses for a .555 winning percentage, and hurled 46 shutouts. Incredibly, 164 of those victories followed his operation and 51 triumphs came after reaching age 40. The three-time 20-game winner boasted a 3.34 ERA and recorded 2,245 strikeouts in 4,710 innings. His career ERA bested National Baseball Hall of Famers Red Ruffing, Mickey Welch, Chief Bender, Red Faber, Vic Willis, Waite Hoyt, and Rollie Fingers. John excelled in several statistical categories. He held the major league record for most years pitched with 26, later surpassed by Ryan. Only Ryan and first baseman Cap Anson played more major league seasons. Among left-handers as of 2013, John ranked first in most seasons with a victory (25), second in games started, third in innings pitched, fifth in shutouts, sixth in victories, tenth in triumphs after age 40, and sixteenth in strikeouts. Altogether, he finished sixth in games started, ninth in wild pitches (187), eighteenth in career innings pitched, and twenty-fourth in victories. John, who was selected to the 1968, 1978, 1979, and 1980 All-Star squads, boasted a 4–1 record and 2.08 ERA in five Championship Series and a 2–1 record and 2.67 ERA in three World Series. "All of his big winning, his pitching in five playoffs and three World Series, came after experimental surgery that saved his career."[49]

John handled television color commentary for the Minnesota Twins, Atlanta Braves, New York Yankees, and ESPN and coached and held front management positions with several minor league teams. The Charlotte, North Carolina, resident promotes Tommy John's Go-Flex joint cream for older athletes, writes a blog for sportable scorecards, educates younger pitchers on taking care of their arms, and serves as a motivational speaker relating his and Travis's dramatic stories.

Since 1974, Tommy John surgery has rescued the careers of hundreds of top athletes. John showed that pitchers could come back from career-threatening surgery. Although sportswriters did not deem his career statistics worthy of National Baseball Hall of Fame consideration, "his ability to endure and come back from adversity again and again when no one gave him a chance, does put him among baseball's all-time elite."[50] His fate rests in the hands of the Veterans Committee now.

John possessed the personal qualities to overcome his traumatic elbow injury and his son's tragic accident. The confident, self-assured competitor exhibited a strong desire to succeed, determination to conquer adversity, and remarkable work ethic. He conceded, "There were times that I thought things wouldn't turn out right. But I never gave up." Dr. Jobe attributed John's recovery to his "great dedication."[51] John, a caring, thoughtful man who places family first, holds strong religious convictions and a deep faith that nothing is impossible with God. Grimsley wrote the classy John "has a deep religious commitment which he shares with his wife, Sally, and he doesn't wear on his sleeve." John wants to be remembered as "a very good pitcher who threw strikes and utilized all of his talents."[52]

# Conclusion: Qualities of Those Who Triumphed Over Adversity

In 1983, Jim Valvano coached North Carolina State to a dramatic 54–52 triumph over the University of Houston for the NCAA basketball title, recording one of the greatest upsets in NCAA Championship history. "His most memorable image is, of course, that of the overjoyed and unrestrained victor, running aimlessly across the court in search of someone to hug in the seconds immediately after the breathtaking conclusion of a thrilling 1983 NCAA title-game victory."[1]

Nine years later, doctors diagnosed Valvano with incurable bone cancer and gave him around a year to live. On February 21, 1993, the tenth anniversary of the dramatic 1983 NCAA title, Valvano told a North Carolina State University audience about his battle with cancer and implored them, "Don't give up. Don't ever give up." Valvano's message resonated with hope, love, and persistence in the battle of and for life.[2]

Valvano delivered a very emotional acceptance speech upon receiving the inaugural Arthur Ashe Courage and Humanitarian Award at the first annual ESPY Awards on March 4, 1993. He encouraged the teary-eyed audience to laugh, think, and cry and announced, with ESPN's support, the formation of the Jimmy V Foundation for Cancer Research, whose motto became "Don't give up. Don't ever give up."[3] Valvano died on April 28 at age 43, but his message of hope, love, and persistence endures.

The 24 athletes profiled in this book heeded Valvano's advice, "Never give up," and represent a resounding triumph of the human spirit over adversity. Each overcame seemingly insurmountable odds to record his or her biggest victory and subsequently attained exceptional athletic accomplishments.

What qualities enabled these athletes to overcome their obstacles and make miraculous comebacks? Fifteen personal qualities distinguished the athletes in their triumphs over adversities. Not all athletes possessed each quality, but a vast majority exhibited many of the 15 qualities. Several of the athletes demonstrated each quality. The fifteen qualities were (1) positive attitude; (2) mental toughness; (3) unyielding passion; (4) competitive drive; (5) courage; (6) strong work ethic; (7) self-discipline; (8) determination; (9) perseverance; (10) confidence; (11) risk-taking; (12) self-critical attitudes; (13) intelligence; (14) resiliency; and (15) spiritual faith.

How did these athletes reflect these various qualities? Although some experienced discouragement at times, the athletes typically possessed a positive attitude and full confidence that they could conquer their medical challenge. Baseball players Jim Abbott and Mordecai Brown did not even consider their adversities stemming from birth or suffered in their childhood as obstacles. Abbott, born with just one hand, became a star high school athlete in three sports, one of the best Big Ten Conference athletes ever, and a major league pitcher, even hurling a no-hitter. Brown, who mangled his right hand in two farm accidents, claimed that pitching with just three fingers gave him an unusual pitch resembling a modern forkball, enhancing his control and effectiveness as a major league pitcher.

Mental toughness epitomized several of the athletes. Tennis player Alice Marble and baseball player Jon Lester notably demonstrated remarkable mental fortitude. Marble, told by doctors that she would never play tennis again after suffering severe anemia, spent two miserable years in a sanitarium. She possessed the mental toughness, however, to recover her tennis skills, stamina, and health, becoming one of the world's greatest singles, doubles, and mixed doubles players. Lester, struck down with non-Hodgkin's lymphoma in the midst of an impressive rookie major league season, exhibited a steely resolve that enabled him to cope with the cancer, restore his pitching strength, return to the Boston Red Sox within a year, and win the clinching game of the 2007 World Series.

Unyielding passion for their sport enabled the athletes to handle their adversities and achieve athletic success. Baseball player Ron Santo and golfer Babe Didrikson Zaharias loved their respective sports so much that they did not let their health issue deter that enthusiasm. Santo, diagnosed with Type 1 diabetes as a teenager, so passionately pursued his baseball dream that he endured the diabetes without letting his teammates or the media know for several years. His enthusiasm for the Chicago Cubs abounded both as a player and as a broadcaster. Zaharias, a superb, all-around athlete, was so driven about returning to competitive golf that she even kept golf clubs in her hospital room to expedite her recovery. The passion motivated her to rejoin the LPGA tournament golf circuit within four months and win several tournaments, including the 1954 U.S. Open.

The athletes demonstrated exceptional competitiveness, the drive to achieve athletic excellence despite facing enormous adversities. Cyclist Greg LeMond and golfer Bobby Jones epitomized the intensity required to attain athletic success. LeMond proved the ultimate competitor after suffering near-fatal gunshot wounds, training rigorously to restore his physical strength and endurance. He fared especially well in the grueling Tour de France, capturing the consecutive titles, and won his second World Road Race. Jones, an intense competitor who miraculously overcame a nearly fatal food disorder as a child, conquered his very fiery temper. He encountered difficulty accepting imperfection and set such high personal standards that he became the era's greatest golfer, reaching the sport's highest pinnacle at age 28 as its only Grand Slam winner.

The 24 stories also are profiles of human courage. Football player Rocky Bleier and track sprinter Wilma Rudolph displayed enormous bravery while overcoming tremendous odds and attained the zenith of their sports. Bleier represented the epitome of courage in rehabilitating from severe leg and foot injuries suffered in South Vietnam and in his heroic struggles to make the Pittsburgh Steelers. The severity of Bleier's injuries would have ended the pro football aspirations of most athletes, but he bravely battled back to achieve pro football stardom and play in four victorious Super Bowls. After wearing braces for several years because of polio, Rudolph valiantly fought back to walk without braces, star in scholastic basketball, become one of the world's best sprinters, and win three Olympic gold medals.

Several figures developed demanding work ethics, which not only helped their rehabilitation, but enabled them to attain athletic excellence. Swimmer Mike Burton, who could no longer participate in contact sports because of a major bicycle accident, exhibited an unprecedented work ethic in practice. He followed coach Sherm Chavoor's rigorous training regimen in practice that required swimming long distances at considerable speed. He always started hard and dared other swimmers to match his pace throughout the race. Golfer Ben Hogan, who suffered near-fatal injuries in a horrendous automobile accident, employed a rigorous work ethic to regain his skills as one of the greatest all-time golfers. He practiced 10 days on the Augusta golf course in 1951 before winning his initial Masters Tournament and captured three of the four major titles in 1953.

Self-discipline also characterized the athletes, most notably swimmers Burton and Gary Hall. Burton revolutionized swimming through enormous self-discipline, implementing Chavoor's arduous swimming regimen in practices to become one of America's greatest long-distance Olympic swimmers. His self-discipline during practices reaped huge dividends, helping him capture three Olympic gold medals. Although a free spirit until being diagnosed with diabetes, Hall became much more disciplined in his life, changed his eating habits, and managed his disease like a scientist. Despite battling depression, he trained more seriously, recorded the fastest times of his swimming career, and won three Olympic gold medals. Hall medaled in all 10 of his Olympic races spanning three Olympics.

Determination abounded in the sagas of the various athletes, who vowed to overcome their adversities regardless of confronting enormous odds. Baseball players Tommy John and Dummy Hoy exhibited extraordinary willpower, focus, and concentration in achieving seemingly insurmountable goals. Doctors gave John just a one percent chance of ever pitching again after the latter tore ligaments in his pitching elbow during his thirteenth major league season. After undergoing risky surgery never performed on a pitcher before, John defied formidable odds by returning to the major leagues an even better hurler than before for thirteen more seasons. Hoy needed to have remarkable concentration on the baseball diamond because of his deafness and helped launch a signal system so he could know when an umpire had called a strike or a ball or notify his fellow outfielders when he was going to catch a fly ball. Tennis player Doris Hart that showed enormous determination, overcoming a crippling leg infection and other physical maladies to win 35 Grand Slam singles, doubles, and mixed doubles titles. Perseverance also enabled the athletes to rebound from their tragedies on the road to athletic success. The inspirational comebacks of baseball player Lou Brissie and football player Bleier illustrate the importance of perseverance in facing personal trials. Brissie, who suffered severe leg injuries in Italy during World War II, persuaded doctors not to amputate his left leg and endured numerous operations to fulfill his dream of becoming a starting pitcher for the Philadelphia Athletics. Bleier, whose leg was shattered in the Vietnam War, underwent an agonizing, strenuous rehabilitation to return to the Pittsburgh Steelers. He became an outstanding blocking back for Franco Harris, playing instrumental roles in four Super Bowl triumphs.

The athletes displayed confidence they would recover from medical adversity to regain athletic success. Cyclist Greg LeMond and basketball player Alonzo Mourning retained assurance that they could overcome personal medical setbacks to reachieve sports glory. LeMond gradually built his confidence following his nearly fatal gunshot wounds, embarking on an intensive training program. He steadily regained his racing form, sufficient physical strength, and endurance, setting the Tour de France record for time trials in 1999 and winning his second and third Tour de Frances. Mourning, who had experienced a very troubled youth, returned to the National Basketball Association after receiving a life-saving kidney transplant and played a valuable supportive role in catapulting the Miami Heat to the 2006 NBA Championship.

Risk-taking often occurred as the athletes continued their athletic endeavors. Boxer Harry Greb and baseball player Abbott proved adventurous spirits, not letting their physical adversities restrict their maneuverability. Greb, already blinded in his right eye in a 1921 boxing match, did not disclose his loss of sight to the media and risked further eye damage by participating in around 90 bouts over the next five years. Greb's risk-taking paid dividends with his winning the light heavyweight and middleweight crowns. Abbott, born with just one hand, remained at risk on the pitcher's mound, vulnerable to sharp line drives that he might not be able to stop. He compensated with very quick reflexes, learning to become an adept fielder.

A self-critical attitude propelled several athletes, notably golfers Jones and Hogan, to reach greater heights. Self-criticism ultimately helped the perfectionist, focused Jones overcome his strident temper and even call a penalty stroke on himself at the 1925 U.S. Open. Jones ultimately became a better golfer by candidly critiquing his own game, capturing 13 major tournaments in eight years and becoming in 1930 the only golfer to record a Grand Slam in the same year. Hogan, the ultimate self-critic, practiced much harder than his contemporaries, driving every ball as far as possible, constantly improving his putting, and correcting his mechanical flaws. He golfed daily into his seventies and possessed an insatiable desire to perfect his game, becoming one of the greatest golfers in the annals of the sport.

The athletes, particularly baseball players Hoy and Brown, possessed the innate intelligence to adapt well to their adversities and convert them into assets. Undeterred by deafness, Hoy developed an effective signal system to communicate with coaches when batting and running the bases and with left fielders and right fielders when playing center field. Hoy's intelligence made him a more complete player as a batter, base runner, and defensive stalwart. Brown, who suffered a mangled right hand in childhood farm accidents, developed a very effective forkball with his three remaining fingers. He utilized his pitching intelligence to become the mainstay of an outstanding Chicago Cubs pitching staff and helped the franchise win its last World Series in its seemingly ill-fated history.

Resiliency enabled the athletes, including track and field decathlete Bill Toomey, wrestler Jeff Blatnick, and basketball star Mourning, to handle their adversities. Toomey displayed remarkable flexibility in coping with his shriveled, partially paralyzed hand from a childhood accident and his shattered kneecap from a motorcycle mishap, competing in the enormously challenging decathlon. He dominated opponents in his strongest events and learned how to use his right hand in the difficult field events, earning an Olympic gold medal in the 1968 decathlon. Blatnick, despite his initial anger at being diagnosed with Hodgkin's disease, adapted well to his changed circumstances and revived his dream of qualifying for the 1984 Greco-Roman Olympic wrestling team. He surpassed that aspiration, becoming the second American to win an Olympic gold medal in Greco-Roman wrestling. Mourning, who titled his autobiography *Resilience*, regained his status as a basketball star after battling with kidney disease and receiving a kidney transplant.

Lastly, several drew upon strong spiritual faith while facing their medical problems. Religious faith especially played instrumental roles in the recoveries of track and field stars Glenn Cunningham and Gail Devers. Cunningham, who was bedridden for two years after the tragic schoolhouse explosion, was inspired by compelling spiritual faith in learning how to walk and run again on the road to becoming a world champion miler and an Olympic silver medalist. He devoted his post-athletic career to helping troubled youth and inspired numerous church and school audiences with his miraculous story. Devers, whose leg was nearly amputated by doctors, found religious faith crucial in battling Graves' disease to become the world's premier hurdler and a three-time Olympic gold medalist.

The athletes, of course, could not have launched their comebacks without the assistance of medical personnel and family. Doctors performed major surgeries on a majority of these athletes, paving the way for their often miraculous comebacks in their respective sports. Caring family support helped the athletes triumph over adversities. The parents of figure skater Scott Hamilton and tennis player Doris Hart provided loving support, enabling the pair to reach their athletic pinnacles. Hamilton's adoptive parents struggled financially so he could train to become a premier figure skater. His mother especially furnished constant emotional support and sacrificed enormously for him before her death from breast cancer. Hart's family proved very supportive in helping her nearly regain normal use of her right leg, moving from St. Louis, Missouri, to Coral Gables, Florida, where she could develop her tennis skills in a warmer climate. Hart's brother, Bud, a knowledgeable tennis player, often lent her valuable advice at tennis tournaments.

Collectively, these athletes not only battled back from major adversities, but typically became exemplary role models outside the athletic arena. Cunningham, Bleier, Blatnick, and Abbott became inspirational motivational speakers, helping others facing similar trials. Santo and Mourning established foundations to help increase public awareness about their diseases and raise financial support for promoting further medical research. Their commitment toward helping others stands out in an age when athletes all too often do not serve as ideal role models.

I hope that these 24 profiles have inspired all readers, especially those who are facing comparable health adversities in your own lives, as much as they would have inspired my older brother and have inspired me. I contracted pneumonia twice as a baby and spent several months in Children's Hospital in Boston. Doctors gave me less than a 10 percent chance of surviving an acute disease that, at that time, was one of the biggest causes of infant and childhood mortality. Through the masterful work of wonderful doctors and nurses, the latest medical technology then available, and the prayers of many wonderful, caring people, I miraculously not only survived that crisis, but am in my eighth decade of what has been a wonderful, productive life.

# Notes

## Preface

1. David L. Porter, *Michael Jordan: A Biography* (Westport, CT: Greenwood, 2007).

## Jeff Blatnick

1. Jeff Blatnick, "If you can win in adversity, you can win anywhere," http://www.jeffblatnick.com/2html-; Lewis H. Carlson and John J. Fogarty, *Tales of Gold* (Chicago: Contemporary, 1987), p. 506.
2. Carlson, *Tales of Gold*, pp. 506, 508.
3. "Interview of Jeff Blatnick," *Opportunities Today* (December 2004), http://www.ihctm.com/OT/December-2004/interview.htm; Carlson, *Tales of Gold*, p. 509.
4. "Interview of Jeff Blatnick"; "AAU Greco-Roman National Championships (1953–1982)," http://www.image.aausports.org/sports/wrestling/.
5. Carlson, *Tales of Gold*, p. 509.
6. Tammy Hine, "Cancer Fails to Dampen Wrestler's Spirit: '84 Gold Medalist Jeff Blatnick Beats Disease, Sets Sights on '88," *Hartford Courant*, November 22, 1986; Steve Springer, "The King Pin," *Los Angeles Times*, August 1, 2004.
7. "AAU Greco-Roman National Championships (1953–1982)"; Springer, "The King Pin."
8. Carlson, *Tales of Gold*, p. 510.
9. Springer, "The King Pin."
10. RPW Staff Writer, "Blatnick has always had his doubters," http://www.intermet wrestle.com/articles/127/; Randy Harvey, "Blatnick Aids Others in Dealing With Fear: Hodgkin's Disease: Olympic champion can tell Lemieux what lies ahead," *Los Angeles Times*, January 18, 1993; Carlson, *Tales of Gold*, pp. 510–511.
11. Carlson, *Tales of Gold*, p. 511; Richard Hoffer, "Jeff Blatnick Is Fighting for His Life Again: Grim Foe Has a New Grip on Gold-Medal Wrestler," *Los Angeles Times*, May 7, 1986.
12. "Awaken the Olympian Within: Stories from America's Greatest Olympic Motivators," http://www99.epinions.com/review/_5014-38824E4-39BC14CB-prodS.
13. NBCOlympics.com history, http://www.2008.nbcolympics.com/wrestling/...newside

120245.html; Springer, "The King Pin"; NBC Olympics.com history.
14. Hine, "Cancer Fails to Dampen Wrestler's Spirit"; Springer, "The King Pin."
15. RPW, "Blatnick has always had his doubters"; "One Happy Dude," *Brandweek* 36 (July 17, 1995), p. 5.
16. Springer, "The King Pin."
17. NBCOlympics.com history; Hine, "Cancer Fails to Dampen Wrestler's Spirit"; Hoffer, "Jeff Blatnick is Fighting for His Life Again."
18. RPW, "Blatnick has always had his doubters"; Los Angeles 84 Foundation, "Official Reports," http://www.la84foundation.org/6oic?OfficialReports/1984v.2.pdf.
19. "Biography — Jeff Blatnick," http://www.hickoksports.com/biograph/blatnick.shtml; Hine, "Cancer Fails to Dampen Wrestler's Spirit"; "1984 Summer Olympics," http://www.databaseolympics.com/gamessport.htm?g:21.
20. "Glory Halleluiah!" *Time* 124 (August 13, 1984); Springer, "The King Pin."
21. Associated Press, "U.S. Olympic Wrestler Jeff Blatnick Says Cancer has Recurred," *Los Angeles Times*, April 5, 1986; William Taaffe, "Bold Strokes on a Big Canvas," *Sports Illustrated* 61 (August 20, 1984); Hoffer, "Jeff Blatnick is Fighting for His Life Again."
22. "Interview of Jeff Blatnick"; Hine, "Cancer Fails to Dampen Wrestler's Spirit."
23. "Glory Halleluiah!" *Time* 124 (August 13, 1984); Jim Koch, "1997 NCAA II Wrestling Hall of Fame Inductees," http://wrestlingusa.com/.../div2halloffame1997.htm/; Carlson, *Tales of Glory*, p. 511; Hine, "Cancer Fails to Dampen Wrestler's Spirit"; Springer, "The King Pin."
24. "One Happy Dude," p. 5; Jeff Blatnick, "If you can win in adversity"; Carlson, *Tales of Glory*, p. 511.
25. Hine, "Cancer Fails to Dampen Wrestler's Spirit."
26. Bob Ottum, "Not At All Pretty, But Almost Perfect," *Sports Illustrated* 61 (August 20, 1984); "1984 Summer Olympics." See "1984 Freestyle Wrestling medal counts," http://www.mcubed.net/oly/summer/years/y1984sfreestylewrestling.shtml.

27. Hoffer, "Jeff Blatnick is Fighting for His Life Again."

28. Hine, "Cancer Fails to Dampen Wrestler's Spirit"; Associated Press, "U.S. Olympic Wrestler"; Hoffer, "Jeff Blatnick is Fighting for His Life Again."

29. "Interview of Jeff Blatnick"; Hoffer, "Jeff Blatnick is Fighting for His Life Again."

30. Hoffer, "Jeff Blatnick is Fighting for His Life Again"; Associated Press, "U.S. Olympic Wrestler"; Hine, "Cancer Fails to Dampen Wrestler's Spirit."

31. Hoffer, "Jeff Blatnick is Fighting for His Life Again."

32. Harvey, "Blatnick Aids Others"; Associated Press, "U.S. Olympic Wrestler"; Randy Harvey, "Blatnick Is Wrestling for His Life. He Has Two Wins That Offset Any Losses on the Mat," *Los Angeles Times*, July 19, 1987.

33. Randy Harvey, "Blatnick Comeback on Hold; Anderson Wins 6 Golds," *Los Angeles Times*, July 17, 1987; Harvey, "Blatnick Is Wrestling for His Life."

34. Harvey, "Blatnick is Wrestling for His Life."

35. United Press International, "Life Remains a Battle for Blatnick," *Los Angeles Times*, August 7, 1988.

36. RPW, "Blatnick has always had his doubters"; "Interview of Jeff Blatnick."

37. Holden Slattery, "Speaker tells Homer students to keep improving," *Cortland Standard*, October 23, 2008. http://cortlandstandard.net/articles/10232008n.html.

38. "Interview of Jeff Blatnick."

39. Mark McGuire, "No Hall for Jeff Blatnick yet (Updated)," July 1, 2009. http://www.blog.timesunion.com/mcguire/no-hall-for-jeff-blatnick-yet/4143/; RPW, "Blatnick has always had his doubters"; "Olympic Gold Medalist Jeff Blatnick Dies at 55," http://espn.go.com/olympics/story/_id/8547815/jeff-blatnick-1984-gold-medal-wrestler-dies.

40. "Interview of Jeff Blatnick"; McGuire, "No Hall for Jeff Blatnick yet."

41. "Jeff Blatnick: Former Olympic Wrestling Great," http://www.brooksinternational.com/Jeff_Blatnick_474/htm; Blatnick, "If you can win in adversity"; Hine, "Cancer Fails to Dampen Wrestler's Spirit."

42. Springer, "The King Pin"; Harvey, "Blatnick Is Wrestling for His Life."

43. Gary Mihoces, "Olympic wrestling gold medalist Jeff Blatnick passes away," http://www.usatoday.com/story/gameon/2012/10/24/olympics-jeff-blatnick-wrestling-cancer-gold-medal-1655393/; Associated Press, "Olympic gold medalist Jeff Blatnick dies," http://wnyt.com/article/stories/s2810721.shtml; USA Wrestling, "1984 Olympic gold medalist Jeff Blatnick dies following complications from heart surgery," http://www.themat.com/sec
tion.ph=section_id=3&page=showarticle*Article ID=25650.

# Jon Lester

1. Peter Richmond, "Jon Lester Is Back in the Game," *Parade* (March 15, 2009).

2. "Jon Lester — Bio," http://www.jockbio.com./Bios/J_Lester/J_Lester_bio.html.

3. Tom Verducci, "Lester's comeback provides a dose of feel-good reality," July 24, 2007 http://sportsillustrated.cnn.com/2007/writers/tomverducci/07/24/redsox.lester/index.html; "Jon Lester — Bio."

4. *2007 Boston Red Sox Media Guide*, pp. 137–138.

5. "Jon Lester — Bio"; *2007 Boston Media Guide*, p. 137.

6. Gordon Edes and Liz Kowalczyk, "Lester diagnosed with cancer," *Boston Globe*, September 2, 2006; Richmond, "Jon Lester."

7. Edes, "Lester diagnosed"; *Boston Globe*, August 25, 2006.

8. "Jon Lester — Bio"; Jim Moore, "Go 2 Guy: Lester went from MLB to cancer ward and back again," *Seattle Post Intelligencer*, February 24, 2007.

9. Edes, "Lester diagnosed"; Verducci, "Lester's comeback."

10. Edes, "Lester diagnosed"; "For the Record," *Sports Illustrated* 105 (September 11, 2006), pp. 22–23.

11. *2007 Boston Media Guide*, p. 137; Ken Davis, "Disease fails to slow Jon Lester's drive to return," *USA Today*, May 15, 2007, pp. 1C-2C.

12. Richmond, "Jon Lester"; Davis, "Disease fails."

13. Davis, "Disease fails"; Edes, "Lester diagnosed."

14. Richmond, "Jon Lester"; Moore, "Go 2 Guy."

15. Richmond, "Jon Lester"; "Jon Lester — Bio"; Davis, "Disease fails."

16. Moore, "Go2 Guy."

17. Davis, "Disease fails."

18. Boston Globe, *So Good! The Incredible Championship Season of the 2007 Red Sox* (Chicago, IL: Triumph Books, 2007), p. 97; Verducci, "Lester's comeback."

19. Jeff Horrigan, "Rally caps work for Sox: Lester's Effort Not For Naught," *Boston Herald*, August 15, 2007.

20. Jeff Horrigan, "Sox pick up Lester: Lefty Scuffles, But Bats, 'Pen Shine," *Boston Herald*, August 22, 2007.

21. *2008 Boston Red Sox Media Guide*; Michael Silverman, "Bullpen opens a 7–11: No Relief for Gagne, Sox as Indians Even Series," *Boston Herald*, October 14, 2007.

22. Michael Silverman, "Masterpiece sends se-

ries back to Hub: Beckett to the Rescue," *Boston Herald*, October 19, 2007.

23. Jeff Horrigan, "How Sweep it is!: Sox scale peak again," *Boston Herald*, October 29, 2007.

24. Horrigan, "How Sweep it is!"; Charlie Doherty, "Profiles in Courage—Jon Lester," November 13, 2009, http://www.suite101.com/content/profileincourage-Jon Lester.

25. Jimmy Golen, "Red Sox's Lester's throws no-hitter," *USA Today*, May 20, 2008, p. 1C; "Series hero Lester throws no-hitter," *Des Moines Register*, May 20, 2008, p. B1.

26. *Baseball America 2009 Almanac* (Durham, NC: Baseball America, 2008), p. 16; Golen, "Red Sox's Lester," p. 1C.

27. *2009 Boston Red Sox Media Guide*.

28. *Boston Herald*, October 2, 2008; *Boston Herald*, October 7, 2008.

29. *Sports Illustrated 2009 Almanac* (New York: Time, Inc., 2008), p. 23.

30. Doherty, "Profiles in Courage."

31. *2010 Boston Red Sox Media Guide*; *Boston Herald*, June 7, 2009.

32. *2010 Boston Red Sox Media Guide*.

33. *Boston Herald*, October 9, 2009.

34. *2011 Boston Red Sox Media Guide*.

35. *Boston Herald*, July 25, 2010; *2011 Boston Red Sox Media Guide*.

36. *2012 Boston Red Sox Media Guide*.

37. Peter Barzilai and Gabe Lacques, "Out-of-control clubhouse set up Red Sox downfall, Globe says," *USA Today*, October 13, 2011, p. 4C; "Lester admits to having 'rally beer' in Red Sox clubhouse," *USA Today*, October 18, 2011, p. 5C.

38. Scott Lauber, "Jon Lester on career-worst season: 'I did what I could,'" http://www. bostonherald.com/blogs/sports/red_sox/index.php/2012/10/02/jon-lester-on-career-worst-season-i-did-what-i-could/; "Red Sox End Dismal Home Campaign," Jon Lester Stats, News, Pictures, Bio, Videos-Boston Red Sox-ESPN, http://espn.go.com/ mlbplayers_/id28487/jon-lester; Dan Dugan, "O my, Jon Lester loses: Baltimore finally beats lefty," September 22, 2012, http://bostonherald.com/sports/baseball/red_sox/view/20220922put _me_in_coach_pedey_still_insists_on_playing.

39. Pat DeCola, "5 Reasons Behind Jon Lester's Shocking 2012 Disappointment," Bleacher Report, August 17, 2012, http://bleacherreport.com/articles/1300987-five-reasons-behind-jon-lesters-shocking-2012-disappointment/; Jen Slothower, "Jon Lester Says John Farrell 'Helped Mold Me Into the Pitcher I Am,' Can Give Him Needed Answers," October 22, 2012, http://www.nesn.com/2012/10/jon-lester-says-john-farrell-helped-mold-me-into-the-pitcher-i-am-can-give-him-needed-answers.html!

40. *Who's Who in Baseball 2013* (New York: Who's Who in Baseball Magazine, 2013), p. 280; "Jon Lester-Bio."

## Babe Didrikson Zaharias

1. Susan E. Cayleff, *Babe: The Life and Legend of Babe Didrikson Zaharias* (Urbana: University of Illinois Press, 1995), p. 218; Jack Newcombe, "The Incomparable Babe Didrikson," *Sport* 14 (December 1959), p. 70.

2. Paul Gallico, "Farewell To The Babe," *Sports Illustrated* 5 (October 8, 1956). For additional information, see Braven Dyer and Frank Finch, "Top Lady Athlete," *Sport* 1 (November 1946), p. 43.

3. Dyer, "Top Lady Athlete," pp. 43–44.

4. Gallico, "Farewell To The Babe." For Didrikson Zaharias's all-around athletic skills, see also Dyer, "Top Lady Athlete," pp. 44–45, 81.

5. Newcombe, "Incomparable Babe Didrikson," pp. 74–75.

6. Don Van Natta Jr., *Wonder Girl: The Magnificent Sporting Life of Babe Didrikson Zaharias* (New York: Little, Brown, 2011), p. 286; Cayleff, *Babe*, p. 204.

7. Van Natta, *Wonder Girl*, p. 287; Cayleff, *Babe*, p. 204.

8. Newcombe, "Incomparable Babe Didrikson," p. 75.

9. Van Natta, *Wonder Girl*, p. 289; Babe Didrikson Zaharias as told to Harry Paxton, *This Life I've Led: My Autobiography* (New York: Dell, 1955), p. 184.

10. Zaharias, *This Life I've Led*, p. 184; Van Natta, *Wonder Girl*, p. 289.

11. Zaharias, *This Life I've Led*, p. 185; Cayleff, *Babe*, p. 205; Van Natta, *Wonder Girl*, p. 290.

12. Zaharias, *This Life I've Led*, pp. 187, 189.

13. Zaharias, *This Life I've Led*, p. 184; Babe Didrikson Zaharias, as told to Booton Herndon, "I'm Not Out of the Rough—Yet," *Cosmopolitan* 135 (October 1953), pp. 79–83; Van Natta, *Wonder Girl*, pp. 293–294.

14. Zaharias, *This Life I've Led*, p. 191; Van Natta, *Wonder Girl*, p. 297.

15. Zaharias, *This Life I've Led*, p. 194; Van Natta, *Wonder Girl*, p. 297.

16. Newcombe, "Incomparable Babe Didrikson," p. 75; Zaharias, *This Life I've Led*, p. 198.

17. Gallico, "Farewell To The Babe"; Van Natta, *Wonder Girl*, p. 295; Cayleff, *Babe*, p. 219.

18. Van Natta, *Wonder Girl*, p. 300; Newcombe, "Incomparable Babe Didrikson," p. 75.

19. Cayleff, *Babe*, pp. 217–218.

20. "The Babe is Back," *Time* 46 (August 10, 1955); Van Natta, *Wonder Girl*, p. 303.

21. Gallico, "Farewell To The Babe"; Van Natta, *Wonder Girl*, p. 303; Newcombe, "Incomparable Babe Didrikson," p. 75.

22. Gallico, "Farewell To The Babe"; Van Natta, *Wonder Girl*, p. 304.

23. Zaharias, *This Life I've Led*, p. 21; Cayleff, *Babe*, p. 226; Van Natta, *Wonder Girl*, pp. 304–305.

24. Zaharias, *This Life I've Led*, p. 205; Van Natta, *Wonder Girl*, p. 305.

25. Cayleff, *Babe*, pp. 224–225; Van Natta, *Wonder Girl*, p. 305.

26. Van Natta, *Wonder Girl*, p. 306; William Oscar Johnson and Nancy P. Williamson, *"Whatta-Gal": The Babe Didrikson Story* (Boston: Little, Brown, 1975), p. 211.

27. Cayleff, *Babe*, p. 226; *New York Times*, February 24, 1954.

28. Cayleff, *Babe*, p. 227.

29. Newcombe, "Incomparable Babe Didrikson," p. 75; Zaharias, *This Life I've Led*, p. 222; Van Natta, *Wonder Girl*, p. 311.

30. Cayleff, *Babe*, p. 227; Zaharias, *This Life I've Led*, p. 209; Nancy Wakeman, *Babe Didrikson Zaharias: Driven to Win* (Minneapolis: Lerner, 2000), p. 99.

31. Newcombe, "Incomparable Babe Didrikson," p. 75; Van Natta, *Wonder Girl*, p. 311; Jim Murray, "The Other Babe," *Los Angeles Times*, 1, 17, BDZ, doc. 11.1.12.18.

32. Zaharias, *This Life I've Led*, p. 210; Van Natta, *Wonder Girl*, p. 312.

33. Van Natta, *Wonder Girl*, p. 314; Cayleff, *Babe*, pp. 239, 230; George Zaharias, "Babe & I," *Look* 20 (December 11, 1956), pp. 92–93.

34. Cayleff, *Babe*, p. 234; Van Natta, *Wonder Girl*, p. 317; Zaharias, *This Life I've Led*, p. 214.

35. Cayleff, *Babe*, p. 231.

36. Gallico, "Farewell To The Babe"; Van Natta, *Wonder Girl*, p. 318.

37. Van Natta, *Wonder Girl*, p. 320; Newcombe, "Incomparable Babe Didrikson," p. 75.

38. Zaharias, *This Life I've Led*, p. 217; Cayleff, *Babe*, p. 234.

39. Zaharias, *This Life I've Led*, pp. 12, 217.

40. Gallico, "Farewell To The Babe"; Van Natta, *Wonder Girl*, p. 326.

41. Cayleff, *Babe*, pp. 238–239, 242; Van Natta, *Wonder Girl*, p. 331.

42. Van Natta, *Wonder Girl*, p. 332; *New York Times*, September 28, 1956, p. 26.

43. For brief summary of her career, see "Mildred Ella Didrikson Zaharias," *The Scribner Encyclopedia of American Lives: Sports Figures*, Vol. 1 (New York: Charles Scribner's Sons, 2002), pp. 231–234. The *1990 Information Please Sports Almanac* (Boston: Houghton Mifflin, 1989) lists her Hall of Fame memberships.

44. Newcombe, "Incomparable Babe Didrikson," p. 51; Gallico, "Farewell To The Babe."

45. Cayleff, *Babe*, pp. 256–257; Van Natta, *Wonder Girl*, p. 326.

46. "Mildred 'Babe' Didrikson Zaharias Courage Award," http://www.asama.org/awards-of-sport/medallion-series/courage/; Cayleff, *Babe*, p. 255.

## Gary Hall Jr.

1. "Gary Hall Jr.," http://www.garyhalljr.com.

2. Johnette Howard, "The Talent Pool," *Sports Illustrated* 84 (April 22, 1996); Jill Lieber, "Hall emerges from darkness," *USA Today*, September 12, 2000, p. 3C.

3. Mike Dodd, "Hall tries to put U.S. back on top in freestyle sprint," *USA Today*, July 25, 1996, p. 8E.

4. Howard, "The Talent Pool."

5. "Gary Hall, Jr. Diabetes Healthcare Consultant," http://www.linkedin.com/pub/gary-hall-jr/11/919/439; Howard, "The Talent Pool."

6. Howard, "The Talent Pool"; Mike Dodd, "Serious Popov wins round one against easygoing rival Hall," *USA Today*, July 23, 1996, p. 3 E.

7. Philip Hersh, "Most Exceptional Games," *1997 Information Please Sports Almanac* (Boston: Houghton Mifflin, 1996), p. 620; Dodd, "Serious Popov," p. 3E.

8. Mike Dodd, "Popov reigns in sprint," *USA Today*, July 26, 1996, p. 3E; Hersh, "Most Exceptional Games," p. 620; *Des Moines Register*, July 27, 1996, p. 1S.

9. "Gary Hall, Jr."

10. Leigh Montville, "Double Take," *Sports Illustrated* 93 (October 2, 2000); Lieber, "Hall emerges," p. 3C.

11. Lieber, "Hall emerges," p. 3C.

12. Karen Allen, "Hall still has the old zip," *USA Today*, August 17, 2000, p. 1C; "Gary Hall, Jr."

13. Lieber, "Hall emerges," p. 3C.

14. Montville, "Double Take."

15. Lieber, "Hall emerges," p. 3C.

16. Lieber, "Hall emerges," p. 3C; "Gary Hall, Jr."

17. Montville, "Double Take."

18. "Hallmark," August 16, 2000, http://www.cnnsi.com.

19. Christine Brennan, "Aussie hero Thorpe provides Olympic lesson with his silver," *USA Today*, September 19, 2000, p. 4E; Montville, "Double Take."

20. Brennan, "Aussie hero Thorpe," p. 4E; http://www/en.wikipedia/org/wiki/GaryHall, Jr.; Montville, "Double Take."

21. Karen Allen, "Dutchman set mark for others to follow," *USA Today*, September 21, 2000, p. 4E; Montville, "Double Take."

22. "Sharing the Gold," *Des Moines Register*, September 23, 2000, p. 46; Karen Allen, "U.S. swim team sets the standard for the future," *USA Today*, September 25, 2000, p. 9E; Montville, "Double Take."

23. *Des Moines Sunday Register*, September 24, 2000, p. 8C; Allen, "U.S. swim team," p. 9E.

24. Kelli Anderson, "Break Out the Bubbly," *Sports Illustrated* 101 (August 30, 2004); Lynn Zin-

ser, "In His Finale, Phelps Takes Away, and Then Gives," *New York Times*, August 21, 2004.

25. Anderson, "Break Out"; Mike Dodd and Vicki Michaels, "Hall: Coach 'made a poor decision,'" *USA Today*, August 20, 2004, p. 6F.

26. Anderson, "Break Out"; Dodd, "Hall," p. 6F.

27. Anderson, "Break Out"; Dodd, "Hall," p. 6F.

28. Zinser, "In His Finale"; Anderson, "Break Out."

29. Zinser, "In His Finale."

30. "Gary Hall, Jr.," *www.linkedin.com*; Zinser, "In His Finale."

## Ron Santo

1. George Von Benko, "Ron Santo: The best NL third sacker of his generation has a legitimate claim to HOF," *Sports Collector's Digest* 24 (August 29, 1997), p. 137; Toni Ginnetti, "Ron Santo a player unlike any other," *Chicago Sun-Times*, December 3, 2010; Fred Katz, "Ron Santo and His Million-Dollar Education," *Sport* 43 (May 1967), pp. 64, 67. For Santo's family background, see Michael G. Glab, "The Slugger," http://www.chicagoreader.com/the-slugger/Content?oid=903469.

2. Glab, "The Slugger"; Von Benko, "Ron Santo," p. 136.

3. Ron Santo, "Ron Santo's Secret on the Field," *Guideposts* (June 2003); Katz, "Ron Santo," p. 64; Ron Santo with Randy Minkoff, *Ron Santo: For Love of Ivy: The Autobiography of Ron Santo* (Chicago: Bonus, 1993), pp. 20, 9–10. See also Glab, "The Slugger."

4. Santo, *Ron Santo*, p. 14; Santo, "Ron Santo's Secret." See also Glab, "The Slugger."

5. Santo, *Ron Santo*, p. 14; Santo, "Ron Santo's Secret."

6. Santo, *Ron Santo*, p. 15.

7. Santo, *Ron Santo*, pp. 16–17; Santo, "Ron Santo's Secret."

8. Jim Brosnan, "Ron Santo Comes of Age," *Sport* 56 (September 1973), p. 71; Ginnetti, "Ron Santo."

9. The Hewitt Interview: Ron Santo, "Positively Focused," *Hewitt magazine online* 9 http://www.hewittassociates.com/Intl/.../magazine/.../interview-hewitt.html.; Santo, Ron Santo, p. 23; Katz, "Ron Santo," p. 67. See also Jeff Santo, This Old Cub, DVD, Sony Pictures Home Entertainment, 2004.

10. Santo, "Ron Santo's Secret"; Santo, *Ron Santo*, p. 27.

11. Van Benko, "Ron Santo," p. 136; Ginnetti, "Ron Santo."

12. Santo, "Ron Santo's Secret"; Santo, *Ron Santo*, pp. 37–38.

13. Santo, *Ron Santo*, pp. 38–40.

14. Santo, "Ron Santo's Secret."

15. Ginnetti, "Ron Santo"; Santo, *Ron Santo*, p. 173.

16. Katz, "Ron Santo," pp. 64–66; Glab, "The Slugger."

17. Glab, "The Slugger"; Brosnan, "Ron Santo Comes of Age," p. 72; Katz, "Ron Santo," p. 64.

18. Brosnan, "Ron Santo Comes of Age," p. 72; Katz, "Ron Santo," p. 68.

19. Brosnan, "Ron Santo Comes of Age," p. 71; Katz, "Ron Santo," p. 68.

20. Santo, "Ron Santo's Secret."

21. Brosnan, "Ron Santo Comes of Age," p. 72; Katz, "Ron Santo," p. 68.

22. Santo, *Ron Santo*, p. 54; Katz, "Ron Santo," p. 68.

23. Santo, *Ron Santo*, p. 56.

24. Katz, "Ron Santo," pp. 63, 68; Von Benko, "Ron Santo," p. 137.

25. Katz, "Ron Santo," p. 68; Santo, *Ron Santo*, p. 59. For Durocher's views on Santo, see Leo Durocher, with Ed Linn, *Nice Guys Finish Last* (New York: Simon and Schuster, 1975), pp. 362–365.

26. Santo, *Ron Santo*, pp. 63–64.

27. Santo, "Ron Santo's Secret"; Santo, *Ron Santo*, p. 61.

28. Santo, "Ron Santo's Secret"; Santo, *Ron Santo*, p. 61.

29. Santo, "Ron Santo's Secret"; Santo, *Ron Santo*, pp. 61–62.

30. Brosnan, "Ron Santo Comes of Age," p. 72.

31. Santo, *Ron Santo*, p. 71; Brosnan, "Ron Santo Comes of Age," p. 72.

32. Santo, *Ron Santo*, pp. 73, 76–78.

33. Brosnan, "Ron Santo Comes of Age," p. 72; Santo, *Ron Santo*, p. 80.

34. Brosnan, "Ron Santo Comes of Age," p. 72.

35. Rick Talley, *The Cubs of '69* (Chicago: Contemporary, 1989); Brosnan, "Ron Santo Comes of Age," p. 72.

36. "Santo Says Young Loses Game," *Chicago Sun-Times*, July 9, 1969; Santo, *Ron Santo*, pp. 96–97.

37. Santo, *Ron Santo*, p. 89; Von Benko, "Ron Santo," p. 137.

38. Santo, *Ron Santo*, pp. 85, 107.

39. Brosnan, "Ron Santo Comes of Age," p. 72.

40. Santo, "Ron Santo's Secret."

41. Ginnetti, "Ron Santo"; The Hewitt Interview: Ron Santo.

42. Katz, "Ron Santo," p. 68.

43. Von Benko, "Ron Santo," p. 136.

44. Ginnetti, "Ron Santo."

45. Glab, "The Slugger"; ESPN Chicago, "Ron Santo, Chicago Cubs announcer, dies at 70," December 3, 2010; Associated Press, "Yes! Yes!: Santo's Hall wish comes to fruition," *Des Moines Register*, December 6, 2011, p. 1C.

46. Bob Nightengale, "After a long, dark winter,

Santo walks in the sunshine," *USA Baseball Weekly*, March 6–12, 2002, p. 5.

47. Ginnetti, "Ron Santo"; Santo, "Ron Santo's Secret."

48. Brosnan, "Ron Santo Comes of Age," p. 71; Santo, "Ron Santo's Secret."

49. Nightengale, "After a long, dark winter," p. 5; ESPN Chicago, "Ron Santo."

50. Ginnetti, "Chicago Cubs great"; Ginnetti, "Ron Santo."

51. "Santo Salute," *USA Today*, August 11, 2011, p. 4C.

52. Associated Press, "Yes! Yes!," *Des Moines Register*, December 6, 2011, p. 4C; Seth Livingstone, "Better late than never for Santo," *USA Today*, December 6, 2011, p. 10C.

53. Associated Press, "Yes! Yes!," *Des Moines Register*, December 6, 2011, p. 4C.

54. Seth Livingstone, "Santo 'always meant to be in Hall of Fame,'" *USA Today Sports Weekly* 10 (December 7–13, 2011), p. 30; Associated Press, "Yes! Yes!," *Des Moines Register,* December 6, 2011, p. 4C.

55. Livingstone, "Better late," *USA Today*, December 6, 2011, p. 10C.

56. Associated Press, "Yes! Yes!," *Des Moines Register*, December 6, 2011, p. 4C; Livingstone, "Santo 'always meant," *USA Today Sports Weekly*, December 7–13, 2011, p. 30.

## Gail Devers

1. Dick Patrick, "Devers never gave up her dream," *USA Today*, August 3, 1992, p. 2A; Kenny Moore, "Gail Force," *Sports Illustrated* 78 (May 10, 1993).

2. Richard Worth, *Gail Devers: Overcoming Adversities* (Philadelphia: Chelsea House, 2001), p. 23; Moore, "Gail Force"; Bill Gutman, *Gail Devers: Overcoming the Odds* (Austin, TX: Raintree Steck-Vaughn Publishers, 1996), p. 11.

3. Gutman, *Devers,* p. 12; Worth, *Devers,* p. 23.

4. Gutman, *Devers,* p. 13; Moore, "Gail Force," pp. 41–43.

5. Worth, *Devers,* p. 28; Kenny Moore, "The Best Is Yet To Come," *Sports Illustrated* 68 (June 6, 1988).

6. Kenny Moore, "Hot Times At The NCAAs," *Sports Illustrated* 68 (June 13, 1988).

7. Gutman, *Devers,* p. 18.

8. Michael Janofsky, "Devers and Christie Get to Dazzle in the Dash," *New York Times,* August 2, 1992, Sect. 8, p. 1; Worth, *Devers,* p. 29; Moore, "Gail Force."

9. Gutman, *Devers,* p. 20; Worth, *Devers,* p. 12; Moore, "Gail Force."

10. Patrick, "Devers never gave up," p. 2A; Worth, *Devers,* pp. 66, 32; Janofsky, "Devers and Christie," p. 1.

11. Gutman, *Devers,* p. 21; Worth, *Devers,* p. 32.

12. Patrick, "Devers never gave up," p. 2A; Worth, *Devers,* p. 67; Gail Devers, "Running for My Life," *Family Circle* 106 (May 18, 1993), pp. 21–23.

13. Kenny Moore, "Dash to Glory," *Sports Illustrated* 77 (August 10, 1992).

14. Gutman, *Devers,* p. 22; Moore, "Gail Force"; Moore, "Dash to Glory."

15. Patrick, "Devers never gave up," p. 2A; Devers, "Running for My Life," pp. 21–23.

16. Gutman, *Devers,* p. 22; Moore, "Dash to Glory"; Janofsky, "Devers and Christie," p. 1.

17. Moore, "Dash to Glory"; *Jet* 82 (August 17, 1992), pp. 51–52.

18. Moore, "Dash to Glory"; Gutman, *Devers,* p. 24; Moore, "Gail Force."

19. Patrick, "Devers never gave up," p. 2A; Worth, *Devers,* p. 68; Moore, "Dash to Glory."

20. Worth, *Devers,* p. 35.

21. Gutman, *Devers,* p. 25; Worth, *Devers,* p. 12.

22. Gutman, *Devers,* pp. 26–27.

23. Devers, "Running," pp. 21–23; Moore, "Dash to Glory."

24. Gutman, *Devers,* pp. 29–30.

25. Moore, "Dash to Glory"; Gutman, *Devers,* p. 8.

26. Janofsky, "Devers and Christie," p. 1; Moore, "Dash to Glory"; Patrick, "Devers never gave up," p. 2A.

27. Gutman, *Devers,* p. 8; Patrick, "Devers never gave up," p. 2A; Janofsky, "Devers and Christie," p. 1.

28. Worth, *Devers,* p. 14; Patrick, "Devers never gave up," p. 2A.

29. Patrick, "Devers never gave up," p. 2A; Gutman, *Devers,* p. 31; Kenny Moore, "Ode to Joy," *Sports Illustrated* 77 (August 17, 1992).

30. Patrick, "Devers never gave up," p. 2A; Moore, "Ode to Joy"; Gutman, *Devers,* p. 32.

31. Moore, "Ode to Joy"; Devers, "Running," pp. 21–23; Moore, "Gail Force."

32. Gutman, *Devers,* p. 32; Worth, *Devers,* pp. 18–19; Janofsky, "Devers and Christie," p. 1.

33. Gutman, *Devers,* p. 36.

34. Moore, "Gail Force"; Worth, *Devers,* p. 58.

35. Gutman, *Devers,* p. 37; "Indoor Dash Queen: World Champion Gail Devers," 46 *Track and Field News* (May 1993).

36. Gutman, *Devers,* p. 38; Ruth Laney, "Controversy Dogs Devers," *Track and Field News* 46 (November 1993), pp. 36–37, 48–49.

37. *New York Times,* August 23, 1993, pp. B9, B13.

38. Gutman, *Devers,* p. 41; James O. Dunaway, "In 100, Devers and Mitchell Are First to the Finish Line," *New York Times,* June 17, 1994; Worth, *Devers,* p. 60.

39. Kenny Moore, "Coming on Strong," *Sports*

*Illustrated* 85 (August 5, 1996); "Fantastic finishes for Bailey, Devers," *Des Moines Sunday Register*, July 28, 1996, p. 1D.

40. Janice Lloyd, "Swede ends Devers' shot at double," *USA Today*, August 1, 1996, p. 1E.

41. "Jones advances, Devers can't finish," *Des Moines Register*, September 28, 2000, p. 5C; Worth, *Devers*, pp. 75, 77.

42. Tim Layden, "Over Life's Hurdles," *Sports Illustrated* 106 (February 12, 2007).

43. Worth, *Devers*, p. 79; Moore, "Gail Force."

44. Worth, *Devers*, pp. 79–80.

45. Devers, "Running," pp. 21–23; Worth, *Devers*, pp. 82–83.

46. USA Track & Field Press Release, "Devers, Greene lead Hall of Fame Class of 2011," November 1, 2011, http://www.usatf.org/News/Devers,-Greene-lead-Hall-of-Fame-Class-of-2011.aspx.

## Alice Marble

1. Alice Marble, *Road to Wimbledon* (New York: Charles Scribner's Sons, 1947), p. 167.

2. "Alice Marble," *The Scribner Encyclopedia of American Lives*, vol. 2 (New York: Charles Scribner's Sons, 1999), p. 603; "Alice Marble," *The Scribner Encyclopedia of American Lives: Sports Figures*, Vol. 2 (New York: Charles Scribner's Sons, 2002), p. 111.

3. "Marble," *SEAL: Sports Figures*, p. 111; Alice Marble with Dale Leatherman, *Courting Danger* (New York: St. Martin's, 1991), pp. 5–6.

4. "Marble," *SEAL*, vol. 2, p. 603.

5. "Marble," *SEAL*, vol. 2, p. 603; Marble, *Courting Danger*, pp. 13–14.

6. "Marble," *SEAL*, vol. 2, p. 604; Marble, *Courting Danger*, pp. 13–14.

7. "Marble," *SEAL: Sports Figures*, p. 112; "Marble," *SEAL*, Vol. 2, p. 604.

8. "Marble," *SEAL*, vol. 2, p. 604; Marble, *Courting Danger*, pp. 17, 20.

9. "Marble," *SEAL*, vol. 2, p. 604; "Marble," *SEAL: Sports Figures*, p. 112.

10. Marble, *Courting Danger*, p. 26.

11. "Marble," *SEAL*, vol. 2, p. 604; "Marble," *SEAL: Sports Figures*, p. 112.

12. Marble, *Courting Danger*, p. 25; Marble, *Road to Wimbledon*, p. 10.

13. Marble, *Courting Danger*, p. 26; Marble, *Road to Wimbledon*, p. 102.

14. Marble, *Courting Danger*, p. 27; Marble, *Road to Wimbledon*, p. 102.

15. Marble, *Courting Danger*, p. 27; Marble, *Road to Wimbledon*, p. 102.

16. Marble, *Road to Wimbledon*, pp. 102–103.

17. Marble, *Courting Danger*, p. 28.

18. Marble, *Road to Wimbledon*, p. 104.

19. Marble, *Courting Danger*, pp. 29–30.

20. Marble, *Road to Wimbledon*, p. 119.

21. Marble, *Road to Wimbledon*, p. 119; Marble, *Courting Danger*, pp. 48–49.

22. "Marble," *SEAL: Sports Figures*, p. 112; Marble, *Road to Wimbledon*, p. 120.

23. Marble, *Courting Danger*, p. 50; Marble, *Road to Wimbledon*, p. 120.

24. Marble, *Courting Danger*, p. 51; Marble, *Road to Wimbledon*, pp. 122–123.

25. "Marble," *SEAL: Sports Figures*, p. 112.

26. "Marble," *SEAL*, vol. 2, p. 604; Marble, *Courting Danger*, p. 57.

27. Marble, *Courting Danger*, pp. 58, 63.

28. "Marble," *SEAL: Sports Figures*, p. 112; Marble, *Courting Danger*, pp. 67–68; Marble, *Road to Wimbledon*, p. 137.

29. Marble, *Courting Danger*, pp. 69, 73; Marble, *Road to Wimbledon*, p. 140.

30. Marble, *Road to Wimbledon*, pp. 144–145.

31. "Marble," *SEAL*, vol. 2, p. 604; Marble, *Road to Wimbledon*, p. 147; Bud Collins and Zander Hollander, eds., *Bud Collins' Tennis encyclopedia* (Detroit: Visible Ink, 1997), p. 593.

32. Marble, *Road to Wimbledon*, p. 155; Marble, *Courting Danger*, p. 89.

33. Marble, *Road to Wimbledon*, p. 156; Collins, *Collins' Tennis Encyclopedia*, p. 593; "Marble," *SEAL: Sports Figures*, p. 112; Marble, *Courting Danger*, pp. 88–89.

34. "Marble," *SEAL: Sports Figures*, p. 112; Collins, *Collins' Tennis Encyclopedia*, pp. 605, 591.

35. Collins, *Collins' Tennis Encyclopedia*, pp. 603, 605.

36. Marble, *Courting Danger*, p. 134.

37. Collins, *Collins' Tennis Encyclopedia*, pp. 591, 593.

38. Marble, *Courting Danger*, pp. 141, 144.

39. Collins, *Collins' Tennis Encyclopedia*, pp. 603, 605; Marble, *Courting Danger*, pp. 147–148; "Marble," *SEAL: Sports Figures*, p. 112.

40. Marble, *Courting Danger*, p. 153.

41. Collins, *Collins' Tennis Encyclopedia*, pp. 591, 593; Marble, *Courting Danger*, p. 155.

42. Collins, *Collins' Tennis Encyclopedia*, pp. 591, 593; "Marble," *SEAL*, vol. 2, p. 604.

43. "Marble," *SEAL: Sports Figures*, p. 113; Marble, *Road to Wimbledon*, p. 167.

44. "Marble," *SEAL*, vol. 2, p. 604.

45. Marble's obituary is in the *New York Times*, December 14, 1990.

46. "Marble," *SEAL: Sports Figures*, p. 111; "Marble," *SEAL*, vol. 2, p. 604.

## Alonzo Mourning

1. Alonzo Mourning with Dan Wetzel, *Resilience: Faith, Focus, Triumph* (New York: Ballantine, 2008); "Alonzo Mourning," *Current Black Biography*, vol. 44 (Detroit: Gale, 2004), p. 125.

2. "Alonzo Mourning," pp. 125–126.

3. *Boy's Life* (January 1989), pp. 26–28.

4. Jack McCallum, "A Season Full of Fight," *Sports Illustrated* 96 (April 1, 2002); Zack Bodendieck et al., eds., *Sporting News Official NBA Register, 2006-07* (St. Louis, MO: The Sporting News, 2006), p. 166.

5. "Alonzo Mourning," p. 126; *Sporting News NBA Register, 2006-07*, p. 166; Alexander Wolff, "Mourning's Glory," *Sports Illustrated* 76 (March 2, 1992), p. 54.

6. "Alonzo Mourning," p. 126; "Alonzo Mourning," http://www.basketball-reference.com/players/m/mournal01.html; Sporting News NBA Register, 2006-07, p. 166; Corrie Anderson et al., eds., *Sporting News Official NBA Guide, 2006-07* (St. Louis, MO: The Sporting News, 2006), p. 110; *New York Times*, May 6, 1993.

7. "Alonzo Mourning," p. 126.

8. McCallum, "A Season Full of Fight"; Jackie McMullan, "Memo to Magic," *Sports Illustrated* 84 (May 13, 1996), p. 19.

9. "Alonzo Mourning," p. 127; McMullan, "Memo to Magic," p. 19.

10. *Sporting News NBA Register, 2006-07*, p. 166; *Sporting News NBA Guide, 2006-07*, p. 407; "Alonzo Mourning," pp. 126–127.

11. "Alonzo Mourning," www.basketball-reference.com; *Sporting News NBA Register, 2006-07*, p. 166.

12. "Alonzo Mourning," www.basketball-reference.com; Craig Carter et al., eds., *Sporting News Official NBA Guide, 2000-2001* (St. Louis, MO: The Sporting News, 2000), pp. 86, 160.

13. Jessie Sholl, "My Life: Alonzo Mourning," http://www.everdayhealth.com/alonzo-mournin.

14. "Alonzo Mourning: NBA star, kidney disease patient and kidney advocate," http://www.davita.com/kidney-disease/motivat; "Mourning & Sean Elliott Talk to BV," http://www.bvwellness.com/…/world-kidney-day-kidney-disease-survivors-alonzo-mourning-and-sea/.

15. "Alonzo Mourning," p. 127; Sholl, "My Life."

16. Sholl, "My Life"; "Alonzo Mourning: NBA star."

17. "Alonzo Mourning: NBA star"; McCallum, "A Season Full of Fight"; "Mourning & Sean Elliott Talk."

18. Sholl, "My Life."

19. McCallum, "A Season Full of Fight."

20. "Alonzo Mourning's All-Star rebound," http://www.men.webmd.com/features/alonzomourning; Sporting News NBA Register, 2006-07, p. 166.

21. McCallum, "A Season Full of Fight."

22. McCallum, "A Season Full of Fight"; "Alonzo Mourning: NBA star"; Craig Carter et al., eds., *Sporting News Official NBA Guide, 2002-2003* (St. Louis, MO: The Sporting News, 2002), p. 80.

23. McCallum, "A Season Full of Fight"; "Alonzo Mourning: NBA Star."

24. "Alonzo Mourning," www.basketball-reference.com; *Sporting News NBA Guide, 2002-2003*, pp. 35, 88, 147.

25. McCallum, "A Season Full of Fight."

26. "Mourning & Sean Elliott Talk."

27. *Sporting News NBA Register, 2006-07*, p. 166; "Retirement necessary after three-year battle," The Associated Press, November 25, 2003.

28. "Alonzo Mourning: NBA star"; "Retirement necessary"; "Doctor: Mourning's labs 'went haywire,'" The Associated Press, November 25, 2003.

29. "Alonzo Mourning," p. 127; "Retirement necessary."

30. "Alonzo Mourning: NBA star"; "Alonzo Mourning's All-Star rebound."

31. Ian Thomsen, "Playstrong," *Sports Illustrated* 103 (December 19, 2005); Ian Thomsen, "Say It Ain't 'Zo," *Sports Illustrated* 101 (November 22, 2004).

32. Thomsen, "Say It Ain't 'Zo."

33. "Alonzo Mourning's All-Star rebound."

34. Thomsen, "Say It Ain't 'Zo."

35. Thomsen, "Say It Ain't 'Zo;" Thomsen, "Playstrong."

36. Thomsen, "Playstrong."

37. *Sporting News NBA Register, 2006-07*, p. 166; "Alonzo Mourning: NBA star."

38. Thomsen, "Playstrong."

39. *Sporting News NBA Guide, 2006-07*, p. 83; Thomsen, "Playstrong."

40. Thomsen, "Playstrong."

41. *Sporting News NBA Register, 2006-07*, p. 166; *Sporting News NBA Guide, 2006-07*, p. 83.

42. Gerry Brown et al., eds., *ESPN Sports Almanac 2008* (New York: ESPN Books, 2007), pp. 363, 367; Sports Illustrated, eds., *Sports Illustrated Sports Almanac 2009* (New York: Sports Illustrated Books, 2008), p. 241; "Heat's Mourning tears knee tendon while playing defense vs. Hawks," http://sports.espn.go.com/nba/news/story?id=3162228.

43. "NBA Heat to Retire Mourning's jersey," http://news.yahoo.com/s/afp/20090301/sp_afp/basketnbaheatmourning_ylt; "Alonzo Mourning," www.basketball-reference.com.

44. Mourning, *Resilience*; "Alonzo Mourning's All-Star rebound."

45. "Alonzo Mourning: NBA star," http://www.charities.com; "Alonzo Mourning's All-Star rebound."

## Wilma Rudolph

1. Wilma Rudolph with Martin Ralbovsky, *Wilma: The Story of Wilma Rudolph* (New York: New American Library, 1977), p. 65; Maureen M. Smith, *Wilma Rudolph: A Biography* (Westport, CT: Greenwood Press, 2006), p. 1.

2. Rudolph, *Wilma*, pp. 17–18.

3. Smith, *Rudolph*, p. 2; Rudolph, *Wilma*, p.

29; David L. Porter, ed., *African-American Sports Greats: A Biographical Dictionary* (Westport, CT: Greenwood Press, 1995), p. 289.

4. Rudolph, *Wilma*, p. 31.

5. *Chicago Tribune*, January 8, 1989; Rudolph, *Wilma*, pp. 31–32, 37.

6. Smith, *Rudolph*, p. 3.

7. Rudolph, *Wilma*, pp. 15, 20.

8. Smith, *Rudolph*, p. 3; Porter, *African-American Sports Greats*, p. 289.

9. Rudolph, *Wilma*, p. 22.

10. Smith, *Rudolph*, p. 4.

11. *Chicago Tribune*, January 8, 1989; Rudolph, *Wilma*, pp. 17, 40.

12. Smith, *Rudolph*, pp. 8–9.

13. Joan Ryan, *Contributions of Women: Sports* (Minneapolis: Dillon, 1956), p. 52.

14. Rudolph, *Wilma*, pp. 62–65.

15. For Temple's training program, see Rudolph, *Wilma*, pp. 67–74.

16. Smith, *Rudolph*, pp. 21, 23; Rudolph, *Wilma*, pp. 76, 79.

17. Rudolph, *Wilma*, pp. 81, 84.

18. Rudolph, *Wilma*, p. 96.

19. Smith, *Rudolph*, p. 37.

20. Rudolph, *Wilma*, p. 98; Dwight Lewis and Susan Thomas, *A Will to Win* (Mt. Juliet, TN: Cumberland, 1983), p. 107.

21. Rudolph, *Wilma*, pp. 98–99; *Chicago Tribune*, January 8, 1989; Anne Janette Johnson, *Great Women in Sports* (Detroit: Visible Ink, 1996), p. 407.

22. Rudolph, *Wilma*, p. 104.

23. Michael D. Davis, *Black American Women in Olympic Track and Field* (Jefferson, NC: McFarland, 1992), p. 114; Smith, *Rudolph*, p. 43.

24. Rudolph, *Wilma*, pp. 110–111, 119.

25. Davis, *Black American Women*, p. 116; Rudolph, *Wilma*, p. 119.

26. Davis, *Black American Women*, p. 117.

27. Davis, *Black American Women*, p. 117; Rudolph, *Wilma*, pp. 121, 124.

28. Rudolph, *Wilma*, pp. 129–130, 132.

29. Rudolph, *Wilma*, pp. 133–135.

30. Rudolph, *Wilma*, p. 135. For overview, see David Maraniss, *Rome 1960: The Summer Olympics that Changed the World* (New York: Simon & Schuster, 2008).

31. Smith, *Rudolph*, p. 58.

32. "The Fastest Female," *Time* 76 (September 19, 1960), pp. 74–75.

33. Lewis, *A Will to Win*, p. 123; Rudolph, *Wilma*, p. 136.

34. Rudolph, *Wilma*, p. 136; Barbara Heilman, "Like Nothing Else in Tennessee," *Sports Illustrated* 13 (November 14, 1960), p. 50.

35. Rudolph, *Wilma*, pp. 139, 143; Smith, *Rudolph*, p. 63.

36. Rudolph, *Wilma*, p. 147; James Murray, "A Big Night for Wilma," *Sports Illustrated* 14 (January 30, 1961), p. 48; Smith, *Rudolph*, pp. 68–69.

37. Smith, *Rudolph*, p. 70; Rudolph, *Wilma*, pp. 151–152.

38. Smith, *Rudolph*, p. 72.

39. Rudolph, *Wilma*, p. 153.

40. Tex Maule, "Whirling Success for the U.S.," *Sports Illustrated* 17 (July 30, 1962), p. 14; Rudolph, *Wilma*, p. 153.

41. Porter, *African American Sports Greats*, p. 290; Smith, *Rudolph*, p. 104. For Rudolph's various activities, see Smith, *Rudolph*, pp. 77–93.

42. Frank Litsky, "Wilma Rudolph, Star of the 1960 Olympics, Dies at 54," *New York Times*, November 19, 1994, p. 53; *Newsday*, October 14, 1990; *Chicago Tribune*, January 8, 1989.

43. Smith, *Rudolph*, p. 104.

44. *Ebony*, February 1984; *Ebony*, January 1992; *Chicago Tribune*, January 8, 1989.

45. Smith, *Rudolph*, p. 101; *Chicago Tribune*, January 8, 1989.

## Scott Hamilton

1. Scott Hamilton with Lorenzo Benet, *Landing It: My Life On and Off the Ice* (New York: Kensington, 1999), p. 312.

2. Bob Ottum, "Wow! Power," *Sports Illustrated* 60 (February 6, 1984); *Washington Post*, January 18, 1984, Sec. D, p. 1.

3. Ottum, "Wow! Power."

4. Ottum, "Wow! Power"; Scott Hamilton, *The Scribner Encyclopedia of American Lives: Sports Figures*, vol. 1 (New York: Charles Scribner's Sons), p. 383.

5. Ottum, "Wow! Power"; "Hamilton," SEAL, p. 383.

6. Hamilton, *Landing It*, pp. 35, 40.

7. Hamilton, *Landing It*, p. 51; *Washington Post*, January 18, 1984, Sec. D, p. 1.

8. Hamilton, *Landing It*, p. 64.

9. Hamilton, *Landing It*, p. 65.

10. Hamilton, *Landing It*, pp. 71–72.

11. Hamilton, *Landing It*, p. 73.

12. *Washington Post*, February 6, 1984, Sec. D, p. 1.

13. Hamilton, *Landing It*, p. 81.

14. Hamilton, *Landing It*, pp. 84–85, 103.

15. Ottum, "Wow! Power"; Hamilton, *Landing It*, pp. 105, 107.

16. Hamilton, *Landing It*, p. 111; Bob Ottum, "Great Scott! What a Doubleheader," *Sports Illustrated* 58 (March 21, 1983).

17. Hamilton, *Landing It*, pp. 125, 128.

18. *Christian Science Monitor*, December 14, 1982.

19. Hamilton, *Landing It*, pp. 139, 149.

20. Ottum, "Great Scott!"; Hamilton, *Landing It*, p. 153.

21. Hamilton, *Landing It*, p. 153; Ottum, "Great Scott!"

22. *New York Times*, March 7, 1983, Sec. C, p. 7; Ottum, "Great Scott!"

23. Ottum, "Wow! Power."

24. Hamilton, *Landing It*, pp. 161–163.

25. Bob Ottum, "Out to Cut Fancy Figures in Sarajevo," *Sports Illustrated* 60 (January 30, 1984); Hamilton, *Landing It*, p. 163; Ottum, "Wow! Power."

26. Bob Ottum, "Notable Triumphs, Wrong Notes," *Sports Illustrated* 60 (February 27, 1984).

27. Ottum, "Notable Triumphs."

28. Ottum, "Notable Triumphs"; Hamilton, *Landing It*, pp. 175–176.

29. Ottum, "Notable Triumphs"; Hamilton, *Landing It*, p. 176.

30. Hamilton, *Landing It*, pp. 177–178.

31. Ottum, "Notable Triumphs"; *Chicago Tribune*, February 17, 1984.

32. Hamilton, *Landing It*, p. 184.

33. *New York Times*, January 16, 1985; "Hamilton," SEAL, p. 384.

34. Hamilton, *Landing It*, pp. 286–305; "Scott Hamilton: Return to the Ice," BIO Channel, March 8, 2010.

35. Hamilton, *Landing It*, pp. 306, 312.

36. Scott Hamilton and Ken Baker, *The Great Eight: How to Be Happy (Even When You Have Every Reason to Be Miserable)* (Nashville: Thomas Nelson, 2008); Jo Ann Schneider Farris, "'The Great Eight' By Olympic Figure Skating Champion Scott Hamilton," http://www.figureskating.about.com/od/figureskatingbooks/p/greateight.htm.

37. *New York Times*, March 7, 1983, Sec. C, p. 7.

## Bobby Jones

1. "Bobby Jones," *Sportscentury*, ESPN, March 12, 1999; Jack Sher, "Bobby Jones Emperor of Golf," *Sport* 7 (August 1949), p. 61; Mark Frost, *The Grand Slam: Bobby Jones, America, and the Story of Golf* (New York: Hyperion, 2004), p. 19.

2. Frost, *The Grand Slam*, p. 19.

3. O.B. Keeler and Grantland Rice, *The Bobby Jones Story* (Atlanta: Tupper & Love, 1953), p. 2.

4. Wells Twombly, *200 Years of Sports in America: A Pageant of a Nation at Play* (New York: McGraw-Hill, 1976), p. 171; Frost, *The Grand Slam*, pp. 19–20.

5. Sher, "Bobby Jones," p. 62; Robert Tyre Jones Jr., *Golf Is My Game* (Garden City, NY: Doubleday, 1960), p. 19.

6. Sidney L. Matthew, *Portrait of a Gentleman: The Life and Times of Bobby Jones* (Chelsea, MI: Sleeping Bear, 1995), p. 8.

7. Matthew, *Portrait*, pp. 10, 14; Jones, *Golf Is My Game*, pp. 84–85.

8. Matthew, *Portrait*, p. 15; Jones, *Golf Is My Game*, pp. 88, 90; Sher, "Bobby Jones," p. 63.

9. Keeler, *Bobby Jones Story*, p. 15; Jones, *Golf Is My Game*, p. 94; Matthew, *Portrait*, pp. 22, 224.

10. Sher, "Bobby Jones," p. 63; Matthew, *Portrait*, p. 21.

11. Sher, "Bobby Jones," p. 63; *New York Times*, December 19, 1971, p. 61.

12. Jones, *Golf Is My Game*, p. 95; Matthew, *Portrait*, pp. 226, 121.

13. Sher, "Bobby Jones," pp. 63–64; Jones, *Golf Is My Game*, p. 96.

14. Sher, "Bobby Jones," p. 64.

15. Jones, *Golf Is My Game*, p. 101.

16. Matthew, *Portrait*, p. 32.

17. Twombly, *200 Years*, p. 171; Matthew, *Portrait*, p. 230.

18. Jones, *Golf Is My Game*, p. 96; *Atlanta Journal*, September 6, 1929.

19. Matthew, *Portrait*, pp. 164, 75. For a comparison with Ben Hogan in the U.S. Opens, see Herbert Warren Wind, "The Age of Hogan," *Sports Illustrated* 2 (June 20, 1955).

20. Matthew, *Portrait*, p. 225.

21. Matthew, *Portrait*, pp. 122, 113, 224.

22. Sher, "Bobby Jones," p. 59; Matthew, *Portrait*, pp. 114–115.

23. Jones, *Golf Is My Game*, pp. 108, 114, 118. For the most detailed account of Jones's remarkable 1930 Grand Slam, see Mark Frost, *The Grand Slam: Bobby Jones, America, and the Story of Golf* (New York: Hyperion, 2004).

24. Sher, "Bobby Jones," p. 65; Jones, *Golf Is My Game*, pp. 128, 131; Matthew, *Portrait*, p. 138.

25. Matthew, *Portrait*, p. 140.

26. Matthew, *Portrait*, pp. 125, 144; Jones, *Golf Is My Game*, pp. 114, 133.

27. Matthew, *Portrait*, p. 145; Jones, *Golf Is My Game*, pp. 136–137.

28. Jones, *Golf Is My Game*, pp. 139, 141; Sher, "Jones," p. 65.

29. Matthew, *Portrait*, p. 152; Jones, *Golf Is My Game*, p. 145.

30. Jones, *Golf Is My Game*, p. 148.

31. Jones, *Golf Is My Game*, pp. 150–151; Sher, "Jones," p. 65.

32. Jones, *Golf Is My Game*, p. 152; Sher, "Jones," p. 65.

33. Jones, *Golf Is My Game*, p. 154.

34. Matthew, *Portrait*, p. 158; Twombly, *200 Years*, p. 174; Jones, *Golf Is My Game*, pp. 156–157.

35. Sher, "Bobby Jones," p. 66; Jones, *Golf Is My Game*, pp. 153, 158.

36. Twombly, *200 Years*, p. 174; Jones, *Golf Is My Game*, p. 158; *New York Times*, September 28, 1930.

37. Keeler, *Bobby Jones Story*, p. 292; Twombly, *200 Years*, p. 170; *New York Times*, September 28, 1930.

38. Jones, *Golf Is My Game*, p. 163; Twombly, *200 Years*, p. 174.

39. Matthew, *Portrait*, p. 199; Jones, *Golf Is My Game*, p. 102.

40. *New York Times*, December 19, 1971, p. 61.

41. Twombly, *200 Years*, p. 170.

42. Twombly, *200 Years*, pp. 170, 174; Jones, *Golf Is My Game*, p. 197.

43. Jones, *Golf Is My Game*, p. 17.

## Doris Hart

1. Doris Hart, *Tennis with Hart* (Philadelphia: J.B. Lippincott, 1956), p. 17; Bud Collins and Zander Hollander, eds., *Bud Collins' Tennis Encyclopedia* (Detroit: Visible Ink, 1997), p. 410.

2. Harry Wismer, "She's a Sweet Hart!," *Sport* 2 (September 1947), p. 32.

3. Hart, *Tennis with Hart*, pp. 12–13.

4. Hart, *Tennis with Hart*, p. 15.

5. Wismer, "Sweet Hart," p. 32; Hart, *Tennis with Hart*, p. 17. Alice Marble, "Lesson in Courage—That's Doris Hart," *American Lawn Tennis* 42 (May 1948), p. 21 lauds Hart's courageous battle.

6. Michelle Kaufman, "Tennis' forgotten past sleeps in South Florida," *Miami Herald*, March 16, 2003; Hart, *Tennis with Hart*, pp. 17–19.

7. Kaufman, "Tennis' forgotten past"; Hart, *Tennis with Hart*, p. 27.

8. Kaufman, "Tennis' forgotten past."

9. Hart, *Tennis with Hart*, p. 20; Kaufman, "Tennis' forgotten past."

10. Wismer, "Sweet Hart," p. 32.

11. Wismer, "Sweet Hart," p. 31; Collins, *Tennis Encyclopedia*, p. 411.

12. Hart, *Tennis with Hart*, p. 35.

13. Wismer, "Sweet Hart," p. 31.

14. Wismer, "Sweet Hart," p. 31; Collins, *Tennis Encyclopedia*, p. 601.

15. Hart, *Tennis with Hart*, pp. 103, 120.

16. "Legendary Tennis Players: 1940's Women Players," http://madeinatlantis.com/tennis/40s_women_tennis_players.htm.

17. Hart, *Tennis with Hart*, p. 166.

18. Hart, *Tennis with Hart*, p. 138; Collins, *Tennis Encyclopedia*, p. 411.

19. Hart, *Tennis with Hart*, pp. 141–142, 145.

20. Andrew Lawrence, "Career Days," *Sports Illustrated* 112 (May 31, 2010).

21. Hart, *Tennis with Hart*, p. 148; Will Grimsley, *Tennis: Its History, People, and Events* (Englewood Cliffs, NJ: Prentice-Hall, 1971), p. 159.

22. Hart, *Tennis with Hart*, pp. 167–168. Connolly, who won nine Grand Slam singles tournaments, defeated Hart in four of those finals. Hart, along with Barbara Scofield, were the only two women to have defeated Connolly in a Grand Slam singles tournament. Hart won her second round match with Connolly at the 1950 U.S. Championships, 6–2, 7–5.

23. Hart, *Tennis with Hart*, p. 180.

24. "The Wonderful World of Sport," *Sports Illustrated* 1 (September 13, 1954); Hart, *Tennis with Hart*, pp. 181–182.

25. Hart, *Tennis with Hart*, pp. 183–184.

26. "Wonderful World of Sport"; "Doris Hart—American Tennis Champion," http://www.all-about-tennis.com/doris-hart.html.

27. Collins, *Tennis Encyclopedia*, p. 603; Hart, *Tennis with Hart*, p. 143.

28. Collins, *Tennis Encyclopedia*, pp. 143, 145, 591, 615.

29. Collins, *Tennis Encyclopedia*, pp. 593, 604, 609, 615; Hart, *Tennis with Hart*, p. 144.

30. Collins, *Tennis Encyclopedia*, pp. 593, 604; Hart, *Tennis with Hart*, p. 189.

31. Hart, *Tennis with Hart*, p. 144.

32. Kaufman, "Tennis' forgotten past"; Collins, *Tennis Encyclopedia*, p. 411.

33. Kaufman, "Tennis' forgotten past"; "Doris Hart—American Tennis Champion"; Collins, *Tennis Encyclopedia*, p. 411.

34. Collins, *Tennis Encyclopedia*, pp. 411–412, 631–633; Kaufman, "Tennis' forgotten past."

35. Kaufman, "Tennis' forgotten past"; "Doris Hart," http://www.tennisfame.com/hall-of-famers/doris-hart."

36. "The 50 Greatest Florida Sports Figures," *Sports Illustrated* 91 (December 27, 1999); Hart, *Tennis with Hart*, p. 184.

## Jim Abbott

1. Lee Jenkins, "Jim Abbott: One-Handed Wonder," *Sports Illustrated* 109 (July 14, 2008), p. 104.

2. Hank Hersch, "That Great Abbott Switch," *Sports Illustrated* 66 (May 25, 1987); Hank Hersch, "Ace of the Angels," *Sports Illustrated* 75 (September 9, 1991). For Abbott's childhood, see Jim Abbott and Tim Brown, *Imperfect: An Improbable Life* (New York: Ballantine, 2012), pp. 47–69, and Bob Bernotas, *Nothing to Prove: The Jim Abbott Story* (New York: Kodansha International, 1995).

3. Johnette Howard, "All I Ever Wanted Was A Shot," *Sport* 80 (March 1989), p. 28; *New York Times*, December 25, 1992.

4. Howard, "All I Ever Wanted," p. 28; *New York Times*, December 25, 1992.

5. Hersch, "That Great Abbott Switch."

6. "Dreaming the Big Dreams," *Time* 133 (March 20, 1989), p. 78; Hersch, "That Great Abbott Switch."

7. Bob Hertzel, "A Real Jim Dandy," *Beckett Baseball Monthly* 10 (June 1993), p. 6; Hersch, "That Great Abbott Switch."

8. Hersch, "That Great Abbott Switch"; Howard, "All I Ever Wanted," p. 289.

9. Hersch, "That Great Abbott Switch." For

Abbott's high school years, see Abbott, *Imperfect*, pp. 73–100.

10. Hersch, "That Great Abbott Switch"; Bill James, *The Baseball Book 1990* (New York: Villard, 1990), p. 169.

11. Howard, "All I Ever Wanted," p. 27; Hersch, "That Great Abbott Switch." For Abbott's University of Michigan experience, see Abbott, *Imperfect*, pp. 118–123, 139.

12. Hersch, "That Great Abbott Switch"; "Jim Abbott," *Current Biography Yearbook 1995* (New York: H.W. Wilson, 1995), p. 2.

13. Howard, "All I Ever Wanted," p. 29.

14. Howard, "All I Ever Wanted," pp. 29, 27.

15. James, *The Baseball Book 1990*, p. 169; Howard, "All I Ever Wanted," p. 29.

16. James, *The Baseball Book 1990*, p. 169; Bruce Anderson, "Angel on the Ascent," *Sports Illustrated* 70 (March 13, 1989), p. 64. For Abbott's Olympic experience, see Abbott, *Imperfect*, pp. 143–153.

17. Anderson, "Angel on the Ascent"; "Dreaming Big Dreams," *Time* 133 (March 20, 1989), p. 78.

18. Rob Brofman, "One for the Angels," *Life* 121 (June 1989), p. 118.

19. Hersch, "Ace of the Angels."

20. Hertzel, "Real Jim Dandy," p. 8; *New York Times*, December 25, 1992.

21. *New York Times*, December 25, 8, 1992.

22. "Jim Abbott," *Current Biography*, 1995, p. 3.

23. Tom Verducci, "A Special Delivery," *Sports Illustrated* 79 (September 13, 1993), pp. 62–63. For Abbott's recollections of each inning of his no-hitter, see Abbott, *Imperfect*, pp. 20–23, 43–46, 70–72, 101–104, 131–133, 158–160, 188–192, 225–228, 256–268.

24. "Yankees' Abbott pitches no-hitter," *Des Moines Sunday Register*, September 5, 1993, p. 1S; Verducci, "Special Delivery," pp. 62–63.

25. *Chicago Tribune*, August 14, 1995.

26. Jack McCallum and Richard O'Brien, "Back in the Game," *Sports Illustrated* 89 (October 5, 1998), p. 35.

27. *The Sporting News Baseball Register 2000 Edition* (St. Louis, MO: The Sporting News, 2000), p. 4.

28. *New York Times*, December 25, 1992; Steve Marantz, "Courage is so much more than playing baseball with one hand," *The Sporting News*, 216 (July 19, 1993), pp. 12–15.

29. Jenkins, "Abbott," p. 103; Brofman, "One for the Angels," p. 118.

30. Jenkins, "Abbott," p. 104; Hertzel, "Real Jim Dandy," p. 8.

31. Abbott, *Imperfect*; Anna Clark, "Former Wolverine, Flint native Jim Abbott's new memoir a candid look at life in baseball," *Detroit Free Press*, April 29, 2012, in http://www.freep.com/article/20220429/FEATURES05/204290391/Former...k-at-life-in-baseball?odyssey=tab%7Cmostpopular%7text%7CFEATURES.

32. Hersch, "Ace of the Angels."

## Dummy Hoy

1. Jonathan Stilwell, "William 'Dummy' Hoy: Proving It Could Be Done," *Bleacher Report*, August 29, 2009.

2. Ralph Berger, "Dummy Hoy," http://www.deafbiography.com/biography/EllsworthHoy.htm; Stephen Jay Gould, Triumph and Tragedy in Mudville: A Lifelong Passion for Baseball (New York: W.W. Norton, 2003), p. 115.

3. Art Kruger, "He Made the Umpires Raise Their Hands: Dummy Hoy," *Baseball Digest* 13 (May 1954), pp. 50–54; Gould, *Triumph and Tragedy*, p. 115.

4. Gould, *Triumph and Tragedy*, p. 116; Berger, "Dummy Hoy."

5. Stilwell, "William 'Dummy' Hoy."

6. Steve Sandy and Richard Miller, "No Dummy: William Ellsworth Hoy," Ohio Historical Society *Timeline* (March-April 2000), p. 49; Gould, *Triumph and Tragedy*, pp. 116, 123.

7. Sandy, "No Dummy," p. 49; "A Brief Overview of Hoy's Career," http://www.dummyhoy.com/bio.htm.

8. Sandy, "No Dummy," p. 49. Stilwell, "William 'Dummy' Hoy"; Bob Brigham, "Dummy Hoy: Forgotten gem on the diamond," *Sports Collectors Digest* 21 (January 14, 1994), p. 40 details the dramatic difference that signals made for Hoy.

9. Gould, *Triumph and Tragedy*, pp. 123–124.

10. Stilwell, "William 'Dummy' Hoy"; Berger, "Dummy Hoy."

11. Berger, "Dummy Hoy."

12. Gould, *Triumph and Tragedy*, pp. 125, 117.

13. "A Brief Overview of Hoy's Career."

14. Gould, *Triumph and Tragedy*, pp. 117–118.

15. Stilwell, "William 'Dummy' Hoy"; Ken Haag, "The silent world of William 'Dummy' Hoy," *Sports Collectors Digest* 21 (January 14, 1994), p. 40. For Hoy's career batting statistics, see Robert L. Tiemann and Mark Rucker, eds., *Nineteenth Century Stars* (Kansas City, MO: Society for American Baseball Research, 1989), p. 64.

16. "A Brief Overview of Hoy's Career"; Gould, *Triumph and Tragedy*, p. 124; Haag, "silent world," p. 40.

17. "Dummy Hoy," http://www.en.wikipedia.org/wiki/Dummy_Hoy.

18. Gould, *Triumph and Tragedy*, p. 124.

19. Lawrence S. Ritter, *The Glory of Their Times* (New York: Macmillan, 1966), pp. 23, 53–54.

20. Stilwell, "William 'Dummy' Hoy."

21. Sandy, "No Dummy," p. 51; Stilwell, "William 'Dummy' Hoy"; Berger, "Dummy Hoy"; "A

capsule biography," http://www.dummyhoy.com/bio.htm.

22. Stilwell, "William 'Dummy' Hoy"; "A Brief Overview of Hoy's Career"; "A capsule biography."

23. "A capsule biography"; Sandy, "No Dummy," p. 51.

24. Sandy, "No Dummy," p. 51; "A Brief Overview of Hoy's Career"; Berger, "Dummy Hoy."

25. "A Brief Overview of Hoy's Career"; Haag, "silent world," p. 40; Stilwell, "William 'Dummy' Hoy"; "Dummy Hoy," en.wikipedia.org.

26. Sandy, "No Dummy," p. 48; Kruger, "He Made the Umpires," pp. 50–54.

27. Dan Krueckeberg, "Take-Charge Cy," *The National Pastime* 4 (Spring 1985), pp. 7–8; "A capsule biography."

28. Berger, "Dummy Hoy"; "A Brief Overview of Hoy's Career"; Brigham, "Dummy Hoy," p. 40.

29. "A Brief Overview of Hoy's Career"; Berger, "Dummy Hoy"; Stilwell, "William 'Dummy' Hoy."

30. Gould, *Triumph and Tragedy*, pp. 122, 128–129.

31. Berger, "Dummy Hoy"; Brigham, "Dummy Hoy," p. 40.

32. Stilwell, "William 'Dummy' Hoy"; Gould, *Triumph and Tragedy*, p. 114.

## Harry Greb

1. Billy Paxton, *The Fearless Harry Greb: Biography of a Tragic Hero of Boxing* (Jefferson, NC: McFarland, 2009), pp. 189–190; Nat Fleischer and Sam Andre, *A Pictorial History of Boxing* (New York: Citadel, 1959), p. 193. See also James R. Fair, *Give Him to the Angels: The Story of Harry Greb* (New York: Smith & Durrell, 1945). Some sources erroneously claim that Greb's last name was Berg. In a 1954 article, *Boxing and Wrestling Magazine* produced Greb's birth certificate clearly showing his last name had always been Greb. "Harry Greb or Harry Berg," *Boxing and Wrestling Magazine* 4 (February 1954).

2. Bert Randolph Sugar and the Editors of *Ring* magazine, *The Great Fights* (New York: Gallery, 1984), p. 55; Fleischer, *Pictorial History*, p. 164.

3. Paxton, *Harry Greb*, p. 36.

4. Jack Cavanaugh, *Tunney: Boxing's Brainiest Champ and His Upset of the Great Jack Dempsey* (New York: Random House, 2006), p. 174.

5. Paxton, *Harry Greb*, p. 96; *Pittsburgh Post*, August 30, 1921.

6. *New York Times*, October 27, 1926.

7. Paxton, *Harry Greb*, p. 101.

8. Paxton, *Harry Greb*, pp. 103, 106, 108, 121.

9. *Pittsburgh Press*, March 22, 1922; *Chicago Daily Tribune*, March 14, 1922.

10. Sugar, *Great Fights*, p. 55.

11. Paxton, *Harry Greb*, pp. 119, 121; Sugar, *Great Fights*, p. 55.

12. Paxton, *Harry Greb*, pp. 122–123; Sugar, *Great Fights*, p. 55.

13. Paxton, *Harry Greb*, pp. 125–126, 196.

14. Sugar, *Great Fights*, pp. 56–57.

15. *New York Times*, February 24, 1923; Sugar, *Great Fights*, p. 57.

16. Sugar, *Great Fights*, p. 57; *Pittsburgh Post*, February 25, 1923; *New York Times*, February 25, 1923.

17. Fleischer, *Pictorial History*, p. 164.

18. Paxton, *Harry Greb*, pp. 131, 139.

19. Paxton, *Harry Greb*, p. 140; *Chicago Tribune*, September 16, 1923; *New York Times*, September 2, 1923.

20. *Pittsburgh Post*, December 4, 1923.

21. Paxton, *Harry Greb*, p. 147; *Pittsburgh Post*, January 19, 1924.

22. Paxton, *Harry Greb*, p. 149; *Pittsburgh Post*, March 25, 1924.

23. Gilbert Odd, "Tough-guy Ted took on Greb the Great," *Boxing News*, July 28, 1989.

24. *Pittsburgh Press*, July 3, 1925; *Pittsburgh Post*, July 3, 1925.

25. *Chicago Daily Tribune*, August 21, 1925.

26. *Pittsburgh Post*, February 27, 28, 1926; Paxton, *Harry Greb*, p. 204.

27. Paxton, *Harry Greb*, p. 210; *Pittsburgh Post*, August 20, 1926.

28. *New York Times*, June 16, 1926; Paxton, *Harry Greb*, p. 210.

29. Grantland Rice, "King of All the Marvels," *Collier's* 77 (February 20, 1926).

30. *Washington Post*, October 24, 1926.

31. *New York Times*, October 27, 1926; Paxton, *Harry Greb*, p. 214.

## Glenn Cunningham

1. Glenn Cunningham with George X. Sand, *Never Quit* (Lincoln, VA: Chosen, 1981), pp. 29, 32. For the explosion, see also Paul J. Kiell, *American Miler: The Life and Times of Glenn Cunningham* (Halcottsville, NY: Breakaway, 2006), pp. 29–36; Darryl Hicks, 1981 Interview with Glenn Cunningham, http://www.mybestyears.com/InterviewSpotlights/CUNNINGHAMGlenn080409.html; Vernon Pizer, "The Man With 8000 Miracles," The Rotarian 108 (February 1966), p. 113, and Edwin V. Burkholder, "Glenn Cunningham and the Four-Minute Mile," Sport 8 (March 1950), p. 63.

2. Cunningham, *Never Quit*, p. 31.

3. "Glenn Cunningham," *Scribner Encyclopedia of American Lives: Sports Figures*, vol. 1 (New York: Charles Scribner's Sons, 2002), p. 206; Hicks 1981 Interview with Cunningham.

4. Cunningham, *Never Quit*, p. 36; Hicks 1981 Interview with Cunningham.

5. Cunningham, *Never Quit*, pp. 44, 46–47. For Floyd's condition, see Kiell, *American Miler*,

pp. 37–44. For Glenn's reaction, see also Hicks 1981 Interview with Cunningham.

6. Pizer, "The Man With 8000 Miracles," p. 113; Cunningham, *Never Quit*, p. 48. For Glenn's painful recovery, see Kiell, *American Miler*, pp. 45–58.

7. Pizer, "The Man With 8000 Miracles," pp. 113–114.

8. Cunningham, *Never Quit*, p. 53.

9. Cunningham, *Never Quit*, pp. 55–56.

10. Cunningham, *Never Quit*, p. 57; *Tri-State News* (Elkhart, KS), March 17, 1988.

11. Isaiah 40:31; Pizer, "The Man With 8000 Miracles," p. 114.

12. Cunningham, *Never Quit*, pp. 61–62, 65.

13. Pizer, "The Man With 8000 Miracles," p. 114; Burkholder, "Glenn Cunningham," p. 63.

14. Cunningham, *Never Quit*, p. 78. Glenn is referred to as Cunningham hereafter.

15. Cunningham, *Never Quit*, p. 82; Burkholder, "Glenn Cunningham," p. 63.

16. Burkholder, "Glenn Cunningham," p. 64; Cunningham, *Never Quit*, pp. 86, 89. For the race, see Kiell, *American Miler*, pp. 85–92, and Hicks 1981 Interview with Cunningham.

17. Burkholder, "Glenn Cunningham," p. 64.

18. Cunningham, *Never Quit*, p. 95.

19. http://www.answers.com/topic/glenn-cun ningham. For Cunningham's career as a runner, see Don Holst and Marcia S. Popp, *American Men of Olympic Track and Field: Interviews with Athletes and Coaches* (Jefferson, NC: McFarland, 2005), pp. 19–34.

20. Cunningham, *Never Quit*, p. 104; Hicks 1981 Interview with Cunningham; David L. Porter, ed., *Biographical Dictionary of American Sports: Outdoor Sports* (Westport, CT: Greenwood, 1988), pp. 445–446. For Glenn's interscholastic track career, see Kiell, *American Miler*, pp. 99–126.

21. Cunningham, *Never Quit*, pp. 114, 116, 119.

22. www.answers.com/cunningham; Cordner Nelson and Roberto Quercetani, *The Milers* (Los Altos, CA: Tafnews Press, 1985).

23. www.answers.com/cunningham; Nelson, *The Milers*.

24. Nelson, *The Milers*.

25. www.answers.com/cunningham.

26. Cunningham, *Never Quit*, pp. 121–123; Barry J. Hugman and Peter Arnold, *The Olympic Games: Complete Track and Field Results 1896–1988* (New York: Facts on File, 1988), pp. 119–120.

27. Cunningham, *Never Quit*, pp. 124–125; Nelson, *The Milers*.

28. Nelson, *The Milers*; www.answers.com/cun ningham.

29. Burkholder, "Glenn Cunningham," p. 64.

30. *Kansas City Times*, March 12, 1938; Burkholder, "Glenn Cunningham," p. 64; Pizer, "The Man with 8000 Miracles," p. 114.

31. *New York Times*, March 6, 1938; Burkholder, "Glenn Cunningham," p. 64; *Kansas City Times*, March 12, 1938.

32. *New York Times*, March 13, 1938.

33. Nelson, *The Milers*; www.answers.com/cun ningham.

34. www.answers.com/cunningham.

35. Porter, *BDAS*, p. 446, Pizer, "The Man With 8000 Miracles," pp. 112–116, and Ken West, "Unforgettable Glenn Cunningham," *Reader's Digest* (1988), pp. 126–130, describe Cunningham's impact on youth at his Cedar Ranch.

## Bill Toomey

1. Sam David International Management, "Bill Toomey," http://www.samdavid international.com/bill_toomey.

2. Christopher Hosford, "30 Years of Progress for the Ultimate 10-Event Man," *Life Extension Magazine* 4 (September 1998); Holst, *American Men*, p. 131.

3. Holst, *American Men*, p. 132; David, "Bill Toomey"; Hosford, "30 Years of Progress"; John Underwood, "Best-kept secrets," *Sports Illustrated* 27 (June 12, 1967).

4. "Bill Toomey: Track and Field," http://www. cubuffs.com/ViewArticle.dbm/%3FDB; Underwood, "Best-kept secrets."

5. "Bill Toomey: Track and Field"; Hosford, "30 Years of Progress."

6. Associated Press, *The Olympic Story: Pursuit of Excellence* (Danbury, CT: Grolier, 1979), p. 287.

7. Underwood, "Best-kept secrets"; Associated Press, *The Olympic Story*, p. 287.

8. Hosford, "30 Years of Progress."

9. Holst, *American Men*, pp. 133–134.

10. Hosford, "30 Years of Progress"; Associated Press, *The Olympic Story*, p. 287.

11. David, "Bill Toomey."

12. Underwood, "Best-kept secrets."

13. David, "Bill Toomey."

14. Holst, *American Men*, p. 133.

15. Underwood, "Best-kept secrets"; David, "Bill Toomey."

16. Underwood, "Best-kept secrets"; David, "Bill Toomey."

17. Holst, *American Men*, p. 132.

18. Cordner Nelson, *Track's Greatest Champions* (Los Altos, CA: Tafnews, 1986), p. 375; Underwood, "Best-kept secrets"; "Bill Toomey: Track and Field."

19. Underwood, "Best-kept secrets."

20. David, "Bill Toomey"; Associated Press, *The Olympic Story*, p. 287.

21. Holst, *American Men*, p. 132; Nelson, *Track's Greatest Champions*, p. 375.

22. "Bill Toomey," USA Track & Field, http// www.usatf.org/halloffame/TF/showBio.a...; John

Underwood, "The Long Long Jump," *Sports Illustrated* 30 (October 28, 1968); David, "Bill Toomey."

23. Associated Press, *The Olympic Story*, p. 287.

24. Associated Press, *The Olympic Story*, p. 287; Underwood, "The Long Long Jump."

25. David, "Bill Toomey"; Howard Cosell and Mickey Herskowitz, *Cosell* (New York: Playboy Press, 1973); Underwood, "The Long Long Jump."

26. Holst, *American Men*, p. 134; Hugman, *The Olympic Games*, p. 248, 255.

27. Nelson, *Track's Greatest Champions*, p. 375; Underwood, "The Long Long Jump"; Hosford, "30 Years of Progress."

28. "Bill Toomey: Track and Field"; "Parade to the Pedestal," *Time* 92 (November 1, 1968).

29. Nelson, *Track's Greatest Champions*, p. 375; Holst, *American Men*, p. 128–129.

30. William F. Reed, "The Ineligible Married Man," *Sports Illustrated* 35 (April 12, 1971); Holst, *American Men*, p. 131.

31. Reed, "The Ineligible Married Man."

32. Reed, "The Ineligible Married Man."

33. Brian Hewitt, "On Track With Bill Toomey: '68 Decathlon Champ Has a Lot on His Mind," *Los Angeles Times*, June 18, 1989.

34. Reed, "The Ineligible Married Man."

35. Reed, "The Ineligible Married Man."

36. Holst, *American Men*, pp. 128–129; David, "Bill Toomey."

37. David, "Bill Toomey"; Bill Toomey and Barry King, *The Olympic Challenge, 1988* (Costa Mesa, CA: Hdl Publishing Company, 1988); Holst, *American Men*, p. 128.

38. David, "Bill Toomey."

39. Holst, *American Men*, p. 129.

40. Hosford, "30 Years of Progress"; "Bill Toomey pleads no contest to DUI," Associated Press News Release, March 26, 2008.

## Three-Finger Brown

1. Mordecai Brown, *How to Pitch Curves* (Chicago: W.D. Boyce, 1913); Cindy Thomson and Scott Brown, *Three-Finger: The Mordecai Brown Story* (Lincoln: University of Nebraska Press, 2006), pp. 7, 11.

2. Terre Haute *Indiana Spectator*, July 21, 1979; Thomson, *Three-Finger*, pp.11–12.

3. Thomson, *Three-Finger*, pp. 11–12.

4. Terre Haute *Indiana Spectator*, July 21, 1979; Thomson, *Three-Finger*, pp. 13, 17; *Terre Haute Tribune*, April 17, 1919.

5. Lee Allen, *The National League Story* (New York: Hill & Wang, 1965), p. 111.

6. Thomson, *Three-Finger*, p. 19; Lowell Reidenbaugh, *Baseball's Hall of Fame: Cooperstown, Where the Legends Live Forever*, rev. ed. (New York: Crescent, 1997), p. 34.

7. Terre Haute *Indiana Spectator*, July 21, 1979; "Mordecai Brown," *Baseball Magazine* 12 (July 1911); Joseph Bennett, "Three-Finger Brown: A Lamb without Blemish," *Philalethes* 52 (June 1998).

8. Thomson, *Three-Finger*, p. 25.

9. *Chicago Tribune*, December 18, 1903; Brown, *How to Pitch Curves*.

10. Thomson, *Three-Finger*, p. 31.

11. *Chicago Tribune*, June 14, 1905.

12. Lee Allen, *The World Series* (New York: G.P. Putnam's Sons, 1969), p. 58; Allen, *National League Story*, p. 111; Hugh S. Fullerton, "The Spring Training: How the Baseball Players Get into Condition," *American Magazine* 23 (April 1910), pp. 783–784; *Chicago Tribune*, July 5, 1906; Thomson, *Three-Finger*, p. 40.

13. *Chicago Tribune*, October 10, 1906.

14. Thomson, *Three-Finger*, p. 43; Larry Burke, *The Baseball Chronicles: A Decade-by-Decade History of the All-American Pastime* (New York: Smithmark, 1995).

15. Frederick G. Lieb, *The Story of the World Series*, rev. ed. (New York: G.P. Putnam's Sons, 1965), pp. 46, 48; Allen, *World Series*, p. 60.

16. Lieb, *Story*, pp. 49–50; Thomson, *Three-Finger*, p. 46.

17. Derek Gentile, *The Complete Chicago Cubs: The Total Encyclopedia of the Team* (New York: Black Dog & Leventhal, 2002), p. 441; Thomson, *Three-Finger*, p. 50.

18. *Chicago Tribune*, September 23, 1908; *New York World*, September 23, 1908.

19. *Chicago Tribune*, October 5, 1908.

20. Thomson, *Three-Finger*, p. 3; Charles C. Alexander, *John McGraw* (Lincoln: University of Nebraska Press, 1988), p. 136; John P. Carmichael, *My Greatest Day in Baseball* (New York: Grosset & Dunlap, 1951), pp. 23–24.

21. Thomson, *Three-Finger*, p. 72; Carmichael, *My Greatest Day*, p. 27.

22. Alexander, *McGraw*, p. 138; Carmichael, *My Greatest Day*, p. 28.

23. Thomson, *Three-Finger*, p. 76; G.H. Fleming, *The Unforgettable Season* (New York: Holt, Rinehart, and Winston, 1981), p. 315.

24. Terre Haute *Indiana Spectator*, July 21, 1979; John J. Evers and Hugh S. Fullerton, *Touching Second: The Science of Baseball* (Chicago: Reilly & Britton, 1910), pp. 257–258.

25. Thomson, *Three-Finger*, p. 51; Lieb, *Story*, p. 60.

26. *Chicago Tribune*, June 2, 9, 1909.

27. Lieb, *Story*, p. 73.

28. *Chicago Tribune*, October 23, 1910.

29. Lieb, *Story*, p. 75; *The Sporting News*, October 27, 1910; Thomson, *Three-Finger*, p. 109.

30. Thomson, *Three-Finger*, p. 122.

31. *New York Times*, July 16, 1913.

32. Harold Seymour, *Baseball: The Golden Age*

(New York: Oxford University Press, 1971), p. 206; *Chicago Tribune*, June 9, 1914.

33. Thomson, *Three-Finger*, pp. 143, 145.
34. Thomson, *Three-Finger*, p. 164.
35. Allen, *National League*, p. 111.
36. Thomson, *Three-Finger*, pp. 173–174, 189.
37. *New York Times*, May 6, 1949; *The Sporting News*, February 13, 1952.

## Mike Burton

1. Randy Peterson, "Accident propelled Burton to Olympic swim gold," *Des Moines Register*, April 15, 1984, pp. 1D, 3D.
2. "Countdown to the Trials," http://www.bt aquatics.org/olympic_trials updates.htm, Peterson, "Accident," pp. 1D, 3D.
3. "Countdown to the Trials"; "Sherm Chavoor, 73, A Swimming Coach," *New York Times*, September 5, 1992. For his impact on Burton, see Sherman Chavoor with Bill Davidson, *The 50-Meter Jungle: How Olympic Gold Medal Swimmers Are Made* (New York: Coward, McCann, Geoghegan, 1973).
4. Peterson, "Accident," p. 3D; Bill Patterson, "Sac-Joaquin Section announces inaugural Hall of Fame class," *Sacramento Bee*, April 21, 2010.
5. David L. Porter, *Biographical Dictionary of American Sports: Basketball and Other Indoor Sports* (Westport, CT: Greenwood, 1989), p. 576. Chavoor, *The 50-Meter Jungle*, outlines Burton's strategy for swimming the distance freestyle events.
6. "Mike Burton (US) 1977 Honor Swimmer," International Swimming Hall of Fame, http://www.ishof.org/Honorees/77/77mburton.html; Bill Mallon and Ian Buchanan, *Quest for Gold: The Encyclopedia of American Olympians* (New York: Leisure, 1984), p. 225; Porter, *Biographical Dictionary*, p. 576.
7. Kim Chapin, "The Times Came For Two Teens," *Sports Illustrated* 26 (April 17, 1967).
8. "Countdown to the Trials"; "Burton & Kolb Named 'World Swimmers' of '66," http//www.magazinesswimmingworld.com.997/spidf//1967 wsoty.pdf; Porter, *Biographical Dictionary*, p. 576.
9. "UD Swimming Crown Held by Indiana," *NCAA News* (May 1970), p. 6; William F. Reed, "Redemption After a False Start," *Sports Illustrated* 32 (April 6, 1970).
10. Richard Rollins, "The Only Year of their Lives," *Sports Illustrated* 29 (August 12, 1968).
11. "Countdown to the Trials"; Michael Scott, "Ingrid," http://www.facebook.com/topic.php?uid=57897846467&topic=9267.
12. Katie Ussin, "Billings Man Recalls Olympic Win," August 12, 2008, http://www.kulr.com/news/local/26897449.html?corder=regular; "Countdown to the Trials"; Bob Ottum, "Fresh, Fair and Golden," *Sports Illustrated* 29 (November 4, 1968).

13. Peterson, "Accident," p. 3D; Cecil M. Colwin," George Haines Talks on Great 'Impact' People," in Cecil M. Colwin, *Swimming Dynamics: Winning Techniques and Strategies* (New York: McGraw Hill, 1999).
14. Peterson, "Accident," p. 3D; Colwin, "George Haines Talks."
15. Colwin, "George Haines Talks"; Ottum, "Fresh, Fair and Golden"; "1968 Summer Olympics, Mexico City, Mexico, Swimming," http://www.databaseOlympics.com.
16. Ottum, "Fresh, Fair and Golden"; "1968 Summer Olympics."
17. Ottum, "Fresh, Fair and Golden."
18. Peterson, "Accident," p. 3D.
19. Colwin, "George Haines Talks"; Jerry Kirshenbaum, "Mark of Excellence," *Sports Illustrated* 37 (August 14, 1972).
20. Jerry Kirshenbaum, "The Golden Moment," *Sports Illustrated* 51 (August 20, 1979); Kirshenbaum, "Mark of Excellence."
21. Kirshenbaum, "The Golden Moment"; Colwin, "George Haines Talks."
22. Colwin, "George Haines Talks."
23. Colwin, "George Haines Talks"; "1972 Summer Olympics, Munich, Germany, Swimming," http://www.databaseOlympics.com; Ussin, "Billings Man."
24. "Mike Burton (USA) 1977 Honor Swimmer." For Spitz, see Jerry Kirshenbaum, "Mexico to Munich: Mark Spitz and the Quest for Gold," *Sports Illustrated* 37 (September 4, 1972), and Jerry Kirshenbaum, "The Golden Days of Mark the Shark," *Sports Illustrated* 37 (September 11, 1972).
25. Jerry Kirshenbaum, "A Sanctuary Violated," *Sports Illustrated* 37 (September 18, 1972). See also *New York Times*, September 6, 1972.
26. Peterson, "Accident," p. 3D.
27. Porter, *Biographical Dictionary*, p. 577.
28. Ussin, "Billings Man"; Peterson, "Accident," p. 3D.

## Ben Hogan

1. Grantland Rice, *The Tumult and the Shouting* (New York: A.S. Barnes, 1954), p. 298; James Dodson, *Ben Hogan: An American Life* (New York: Broadway, 2004), pp. 35–52.
2. Curt Sampson, *Hogan* (Nashville: Rutledge Hill, 1996), p 19; Dodson, *Ben Hogan*, p. 61.
3. Herbert Warren Wind, *The Story of American Golf*, 3rd rev. ed. (New York: Alfred A. Knopf, 1975), p. 366; Dodson, *Ben Hogan*, p. 77.
4. Herbert Warren Wind, "The Age of Hogan," *Sports Illustrated* 2 (June 20, 1955); Dodson, *Ben Hogan*, p. 105; Will Grimsley, "Sport's Hall of Fame: Bantam Ben Hogan," *Sport* 32 (November 1961), p. 82.

5. Dodson, *Ben Hogan*, p. 109; Grimsley, "Bantam Ben," p. 82.

6. Dodson, *Ben Hogan*, pp. 117, 139, 141.

7. Wind, "The Age of Hogan"; Rice, *Tumult and the Shouting*, p. 298.

8. Wind, "The Age of Hogan"; Rice, *Tumult and the Shouting*, p. 299.

9. Wind, "The Age of Hogan."

10. Sampson, *Hogan*, p. 102; Wind, "The Age of Hogan."

11. Wind, *American Golf*, p. 369; Dodson, *Ben Hogan*, p. 225.

12. Sampson, *Hogan*, p. 112; "Little Ice Water," *Time* 53 (January 10, 1949).

13. Sampson, *Hogan*, p. 115; Dodson, *Ben Hogan*, p. 238.

14. Grimsley, "Bantam Ben," p. 69; Dodson, *Ben Hogan*, p. 239; Sampson, *Hogan*, p. 116.

15. Dodson, *Ben Hogan*, pp. 241, 240; Grimsley, "Bantam Ben," p. 69.

16. Grimsley, "Bantam Ben," p. 69; Sampson, *Hogan*, p. 117.

17. Dodson, *Ben Hogan*, p. 250.

18. Dodson, *Ben Hogan*, pp. 251–252; Wind, *American Golf*, p. 354.

19. Grimsley, "Bantam Ben," pp. 69, 81–82.

20. Wind, *American Golf*, p. 356.

21. Sampson, *Hogan*, p. 133.

22. Dodson, *Ben Hogan*, p. 276.

23. Sampson, *Hogan*, p. 135; Grimsley, "Bantam Ben," p. 83.

24. Sampson, *Hogan*, pp. 135, 141–142.

25. Dodson, *Ben Hogan*, p. 292; Sampson, *Hogan*, p. 143.

26. Dodson, *Ben Hogan*, p. 301; Wind, *American Golf*, p. 360.

27. Sampson, *Hogan*, p. 147; Grimsley, "Bantam Ben," p. 83.

28. Dodson, *Ben Hogan*, p. 313; Wind, *American Golf*, p. 360; Sampson, *Hogan*, p. 150.

29. Wind, *American Golf*, pp. 361–362; Sampson, *Hogan*, p. 151.

30. Wind, *American Golf*, pp. 362–363.

31. Sampson, *Hogan*, pp. 156–157; Dodson, *Ben Hogan*, pp. 320, 323.

32. Grimsley, "Bantam Ben," pp. 83, 71; Wind, "The Age of Hogan."

33. Dodson, *Ben Hogan*, p. 336; Wind, *American Golf*, p. 378.

34. Dodson, *Ben Hogan*, p. 348.

35. Wind, "The Age of Hogan"; Dodson, *Ben Hogan*, p. 348; Wind, *American Golf*, pp. 378–379.

36. Dodson, *Ben Hogan*, pp. 365, 369; Wind, *American Golf*, p. 379.

37. For a brief explanation of the Grand Slam situation, see Peter Alliss, *Who's Who of Golf* (Englewood Cliffs, NJ: Prentice-Hall, 1983).

38. Grimsley, "Bantam Ben," p. 83; Wind, "The Age of Hogan."

39. Wind, *American Golf*, p. 380; Wind, "The Age of Hogan"; Dodson, *Ben Hogan*, p. 375.

40. Dodson, *Ben Hogan*, pp. 383–384; Wind, *American Golf*, pp. 380, 384.

41. Dodson, *Ben Hogan*, pp. 387, 389–390, 393–394; Wind, *American Golf*, p. 384.

42. Wind, *American Golf*, p. 384.

43. Dodson, *Ben Hogan*, p. 393; Grimsley, "Bantam Ben," pp. 69, 84.

44. Wind, *American Golf*, p. 386; Wind, "The Age of Hogan."

45. Dodson, *Ben Hogan*, p. 411; Grimsley, "Bantam Ben," p. 84.

46. For the final round, see Herbert Warren Wind, "Jack The Giant Killer," *Sports Illustrated* 2 (June 27, 1955) and Herbert Warren Wind, "When The News Arrived," *Sports Illustrated* 2 (June 27, 1955).

47. Wind, "Jack the Giant Killer"; Wind, "When the News Arrived."

48. Grimsley, "Bantam Ben," p. 84; Wind, "When the News Arrived."

49. Grimsley, "Bantam Ben," p. 69.

50. Grimsley, "Bantam Ben," p. 69; Wind, "The Age of Hogan."

51. "Ben Hogan," *The Scribner Encyclopedia of American Lives: Sports Figures*, vol. 1 (New York: Charles Scribner's Sons, 2002), p. 422; Sampson, *Hogan*, p. 247; Grimsley, "Bantam Ben," p. 82.

52. Ben Hogan, *Power Golf* (New York: A.S. Barnes, 1948); Ben Hogan, *Five Lessons: The Modern Fundamentals of Golf* (New York: A.S. Barnes, 1957); *New York Times*, July 26, 1997.

## Greg LeMond

1. Franz Lidz, "Greg LeMond," *Sports Illustrated* 81 (September 19, 1994); Bob Ottum, "Climbing Clear Up To The Heights," *Sports Illustrated* 61 (September 3, 1984). Greg LeMond and Kent Gordis, *Greg LeMond's Complete Book of Bicycling* (New York: Putnam, 1987) provides insight into LeMond's life and early development as a cyclist.

2. E.M. Swift, "Le Grand LeMond," *Sports Illustrated* 71 (December 25, 1989).

3. Ralph Hickok, *A Who's Who of Sports Champions* (Boston: Houghton Mifflin, 1995), p. 473; Swift, "Le Grand LeMond."

4. Ottum, "Climbing Clear Up."

5. E.M. Swift, "An American Takes Paris," *Sports Illustrated* 65 (August 4, 1986).

6. "A Grand Tour for an American," *Time* 128 (August 11, 1986), p. 56; *New York Times*, July 28, 1986, p. 12.

7. Swift, "An American Takes Paris."

8. Franz Lidz, "Vive LeMond!" *Sports Illustrated* 71 (July 31, 1989); Swift, "Le Grand LeMond."

9. Samuel Abt, *LeMond: The Incredible Comeback of an American Hero* (New York: Random House, 1990), pp. 111–112; Swift, "Le Grand LeMond."

10. Abt, *LeMond*, pp. 113, 115.

11. Lidz, "Greg LeMond"; *New York Times Magazine*, June 5, 1988.

12. *New York Times Magazine*, June 5, 1988.

13. Abt, *LeMond*, p. 121.

14. *New York Times Magazine*, June 5, 1988.

15. Abt, *LeMond*, pp. 133–136, 141.

16. Lidz, "Greg LeMond"; Abt, *LeMond*, p. 149.

17. Abt, *LeMond*, p. 159; Lidz, "Vive LeMond!"

18. Abt, *LeMond*, pp. 161, 169, 175–177.

19. Abt, *LeMond*, p. 182; *New York Times*, July 24, 1989.

20. Lidz, "Vive LeMond!"

21. Abt, *LeMond*, pp. 187, 191; *USA Today*, July 24, 1989; Lidz, "Vive LeMond!"

22. Lidz, "Vive LeMond!"; Abt, *LeMond*, p. 191.

23. Abt, *LeMond*, pp. 192–193; *USA Today*, July 24, 1989.

24. Lidz, "Vive LeMond!"

25. Abt, *LeMond*, p. 193; Lidz, "Greg LeMond."

26. Abt, *LeMond*, p. 198.

27. Abt, *LeMond*, p. 196. For accounts of LeMond's exploits in the Tour de France and World Racing Championships, see *Velonews* staff, ed., *Bicycle Racing in the Modern Era* (Boulder, CO: Velo, 1997) and John Wilcockson, *John Wilcockson's World of Cycling* (Boulder, CO: Velo, 1998).

28. Swift, "Le Grand LeMond"; Mike Meserole, ed., *The 1991 Information Please Sports Almanac* (Boston: Houghton Mifflin, 1990), p. 471.

29. Leigh Montville, "Triumph," *Sports Illustrated* 73 (July 30, 1990); Lidz, "Greg LeMond."

30. Alexander Wolff, "Tour De Courage," *Sports Illustrated* 75 (August 5, 1991).

31. Samuel Abt, *A Season in Turmoil* (Boulder, CO: Velo, 1995) details LeMond's disappointing final year of cycling.

32. "All-Time Top 100 Rider Biographies," http://www.cyclinghalloffame.com/riders/alltime100.asp; LeMond and Gordis, Greg LeMond's Complete Book; Lidz, "Greg LeMond."

## Lou Brissie

1. Joe O'Loughlin, "Lou Brissie is an All-American," *Baseball Digest* 64 (June 2005); Bill Nowlin, "Lou Brissie," The Baseball Biography Project, http://www.bioproj.sabr.org/biorproj.cfm?a=r&v=i&bid=2617&pid.

2. Ira Berkow, *The Pitcher Was a Corporal: The Courage of Lou Brissie* (Chicago: Triumph, 2009), pp. 5, 52; Nowlin, "Lou Brissie."

3. Berkow, *Brissie*, p. 8.

4. Nowlin, "Lou Brissie."

5. Connie Mack, *Connie Mack's Baseball Book* (New York: Alfred A. Knopf, 1950), p. 43; Berkow, *Brissie*, p. 10.

6. Berkow, *Brissie*, p. 15; O'Loughlin, "Lou Brissie is an All-American."

7. Nowlin, "Lou Brissie"; Paul Green, "Lou Brissie," *Sports Collectors Digest* 12 (January 4, 1985), p. 135.

8. Nowlin, "Lou Brissie"; Berkow, *Brissie*, pp. 24–25.

9. Berkow, *Brissie*, pp. 31, 30, 40–41; Nowlin, "Lou Brissie."

10. Berkow, *Brissie*, pp. 42, 62; Nowlin, "Lou Brissie."

11. Berkow, *Brissie*, p. 68; Green, "Lou Brissie," p. 139.

12. Berkow, *Brissie*, p. 74; *The Sporting News*, March 1947.

13. Nowlin, "Lou Brissie"; *The Sporting News Baseball Guide and Record Book 1948* (St. Louis, MO: Charles C. Spink & Son, 1948), p. 280.

14. Nowlin, "Lou Brissie"; Berkow, *Brissie*, p. 88.

15. Nowlin, "Lou Brissie"; Berkow, *Brissie*, p. 98.

16. Berkow, *Brissie*, p. 95; Nowlin, "Lou Brissie."

17. Mack, *Baseball Book*, p. 43; Nowlin, "Lou Brissie."

18. Ted Williams with John Underwood, *My Turn at Bat: The Story of My Life* (New York: Simon and Schuster, 1969), p. 16; Nowlin, "Lou Brissie."

19. Berkow, *Brissie*, pp. 102–103, 106; Mack, *Baseball Book*, p. 44.

20. *The Sporting News Baseball Guide and Record Book 1949* (St. Louis, MO: Charles C. Spink & Son, 1949), pp. 15, 30; Nowlin, "Lou Brissie"; Berkow, *Brissie*, p. 125. For season highlights, see David Kaiser, *The 1948 American League Pennant Race* (Amherst: University of Massachusetts Press, 1998).

21. Berkow, *Brissie*, p. 133; Rich Westcott, "Lou Brissie," Philadelphia Athletics Historical Society, Hatboro, PA.

22. *The Sporting News Baseball Guide and Record Book 1950* (St. Louis, MO: Charles Spink & Son, 1950), pp. 13, 29; *Washington Post*, August 11, 1949.

23. *New York Times*, August 19, 1950.

24. Berkow, *Brissie*, p. 158; *The Sporting News Baseball Guide and Record Book 1951* (St. Louis, MO: Charles Spink & Son, 1951), p. 34.

25. *New York Times*, May 1, 1951; Berkow, *Brissie*, pp. 167–168.

26. Berkow, *Brissie*, p. 175; *The Sporting News Baseball Guide and Record Book 1952* (St. Louis, MO: Charles Spink & Son, 1952), pp. 34–35.

27. Green, "Brissie," p. 152.

28. *New York Times*, August 28, 1952; *The Sporting News Baseball Guide and Record Book 1953* (St. Louis, MO: Charles Spink & Son, 1953), pp. 35–36.

29. Berkow, *Brissie*, pp. 195, 197, 199, 207.

30. Nowlin, "Lou Brissie"; *1954 Who's Who in Baseball*, 39th ed. (New York: Who's Who in Baseball Magazine, 1954); Berkow, *Brissie*, p. 208.

31. Berkow, *Brissie*, pp. 206, 203.

32. For Brissie's post–major league career, see Nowlin, "Lou Brissie."

33. Nowlin, "Lou Brissie"; Berkow, *Brissie*, p. 227.

34. Green, "Brissie," p. 156; Grantland Rice, "My Rookie Team of '48," *Sport* 5 (September 1948), p. 84.

# Rocky Bleier

1. Mark Mandarich, "Q & A with Robert 'Rocky' Bleier," *Sports Collectors Digest* 22 (June 30, 1995), p. 140; Rocky Bleier with Terry O'Neal, *Fighting Back* (New York: Stein & Day, 1976), p. 20.

2. Mandarich, "Q & A," p. 140.

3. Mandarich, "Q & A," p. 140; Joe Hoppel et al., eds., *College Football's Twenty-Five Greatest Teams* (St. Louis, MO: The Sporting News, 1988) ranked the 1966 Notre Dame squad eleventh among college football's greatest teams.

4. Bleier, *Fighting Back*, pp. 46–47.

5. Mandarich, "Q & A," p. 140; Bleier, *Fighting Back*, pp. 51, 53–54.

6. Bleier, *Fighting Back*, pp. 53, 61, 70; Mandarich, "Q & A," p. 140.

7. Bleier, *Fighting Back*, p. 68.

8. Erik Brady, "Generation's sports icons are feeling their age," *USA Today*, November 17, 2010, p. 2A. For an account of the ambush, see Rocky Bleier and Terry O'Neil, "Rocky Bleier's War," *Sports Illustrated* 42 (June 9, 1975) and Bleier, *Fighting Back*, pp. 99–111.

9. Bleier, "Bleier's War"; Brady, "Generation's," p. 2A.

10. Bleier, "Bleier's War."

11. Bleier, "Bleier's War."

12. Bleier, *Fighting Back*, p. 116.

13. Bleier, *Fighting Back*, p. 13; Mandarich, "Q & A," p. 140.

14. Bleier, *Fighting Back*, pp. 13, 125–126.

15. "Rocky Bleier—'The Good Soldier,'" http://www.pittsburghsteelers.co.uk/steelers/.../rocky%20bleier.htm.

16. Mandarich, "Q & A," p. 140.

17. Bleier, *Fighting Back*, pp. 132, 13.

18. "The Good Soldier."

19. "The Good Soldier."

20. "The Good Soldier"; Bleier, *Fighting Back*, p. 141.

21. Bleier, *Fighting Back*, pp. 144, 146, 148.

22. Bleier, *Fighting Back*, pp. 152–154.

23. Bleier, *Fighting Back*, pp. 14, 155.

24. Bleier, *Fighting Back*, pp. 164, 166, 187.

25. Mandarich, "Q & A," p. 140; "The Good Soldier."

26. "Rocky Bleier: Purple Heart and Bronze Star," *Sports Illustrated* 45 (December 6, 1976); Mandarich, "Q & A," p. 140; "Rocky Bleier: Purple Heart."

27. "The Good Soldier."

28. "The Good Soldier"; Bleier, *Fighting Back*, p. 181.

29. Mandarich, "Q & A," p. 140; "The Good Soldier."

30. Bleier, *Fighting Back*, pp. 182, 187.

31. Bob Carroll et al., eds., *Total Football* (New York: HarperCollins Publishers, 1997), p. 536; Bleier, *Fighting Back*, p. 186.

32. Bleier, *Fighting Back*, p. 187.

33. Bleier, *Fighting Back*, pp. 211–212, 214.

34. Bleier, *Fighting Back*, pp. 215, 217.

35. Bleier, *Fighting Back*, pp. 219, 14.

36. Carroll, *Total Football*, pp. 536, 82.

37. Carroll, *Total Football*, pp. 82, 153–155, 536.

38. Dan Jenkins, "What a Passing Parade!" *Sports Illustrated* 50 (January 29, 1979); "The Good Soldier."

39. Jenkins, "What a Passing Parade"; Mandarich, "Q & A," p. 140.

40. Carroll, *Total Football*, pp. 109–110, 536, 82, 156–157.

41. Mandarich, "Q & A," p. 140.

42. Carroll, *Total Football*, p. 536.

43. "Rocky Bleier: Purple Heart"; "The Good Soldier"; Rick Telander, "Local Boy Makes Good," *Sports Illustrated* 65 (August 11, 1986).

44. Doug Russell, "Solid as a Rock," March 1, 2012, http://www.onmilwaukee.com/sports/articles/rockybleier.htm!?page=2; Mandarich, "Q & A," p. 141.

# Tommy John

1. Nolan Ryan with Mickey Herskowitz, *Kings of the Hill* (New York: HarperCollins Publishers, 1992), p. 173; Sally and Tommy John, *The Sally and Tommy John Story: Our Life in Baseball* (New York: Macmillan, 1983), p. 54.

2. Tommy John Interview, Bob Feller Museum, Van Meter, IA, October 23, 2010; Will Grimsley, "Tommy John oozes with class," *Des Moines Register*, August 21, 1981, p. 1S.

3. John, *Sally and Tommy John Story*, pp. 65–66, 72–73.

4. John Interview, October 23, 2010; Ryan, *Kings*, p. 174.

5. John, *Sally and Tommy John Story*, p. 129.

6. John, *Sally and Tommy John Story*, p. 195; Michael Fallon, "Tommy John," The Baseball Biography Project, Society for American Baseball Research, http://bioproj.sabr.org/bioproj.cfm?a=v&v=1&bid=3834&pld=6969.

7. John, *Sally and Tommy John Story*, pp. 201, 210, 131.

8. Fallon, "Tommy John"; John, *Sally and Tommy John Story*, p. 132.

9. Ron Fimrite, "Stress, Strain, and Pain," *Sports Illustrated* 49 (August 14, 1978); John, *Sally and Tommy John Story*, p. 133.

10. John, *Sally and Tommy John Story*, p. 134; Fimrite, "Stress, Strain, and Pain."

11. John, *Sally and Tommy John Story*, pp. 134–135; Randy Schultz, "Tommy John: The right-handed left-hander," *Sports Collectors Digest* 22 (October 6, 1995), p. 170.

12. Fallon, "Tommy John"; Tommy John, with Dan Valenti, *T.J.: My 26 Years in Baseball* (New York: Bantam, 1991), p. 129.

13. John, *Sally and Tommy John Story*, pp. 136–137; John Interview, October 23, 2010; Dave Nightingale, "The Oldest Lefty of Them All," *The Sporting News* (May 22, 1989), p. 10.

14. John Interview, October 23, 2010; Fallon, "Tommy John."

15. Fimrite, "Stress, Strain, and Pain"; Fallon, "Tommy John"; Schultz, "Tommy John," p. 170; John, *Sally and Tommy John Story*, p. 139.

16. Schultz, "Tommy John," p. 170; John, *Sally and Tommy John Story*, p. 141.

17. John, *T.J.*, p. 183; Fallon, "Tommy John."

18. John, *Sally and Tommy John Story*, pp. 142–143.

19. John, *Sally and Tommy John Story*, pp. 141–142; John Interview, October 23, 2010.

20. John, *T.J.*, pp. 184–185; John, *Sally and Tommy John Story*, pp. 147–148.

21. John, *Sally and Tommy John Story*, p. 148.

22. John Interview, October 23, 2010; John, *Sally and Tommy John Story*, p. 151.

23. John Interview, October 23, 2010.

24. John, *Sally and Tommy John Story*, p. 153; Schultz, "Tommy John," p. 170.

25. Grimsley, "Tommy John oozes," p. 1S; Schultz, "Tommy John," p. 170.

26. William F. McNeill, *The Dodgers Encyclopedia* (Champaign, IL: Sports Publishing, 1997), p. 215; John Interview, October 23, 2010; John, *Sally and Tommy John Story*, pp. 160–161.

27. John, *Sally and Tommy John Story*, p. 160; McNeill, *Dodgers Encyclopedia*, p. 215.

28. John Interview, October 23, 2010; McNeil, *Dodgers Encyclopedia*, p. 216; Schultz, "Tommy John," p. 170.

29. John Interview, October 23, 2010; John, *Sally and Tommy John Story*, p. 160.

30. McNeill, *Dodgers Encyclopedia*, p. 219; John, *Sally and Tommy John Story*, p. 161; Fallon, "Tommy John."

31. Fallon, "Tommy John"; John, *Sally and Tommy John Story*, pp. 162–163.

32. McNeill, *Dodgers Encyclopedia*, p. 221; *Offi-cial Baseball Guide for 1979* (St. Louis, MO: The Sporting News, 1979), p. 254.

33. John, *Sally and Tommy John Story*, p. 163; McNeill, *Dodgers Encyclopedia*, pp. 222, 224.

34. John, *Sally and Tommy John Story*, p. 164; Fallon, "Tommy John"; Mark Gallagher and Walter LeConte, *The Yankee Encyclopedia*, 5th ed. (Champaign, IL: Sports Publishing, 2001), pp. 414, 131.

35. Gallagher, *The Yankee Encyclopedia*, pp. 418, 459–460.

36. John, *Sally and Tommy John Story*, pp. 19–21.

37. John, *Sally and Tommy John Story*, p. 42; Gallagher, *The Yankee Encyclopedia*, p. 418.

38. Fallon, "Tommy John"; John, *Sally and Tommy John Story*, pp. 119–120, 237.

39. John Interview, October 23, 2010; Ryan, *Kings*, p. 174.

40. Gallagher, *The Yankee Encyclopedia*, pp. 131, 522–523.

41. Fallon, "Tommy John"; John, *Sally and Tommy John Story*, p. 247; Gallagher, *The Yankee Encyclopedia*, p. 131; Schultz, "Tommy John," p. 170.

42. Nightingale, "Oldest Lefty," p. 10.

43. Gallagher, *The Yankee Encyclopedia*, p. 132; Nightingale, "Oldest Lefty," p. 10.

44. Nightingale, "Oldest Lefty," p. 10; Gallagher, *The Yankee Encyclopedia*, p. 132.

45. John Interview, October 23, 2010; Nightingale, "Oldest Lefty," p. 10.

46. Schultz, "Tommy John," p. 170.

47. Ryan, *Kings*, pp. 172–173; Fallon, "Tommy John"; John Interview, October 23, 2010.

48. Fallon, "Tommy John."

49. Ryan, *Kings*, p. 173; Fallon, "Tommy John"; Lyle Spatz, ed., *The SABR Baseball List and Record Book* (New York: Scribner, 2007), pp. 193–281; Ryan, *Kings*, p. 173.

50. Fallon, "Tommy John."

51. Schultz, "Tommy John," p. 170; Nightingale, "Oldest Lefty," p. 10.

52. Grimsley, "Tommy John oozes," p. 1S; John Interview, October 23, 2010.

## Conclusion

1. Peter C. Bjarkman, *The Biographical History of Basketball* (Chicago: Masters, 2000), p. 510.

2. Julie-Ann Amos, "Jim Valvano and the V Foundation 74," http://www.hubpages.com/hub/Jim-Valvano.

3. The V Foundation for Cancer Research, "Remembering Jim — ESPY Awards Speech," http://www.jimmyv.org/remembering-jim/espy-awards-speech.html. For Valvano's battle with cancer, see Adrian Wojnarowski, *Jimmy V: The Life and Death of Jim Valvano* (New York: Gotham, 2008).

# Bibliography

## Books

Abbott, Jim, and Tim Brown. *Imperfect: An Improbable Life.* New York: Ballantine, 2012.

Abt, Samuel. *LeMond: The Incredible Comeback of an American Hero.* New York: Random House, 1990.

_____. *A Season in Turmoil.* Boulder, CO: Velo, 1995.

Alexander, Charles C. *John McGraw.* Lincoln: University of Nebraska Press, 1988.

Allen, Lee. *The National League Story.* New York: Hill & Wang, 1965.

_____. *The World Series.* New York: G.P. Putnam's Sons, 1969.

Allis, Peter. *Who's Who of Golf.* Englewood Cliffs, NJ: Prentice Hall, 1983.

Associated Press. *The Olympic Story: Pursuit of Excellence.* Danbury, CT: Grolier, 1979.

*Baseball America Almanac 2009.* Durham, NC: Baseball America, 2008.

Berkow, Ira. *The Pitcher Was a Corporal: The Courage of Lou Brissie.* Chicago: Triumph, 2009.

Bernotas, Bob. *Nothing to Prove: The Jim Abbott Story.* New York: Kodansha International, 1995.

Bjarkman, Peter C. *The Biographical History of Basketball.* Chicago: Masters, 2000.

Bleier, Rocky, with Terry O'Neal. *Fighting Back.* New York: Stein & Day, 1976.

Boston Globe. *So Good! The Incredible Championship Season of the 2007 Boston Red Sox.* Chicago: Triumph, 2007.

*Boston Red Sox Media Guide, 2007–2012.*

Brown, Mordecai. *How to Pitch Curves.* Chicago: W.D. Boyce, 1913.

Burke, Larry. *The Baseball Chronicles: A Decade-by-Decade History of the All-American Pastime.* New York: Smithmark, 1995.

Carlson, Lewis H., and John J. Fogarty. *Tales of Gold.* Chicago: Contemporary, 1987.

Carmichael, John P. *My Greatest Day in Baseball.* New York: Grosset & Dunlap, 1951.

Carroll, Bob, et al. *Total Football.* New York: HarperCollins, 1997.

Cavanaugh, Jack. *Tunney: Boxing's Brainiest Champ and His Upset of the Great Jack Dempsey.* New York: Random House, 2006.

Cayleff, Susan E. *Babe: The Life and Legend of Babe Didrikson Zaharias.* Urbana: University of Illinois Press, 1995.

Chavoor, Sherman, with Bill Davidson. *The 50-Meter Jungle: How Olympic Gold Medal Swimmers Are Made.* New York: Coward, McCann, Geoghegan, 1973.

Collins, Bud, and Zander Hollander, eds. *Bud Collins' Tennis Encyclopedia.* Detroit: Visible Ink, 1997.

Colwin, Cecil M. *Swimming Dynamics: Winning Techniques and Strategies.* New York: McGraw Hill, 1999.

Cosell, Howard, and Mickey Herskowitz. *Cosell.* New York: Playboy Press, 1973.

Cunningham, Glenn, with George X. Sand. *Never Quit.* Lincoln, VA: Chosen, 1981.

*Current Biography Yearbook 1995.* New York: H.W. Wilson, 1995.

*Current Black Biography*, vol. 44. Detroit: Gale, 2004.

Davis, Michael D. *Black American Women in Olympic Track and Field.* Jefferson, NC: McFarland, 1992.

Dodson, James. *Ben Hogan: An American Life.* New York: Broadway, 2004.

Durocher, Leo, with Ed Linn. *Nice Guys Finish Last.* New York: Simon & Schuster, 1975.

*ESPN Sports Almanac 2000; 2001; 2002; 2003; 2004; 2006; 2008.*

Evers, John J., and Hugh S. Fullerton. *Touching Second: The Science of Baseball.* Chicago: Reilly & Britton, 1910.

Fair, James R. *Give Him to the Angels: The Story of Harry Greb.* New York: Smith and Durrell, 1946.

Fleischer, Nat, and Sam Andre. *A Pictorial History of Boxing.* New York: Citadel, 1959.

Fleming, G.H. *The Unforgettable Season.* New York: Holt, Rinehart, and Winston, 1981.

Frost, Mark. *The Grand Slam: Bobby Jones, America, and the Story of Golf.* New York: Hyperion, 2004.

Gallagher, Mark, and Walter LeConte. *The Yankee Encyclopedia.* 5th ed. Champaign, IL: Sports Publishing, 2001.

Gentile, Derek. *The Complete Chicago Cubs: The Total Encyclopedia of the Team.* New York: Black Dog & Leventhal, 2002.

Gould, Stephen Jay. *Triumph and Tragedy in Mudville: A Lifelong Passion for Baseball.* New York: W.W. Norton, 2003.

Grimsley, Will. *Tennis: Its History, People, and Events.* Englewood Cliffs, NJ: Prentice-Hall, 1971.

Gutman, Bill. *Gail Devers: Overcoming the Odds.* Austin, TX: Raintree Steck-Vaughn, 1996.

Hamilton, Scott, with Lorenz Benet. *Landing It: My Life On and Off the Ice.* New York: Kensington, 1999.

Hart, Doris. *Tennis with Hart.* Philadelphia: J.B. Lippincott, 1955.

Hickok, Ralph. *A Who's Who of Sports Champions.* Boston: Houghton Mifflin, 1995.

Hogan, Ben. *Five Lessons: The Modern Fundamentals of Golf.* New York: A.S. Barnes, 1957.

_____. *Power Golf.* New York: A.S. Barnes, 1948.

Holst, Don, and Marcia S. Popp. *American Men of Track and Field: Interviews with Athletes and Coaches.* Jefferson, NC: McFarland, 2005.

Hoppel, Joe, et al. *College Football's Twenty-Five Greatest Teams.* St. Louis, MO: The Sporting News, 1988.

Hugman, Barry J., and Peter Arnold. *The Olympic Games: Complete Track and Field Results 1896–1988.* New York: Facts on File, 1988.

*The Information Please Sports Almanac, 1991, 1997.* Boston: Houghton Mifflin, 1991, 1997.

James, Bill. *The Baseball Book 1990.* New York: Villard, 1990.

John, Sally, and Tommy John. *The Sally and Tommy John Story: Our Life in Baseball.* New York: Macmillan, 1983.

John, Tommy. *TJ: My 26 Years in Baseball.* New York: Bantam, 1991.

Johnson, Anne Janette. *Great Women in Sports.* Detroit: Visible Ink, 1996.

Johnson, William Oscar, and Nancy P. Williamson. *"Whatta-Gal": The Babe Didrikson Story.* Boston: Little, Brown, 1975.

Jones, Robert Tyre, Jr. *Golf Is My Game.* Garden City, NY: Doubleday, 1960.

Kaiser, David. *The 1948 American League Pennant Race.* Amherst: University of Massachusetts Press, 1998.

Keeler, O.B., and Grantland Rice. *The Bobby Jones Story.* Atlanta: Tupper & Love, 1953.

LeMond, Greg, and Kent Gordis. *Greg LeMond's Complete Book of Bicycling.* New York: Putnam, 1987.

Lewis, Dwight, and Susan Thomas. *A Will to Win.* Mt. Juliet, TN: Cumberland, 1983.

Lieb, Frederick G. *The Story of the World Series.* Rev. ed. New York: G.P. Putnam's Sons, 1965.

Mack, Connie. *Connie Mack's Baseball Book.* New York: Alfred A. Knopf, 1950.

Mallon, Bill, and Ian Buchanan. *Quest for Gold: The Encyclopedia of American Olympians.* New York: Leisure, 1984.

Maraniss, David. *Rome 1960: The Olympics that Changed the World.* New York: Simon & Schuster, 2008.

Marble, Alice. *Road to Wimbledon.* New York: Charles Scribner's Sons, 1947.

_____, with Dale Leatherman. *Courting Danger.* New York: St. Martin's Press, 1991.

Matthew, Sidney L. *Portrait of a Gentleman: The Life and Times of Bobby Jones.* Chelsea, MI: Sleeping Bear, 1995.

McNeil, William F. *The Dodger Encyclopedia.* Champaign, IL: Sports Publishing, 1997.

Mourning, Alonzo, with Dan Wetzel. *Resilience: Faith, Focus, Triumph.* New York: Ballantine, 2008.

Nelson, Cordner. *Track's Greatest Champions.* Los Altos, CA: Tafnews, 1986.

_____, and Roberto Quercetani. *The Milers.* Los Altos, CA: Tafnews, 1985.

Paxton, Billy. *The Fearless Harry Greb: Biography of a Tragic Hero of Boxing.* Jefferson, NC: McFarland, 2009.

Porter, David L. *Michael Jordan: A Biography.* Westport, CT: Greenwood, 2007.

_____, ed. *African American Sports Greats: A Biographical Dictionary.* Westport, CT: Greenwood, 1995.

_____, ed. *Biographical Dictionary of American Sports: Basketball and Other Indoor Sports.* Westport, CT: Greenwood, 1989.

_____, ed. *Biographical Dictionary of American Sports: Outdoor Sports.* Westport, CT: Greenwood, 1988.

Reidenbaugh, Lowell. *Baseball's Hall of Fame: Cooperstown, Where the Legends Live Forever.* Rev. ed. New York: Crescent, 1997.

Rice, Grantland. *The Tumult and the Shouting.* New York: A.S. Barnes, 1954.

Ritter, Lawrence S. *The Glory of their Times*. New York: Macmillan, 1966.

Rudolph, Wilma, with Martin Ralbovsky, *Wilma: The Story of Wilma Rudolph*. New York: New American Library, 1977.

Ryan, Joan. *Contributions of Women: Sports*. Minneapolis: Dillon, 1956.

Ryan, Nolan, with Mickey Herskowitz. *Kings of the Hill*. New York: HarperCollins 1992.

Sampson, Curt. *Hogan*. Nashville: Rutledge Hill, 1996.

Santo, Ron, with Randy Minkoff. *Ron Santo: For Love of Ivy: The Autobiography of Ron Santo*. Chicago: Bonus, 1993.

*The Scribner Encyclopedia of American Lives*. 2 vols. New York: Charles Scribner's Sons, 1999.

*The Scribner Encyclopedia of American Lives: Sports Figures*. 2 vols. New York: Charles Scribner's Sons, 2002.

Seymour, Harold, and Dorothy Seymour Mills. *Baseball: The Golden Age*. New York: Oxford University Press, 1971.

Smith, Maureen M. *Wilma Rudolph: A Biography*. Westport, CT: Greenwood, 2006.

Spatz, Lyle, ed. *The SABR Baseball List and Record Book*. New York: Scribner, 2007.

*The Sporting News Baseball Guide and Record Book 1948–1953*. St. Louis, MO: Charles C. Spink & Son, 1948–1953.

*The Sporting News Baseball Register 2000 Edition*. St. Louis, MO: The Sporting News, 2000.

*The Sporting News Official Baseball Guide 1979*. St. Louis, MO: The Sporting News, 1979.

*Sporting News Official NBA Guide, 2000–2001, 2002–2003, 2006–07*. St. Louis, MO: The Sporting News, 2000, 2002, 2006.

*Sporting News Official NBA Register, 2006–07*. St. Louis, MO: The Sporting News, 2006.

*Sports Illustrated Almanac 2001, 2003, 2004, 2005, 2006, 2009, 2010*. New York: Time, Inc., 2000, 2002–2005, 2008–2009.

Sugar, Bert Randolph, and the editors of *Ring* magazine. *The Great Fights*. New York: Gallery, 1984.

Talley, Rick. *The Cubs of '69*. Chicago: Contemporary, 1989.

Thomson, Cindy, and Scott Brown. *Three-Finger: The Mordecai Brown Story*. Lincoln: University of Nebraska Press, 2006.

Tieman, Robert L., and Mark Rucker, eds. *Nineteenth Century Stars*. Kansas City, MO: Society for American Baseball Research, 1989.

Toomey, Bill, and Barry King. *The Olympic Challenge, 1988*. Costa Mesa, CA: Hdl Publishing Company, 1988.

Twombly, Wells. *200 Years of Sports in America: A Pageant of a Nation at Play*. New York: McGraw-Hill, 1976.

Van Natta, Don, Jr. *Wonder Girl: The Magnificent Sporting Life of Babe Didrikson Zaharias*. New York: Little, Brown, 2011.

*Velonews* staff, ed. *Bicycle Racing in the Modern Era*. Boulder, CO: Velo, 1997.

Wakeman, Nancy. *Babe Didrikson Zaharias: Driven to Win*. Minneapolis: Lerner, 2000.

*Who's Who in Baseball 1954, 2013*, 39th and 98th eds. New York: Who's Who in Baseball Magazine, 1954, 2013.

Wilcockson, John. *John Wilcockson's World of Cycling*. Boulder, CO: Velo, 1998.

Williams, Ted, with John Underwood. *My Turn at Bat: The Story of My Life*. New York: Simon & Schuster, 1969.

Wind, Herbert Warren. *The Story of American Golf*. 3rd rev. ed. New York: Alfred A. Knopf, 1975.

Wojnarowski, Adrian. *Jimmy V: The Life and Death of Jim Valvano*. New York: Gotham, 2008.

Worth, Richard. *Gail Devers: Overcoming Adversities*. Philadelphia: Chelsea House, 2001.

Zaharias, Babe Didrikson, as told to Harry Paxton. *This Life I've Led: My Autobiography*. New York: Dell, 1955.

## Magazine Articles

Anderson, Bruce. "Angel on the Ascent." *Sports Illustrated* 70 (March 13, 1989).

Anderson, Kelli. "Break Out the Bubbly." *Sports Illustrated* 101 (August 30, 2004).

"The Babe Is Back." *Time* 42 (August 10, 1953).

Bennett, Joseph. "Three-Finger Brown: A Lamb Without Blemish." *Philathes* 51 (June 1998).

Bleier, Rocky, and Terry O'Neil. "Rocky Bleier's War." *Sports Illustrated* 42 (June 9, 1975).

Brigham, Bob. "Dummy Hoy: Forgotten Gem on the Diamond." *Sports Collectors Digest* 21 (January 14, 1994).

Brofman, Rob. "One for the Angels." *Life* 121 (June 1989).

Brosnan, Jim. "Ron Santo Comes of Age." *Sport* 56 (September 1973).

Burkholder, Edwin V. "Glenn Cunningham and the Four-Minute Mile." *Sport* 8 (March 1950).

Chapin, Kim. "The Times Came for Two Teens." *Sports Illustrated* 26 (April 17, 1967).

DeCola, Pat. "5 Reasons Behind Jon Lester's Shocking 2012 Disappointment." *Bleacher Report* (August 17, 2012).

Devers, Gail. "Running for My Life." *Family Circle* 106 (May 18, 1993).

"Dreaming of Big Dreams." *Time* 133 (March 20, 1989).

Dyer, Braven, and Frank Finch. "Top Lady Athlete." *Sport* 1 (November 1946).

"The Fastest Female." *Time* 76 (September 19, 1960).

"The Fifty Greatest Florida Sports Figures." *Sports Illustrated* 91 (December 27, 1999).

Fimrite, Ron. "Stress, Strain, and Pain." *Sports Illustrated* 49 (August 14, 1978).

"For the Record." *Sports Illustrated* 105 (September 11, 2006).

Fullerton, Hugh S. "The Spring Training: How the Baseball Players Get into Condition." *American Magazine* 23 (April 1910).

Gallico, Paul. "Farewell to the Babe." *Sports Illustrated* 5 (October 8, 1956).

"Glory Halleluiah!" *Time* 124 (August 13, 1984).

"A Grand Tour for an American." *Time* 128 (August 11, 1986).

"Great Olympic Moments: Wilma Rudolph — Rome 1960." *Ebony* 47 (January 1992).

Green, Paul. "Lou Brissie." *Sports Collectors Digest* 12 (January 4, 1985).

Grimsley, Will. "Sport's Hall of Fame: Bantam Ben Hogan." *Sport* 32 (November 1961).

Haag, Ken. "The Silent World of William 'Dummy' Hoy." *Sports Collectors Digest* 21 (January 14, 1994).

"Harry Greb or Harry Berg." *Boxing and Wrestling Magazine* 4 (February 1954).

Heilman, Barbara. "Like Nothing Else in Tennessee." *Sports Illustrated* 13 (November 14, 1960).

Hersch, Hank. "Ace of the Angels." *Sports Illustrated* 75 (September 9, 1991).

_____. "That Great Abbott Switch." *Sports Illustrated* 66 (May 25, 1987).

Hertzel, Bob. "A Real Jim Dandy." *Beckett Baseball Monthly* 10 (June 1993).

Hosford, Christopher. "30 Years of Progress for the Ultimate 10-Event Man." *Life Extension Magazine* 4 (September 1998).

Howard, Johnette. "All I Ever Wanted Was a Shot." *Sport* 80 (March 1989).

_____. "The Talent Pool." *Sports Illustrated* 84 (April 22, 1996).

"Indoor Dash Queen: World Champion Gail Devers." *Track and Field News* 46 (November 1993).

Jenkins, Dan. "What a Passing Parade!" *Sports Illustrated* 50 (January 29, 1979).

Jenkins, Lee. "Jim Abbott: One-Handed Wonder." *Sports Illustrated* 109 (July 14, 2008).

Katz, Fred. "Ron Santo and His Million-Dollar Education." *Sport* 43 (May 1967).

Kirshenbaum, Jerry. "The Golden Days of Mark the Shark." *Sports Illustrated* 37 (September 11, 1972).

_____. "The Golden Moment." *Sports Illustrated* 51 (August 20, 1979).

_____. "Mark of Excellence." *Sports Illustrated* 37 (August 14, 1972).

_____. "Mexico to Munich: Mark Spitz and the Quest for Gold." *Sports Illustrated* 37 (September 4, 1972).

_____. "A Sanctuary Violated." *Sports Illustrated* 37 (September 18, 1972).

Krueckeberg, Dan. "Take-Charge Cy." *The National Pastime* 4 (Spring 1985).

Kruger, Art. "He Made the Umpires Raise Their Hands: Dummy Hoy." *Baseball Digest* 13 (May 1954).

Laney, Ruth. "Controversy Dogs Devers." *Track and Field News* 46 (November 1993).

Lawrence, Andrew. "Career Days." *Sports Illustrated* 112 (May 31, 2010).

Layden, Tim. "Over Life's Hurdles." *Sports Illustrated* 106 (February 12, 2007).

Lidz, Franz. "Greg LeMond." *Sports Illustrated* 81 (September 19, 1994).

_____. "Vive LeMond!" *Sports Illustrated* 71 (July 31, 1989).

"Little Ice Water." *Time* 53 (January 10, 1949).

Mandarich, Mark. "Q & A with Robert 'Rocky' Bleier." *Sports Collectors Digest* 22 (June 30, 1995).

Marble, Alice. "Lesson in Courage — That's Doris Hart." *American Lawn Tennis* 42 (May 1948).

Maule, Tex. "Whirling Success for the U.S." *Sports Illustrated* 17 (July 30, 1962).

McCallum, Jack. "A Season Full of Fight." *Sports Illustrated* 96 (April 1, 2002).

_____, and Richard O'Brien. "Back in the Game." *Sports Illustrated* 89 (October 5, 1998).

McMullan, Jackie. "Memo to Magic." *Sports Illustrated* 84 (May 13, 1996).

Montville, Leigh. "Double Take." *Sports Illustrated* 93 (October 2, 2000).

_____. "Triumph." *Sports Illustrated* 73 (July 30, 1990).

Moore, Kenny. "The Best Is Yet to Come." *Sports Illustrated* 68 (June 6, 1988).

_____. "Coming on Strong." *Sports Illustrated* 85 (August 5, 1996).

_____. "Dash to Glory." *Sports Illustrated* 77 (August 10, 1992).

_____. "Gail Force." *Sports Illustrated* 78 (May 10, 1993).

_____. "Hot Times at the NCAAs." *Sports Illustrated* 68 (June 13, 1988).

_____. "Ode to Joy." *Sports Illustrated* 77 (August 17, 1992).

"Mordecai Brown." *Baseball Magazine* 12 (July 1911).

Murray, James. "A Big Night for Wilma." *Sports Illustrated* 14 (January 30, 1961).

Newcombe, Jack. "The Incomparable Babe Didrikson." *Sport* 14 (December 1959).

Odd, Gilbert. "Tough-Guy Ted Took on Greb the Great." *Boxing News* (July 28, 1989).

O'Loughlin, Joe. "Lou Brissie Is an All-American." *Baseball Digest* 64 (June 2005).

"One Happy Dude." *Brandweek* 36 (July 17, 1995).

Ottum, Bob. "Climbing Clear Up to the Heights." *Sports Illustrated* 61 (September 3, 1984).

_____. "Fresh, Fair and Golden." *Sports Illustrated* 29 (November 4, 1968).

_____. "Great Scott! What a Doubleheader." *Sports Illustrated* 58 (March 21, 1983).

_____. "Not At All Pretty, but Almost Perfect." *Sports Illustrated* 61 (August 20, 1984).

_____. "Notable Triumphs, Wrong Notes." *Sports Illustrated* 60 (February 27, 1984).

_____. "Out to Cut Fancy Figures in Sarajevo." *Sports Illustrated* 60 (January 30, 1984).

_____. "Wow! Power." *Sports Illustrated* 60 (February 6, 1984).

"Parade to the Pedestal." *Time* 92 (November 1, 1968).

Pizer, Vernon. "The Man with 8000 Miracles." *The Rotarian* 108 (February 1966).

Reed, William F. "The Ineligible Married Man." *Sports Illustrated* 35 (April 12, 1971).

_____. "Redemption After a False Start." *Sports Illustrated* 32 (April 6, 1970).

Rice, Grantland. "King of All the Marvels." *Collier's* 77 (February 20, 1926).

_____. "My Rookie Team of '48." *Sport* 5 (September 1948).

Richmond, Peter. "Jon Lester Is Back in the Game." *Parade* (March 15, 2009).

"Rocky Bleier: Purple Heart and Bronze Star." *Sports Illustrated* 45 (December 6, 1976).

Rollins, Richard. "The Only Year of their Lives." *Sports Illustrated* 29 (August 12, 1968).

Sandy, Steve, and Richard Miller. "No Dummy: William Ellsworth Hoy." Ohio Historical Society *Timeline* (March-April 2000).

Santo, Ron. "Ron Santo's Secret on the Field." *Guideposts* (June 2003).

Schultz, Randy. "Tommy John: The Right-Handed Left-Hander." *Sports Collectors Digest* 22 (October 6, 1995).

Sher, Jack. "Bobby Jones Emperor of Golf." *Sport* 7 (August 1949).

Stilwell, Jonathan. "William 'Dummy' Hoy Proving It Could Be Done." *Bleacher Report* (August 25, 2009).

Swift, E.M. "An American Takes Paris." *Sports Illustrated* 65 (August 4, 1986).

_____. "Le Grand LeMond." *Sports Illustrated* 71 (December 25, 1989).

Taafe, William. "Bold Strokes on a Big Canvas." *Sports Illustrated* 61 (August 20, 1984).

Telander, Rick. "Local Boy Makes Good." *Sports Illustrated* 65 (August 11, 1986).

Thomsen, Ian. "Playstrong." *Sports Illustrated* 103 (December 19, 2005).

_____. "Say It Ain't 'Zo." *Sports Illustrated* 101 (November 22, 2004).

"UD Swimming Crown Held by Indiana." *NCAA News* (May 1970).

Underwood, John. "Best-Kept Secrets." *Sports Illustrated* 27 (June 12, 1967).

_____. "The Long Long Jump." *Sports Illustrated* 30 (October 28, 1968).

Verducci, Tom. "A Special Delivery." *Sports Illustrated* 79 (September 13, 1993).

Von Benko, George. "Ron Santo: The Best NL Third Sacker of His Generation Has a Legitimate Claim to HOF." *Sports Collectors Digest* 24 (August 29, 1997).

West, Ken. "Unforgettable Glenn Cunningham." *Reader's Digest* (1988).

Westcott, Rich. "Lou Brissie." Philadelphia Athletics Historical Society, Hatboro, PA.

"Whatever Happened to Wilma Rudolph?" *Ebony* 39 (February 1984).

Wind, Herbert Warren. "The Age of Hogan." *Sports Illustrated* 2 (June 20, 1955).

_____. "Jack the Giant Killer." *Sports Illustrated* 2 (June 27, 1955).

_____. "When the News Arrived." *Sports Illustrated* 2 (June 27, 1955).

Wismer, Harry. "She's a Sweet Hart!" *Sport* 2 (September 1947).

Wolff, Alexander. "Mourning's Glory." *Sports Illustrated* 76 (March 2, 1992).

_____. "Tour de Courage." *Sports Illustrated* 75 (August 5, 1991).

"The Wonderful World of Sport." *Sports Illustrated* 1 (September 13, 1954).

Zaharias, Babe Didrikson, as told to Booton Herndon. "I'm Not Out of the Rough — Yet!" *Cosmopolitan* 135 (October 1953).

Zaharias, George. "Babe & I." *Look* 20 (December 11, 1956).

## Newspapers / New Services

Associated Press News Release, November 25, 2003; March 26, 2008.

*Atlanta Journal*, September 6, 1929.

*Boston Globe*, August 25, 2006; September 2, 2006.

*Boston Herald*, August 15, 2007; August 22, 2007; October 14, 2007; October 19, 2007; October 29, 2007; October 2, 2008; October 7, 2008; June 7, 2009; October 9, 2009; July 5, 2010; September 22, 2012.

*Chicago Sun-Times*, July 9, 1969; December 3, 2010.

*Chicago Tribune*, December 18, 1903; June 14, 1905; July 5, 1906; October 10, 1906; September 23, 1908; October 5, 1908; June 2, 1909; June 9, 1909; October 23, 1910; October 27, 1910; June 9, 1914; March 14, 1922; September 16, 1923; August 21, 1925; February 17, 1984; January 8, 1989; August 14, 1995.

*Christian Science Monitor*, December 14, 1982.

*Cortland Standard*, October 23, 2008.

*Detroit Free Press*, April 12, 2012; April 29, 2012.

ESPN Chicago, December 3, 2010.

*Hartford Courant*, November 22, 1986.

*Indiana Spectator* (Terre Haute), July 21, 1979.

*Kansas City Times*, March 12, 1938.

*Los Angeles Times*, April 5, 1986; May 7, 1986; July 19, 1987; August 7, 1988; June 18, 1989; January 18, 1993; August 1, 2004.

*Miami Herald*, March 16, 2003.

*New York Times*, July 16, 1913; February 24–25, 1923; September 2, 1923; June 16, 1926; August 27, 1926; October 27, 1926; September 28, 1930; March 6, 1938; March 13, 1938; May 6, 1949; August 19, 1950; May 1, 1951; August 28, 1952; February 24, 1954; September 28, 1956; December 19, 1971; September 6, 1972; March 7, 1983; January 16, 1985; July 28, 1986; June 5, 1988; December 14, 1990; August 2, 1992; September 5, 1992; December 8, 1992; December 25, 1992; May 6, 1993; August 23, 1993; June 17, 1994; November 19, 1994; July 26, 1997; September 28, 2000; August 21, 2004.

*New York World*, September 23, 1908.

*Newsday*, October 14, 1990.

*Oskaloosa Herald*, August 23, 2010.

*Pittsburgh Post*, August 30, 1921; February 25, 1923; December 4, 1923; January 19, 1924; March 25, 1924; July 3, 1925; February 27, 28, 1926; August 20, 1926.

*Pittsburgh Press*, March 22, 1922; July 3, 1922.

*Sacramento Bee*, April 21, 2010.

*Seattle Post-Intelligencer*, February 24, 2007.

*The Sporting News*, October 27, 1910; March 1947; February 13, 1952; May 22, 1989; July 19, 1993.

*Terre Haute Tribune*, April 17, 1919.

*Tri-State News* (Elkhart, KS), March 17, 1988.

*USA Baseball Weekly*, March 6–12, 2002.

*USA Sports Weekly*, December 7–13, 2011.

*USA Today*, July 24, 1989; August 3, 1992; July 15, 1996; July 23, 1996; July 25–26, 1996; August 1, 1996; August 17, 2000; September 12, 2000; September 19, 2000; September 21, 2000; September 25, 2000; August 20–21, 2004; May 15, 2007; May 20, 2008; November 17, 2010; August 11, 2011; October 13, 2011; October 18, 2011; December 6, 2011; February 14, 2012; June 12, 2012.

*Washington Post*, October 24, 1926; August 11, 1949; January 18, 1984.

## Interviews

Tommy John, Bob Feller Museum, Van Meter, Iowa, October 23, 2010.

## Television Programs

"Bobby Jones." *Sportscentury*, ESPN, March 12, 1999.

Santo, Jeff. *This Old Cub*, DVD, Sony Pictures Home Entertainment, 2004.

*Scott Hamilton: Return to the Ice*, BIO Channel, March 8, 2010.

## Web Sites

all-about-tennis.com.
answers.com.
asama.org
basketball-reference.com.
bioproj.sabr.org.
bostonherald.com
brooksinternational.com.
btaquatics.org.
bvwellness.com.
charities.com.
chicagoreader.com.
cnnsi.com.
cubuffs.com.
cyclingfan.net.
cyclinghalloffame.com.
databaseolympics.com
davita.com.
deafbiography.com.
dummyhoy.com.
ecac.org.

espn.go.com
everydayhealth.com.
figureskating.about.com.
freep.com.
garyhalljr.com.
hewittassociates.com.
hickoksports.com.
hubpages.com.
ihctm.com.
image.aausports.org.
intermetwrestle.com.
ishof.org.
jeffblatnick.com.
jimmyv.org.
jockbio.com.
kulr8.com
la84foundation.org.
linkedin.com.
madeinatlantis.com.
magazinesswimmingworld.com.
mcubed.net.

men.webmd.com.
NBCOlympics.com.
nesn.com
news.yahoo.com.
99.epinions.com.
onmilwaukee.com.
pittsburghsteelers.com.
rockybleier.com
samdavidinternational.com.
sportsillustrated.cnn.com.
sports.espn.go.com.
suite101.com.
tennisfame.com.
themat.com
timesunion.com.
2008.nbcolympics.com.
usatf.org.
usatoday.com
wnyt.com
wrestlingusa.com.

# Index